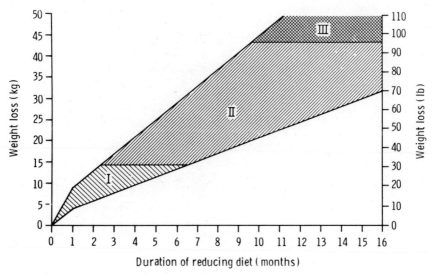

Fig. 9.1 Range of desirable rate of weight loss in obese patients in order to achieve loss of the appropriate 75% fat : 25% fat-free tissue. Younger and taller patients may achieve rates at upper limit of range: older and shorter patients will probably be near lower limit of range. Shaded areas show the length of treatment required for patients in grade I, II or III to reach $W/H^2 = 25$. For explanation of grades see Figure 1.1

Obesity and Related Diseases

Obesity and Related Diseases

J. S. Garrow MD, PhD, FRCP

Rank Foundation Professor of Human Nutrition, University of London, St Bartholomew's Hospital Medical School, London; *Formerly* Head, Nutrition Research Group, Clinical Research Centre, Harrow

CHURCHILL LIVINGSTONE
EDINBURGH LONDON MELBOURNE AND NEW YORK 1988

CHURCHILL LIVINGSTONE
Medical Division of Longman Group UK Limited

Distributed in the United States of America by
Churchill Livingstone Inc., 1560 Broadway, New
N.Y. 10036, and by associated companies, branches
and representatives throughout the world.

First published as *Treat Obesity Seriously* 1981

ISBN 0-443-03798-1

British Library Cataloguing in Publication Data
Garrow, J.S.
    Obesity and related diseases. — [2nd ed].
    1. Obesity
    I. Title   II. Garrow, J.S. Treat obesity
    seriously
    616.3'98   RC628

Library of Congress Cataloging-in-Publication Data
Garrow, J.S.
    Obesity and related diseases.
    Rev. ed. of: Treat obesity seriously. 1981.
    Bibliography: p.
    Includes indexes.
    1. Obesity — Treatment. I. Garrow, J.S.
Treat obesity seriously. II. Title. [DNLM:
1. Obesity. WD 210 G342t]
RC628.G38 1988 616.3'98   87-14631

Produced by Longman Group (FE) Ltd
Printed in Hong Kong

Preface

This book brings up to date and extends the work reviewed in two previous monographs: *Energy Balance and Obesity in Man* (1978) and *Treat Obesity Seriously* (1981). In the last decade there have been many books and symposia published which deal with various aspects of human obesity. However, there is no book which offers an organised and critical view of the whole field of human obesity — the techniques for studying body composition and energy intake and expenditure; the definition, prevalence and epidemiology of obesity; the associated diabetes and cardiovascular diseases; the many factors involved in the aetiology of obesity; the options for treatment, how they should be chosen and applied in different clinical situations, and what steps can be taken to prevent obesity. Ideally the basic scientist working on the biochemistry, physiology or psychology of energy metabolism should also know about the epidemiology and clinical consequences of obesity, just as the clinician should be aware of the scientific basis of the disorder and of the procedures which are advocated for treatment. Health educators wish to prevent obesity, but they are unlikely to succeed in this objective without a sound understanding of the aetiology and natural history of the disease, and the disabilities which are likely to arise if the obesity is left unchecked.

Since I have been working in both the scientific and clinical aspects of this field for more than 20 years I have tried to present a large mass of information, gleaned from the literature and from personal experience, in a form which will be a useful and reliable guide to all those who need to understand human obesity. No doubt experts in particular fields will think my treatment of their special interest is inadequate or even inaccurate: it is unlikely that the work of all of the 1200 investigators cited here is treated exactly as they would have wished.

Perhaps it is rash to attempt a monograph on so wide a field, although the effect of writing it is at least to educate the author. I must rely on the position well stated by John Arbuthnot, MD FRS, the Scottish polymath, wit and friend of Alexander Pope and Dr Samuel Johnson, in the preface to his Essay Concerning the Nature of Aliments (1731):

'I do not presume to instruct the Gentlemen of my own Profession; and if any of them shall instruct me better, I declare before-hand that I am very willing to be convinc'd: I will not defend any Mistake, and at the same time do not think my self oblig'd to answer every frivolous Objection.'

Harrow, 1987   J. S. G.

Acknowledgements

I am most grateful to many colleagues at the Clinical Research Centre, particularly in the Nutrition Research Group, Division of Bioengineering, and the Hospital Dietetic Department, for much help and advice with the work described in this book. In particular I thank Drs David Halliday, Sree Nair and Paul Pacy; Mrs Margot Hattam who helped with preparation of the typescript; and Joan Webster, without whom it would not have been completed on time.

I also thank my family for their support: Katharine, Jennifer & Nick, Margaret & Paul, Diana & Tim, and Alan: W/H^2 22 ± 2, who have no need for the advice in this book.

J.S.G.

Contents

1

Health implications of obesity

Ten years ago a study group set up jointly by the UK Department of Health and the UK Medical Research Council started their report thus: 'We are unanimous in our belief that obesity is a hazard to health and a detriment to well-being. It is common enough to constitute one of the most important medical and public health problems of our time, whether we judge importance by a shorter expectation of life, increased morbidity, or cost to the community in terms of both money and anxiety' (James 1976). This passage was quoted in the proceedings of a conference on Obesity in America with the comment that it succinctly summarised the situation in the USA also (Bray 1979).

1.a A WORKING DEFINITION OF OBESITY: GRADES 0–III

Before we can agree or disagree with the views expressed above it is necessary to have a working definition of 'obesity'. An abstract definition is that obesity is a condition in which the fat stores are excessive, but this begs two questions: how do you know how much fat an individual has stored? and how much is excessive? Methods by which the fat stores of a living person can be measured are discussed in detail in Chapter 3, but they are all too complex for use in epidemiological studies, so we have to rely on less direct estimates of fatness to relate obesity to mortality and morbidity. Fortunately there is a simple index which will serve well for his purpose, namely W/H^2, where W is body weight (kg) and H is height (m).

It was the Belgian astronomer Quetelet who founded the science of anthropometry more than 100 years ago. He observed 'Nous trouverons que les poids, chez les individus developpes et de hauteurs differentes, sont a peu pres comme les carres de tailles.' (Quetelet 1869). So in normal adults the ratio of weight to the square of height is roughly constant, and a person with a high W/H^2 ratio is over-weight-for-height. This ratio was adopted by Keys et al (1972b) and perhaps rather ungraciously renamed body mass index (BMI). Out of respect for our European anthopometric forefathers it will here be called Quetelet's index (QI). The relation of this index to body fat is considered later (see Chapter 3.f.).

Obesity, like baldness, is a matter of degree. To simplify discussion of the health hazards of obesity the following grades of obesity, defined by ranges of QI will be used (Garrow 1981):

Grade III W/H^2 >40
Grade II W/H^2 30–40
Grade I W/H^2 25–29.9
Grade 0 W/H^2 20–24.9

Figure 1.1 is designed to make it easier to calculate the grade appropriate to a given patient. It is also useful when explaining to a patient

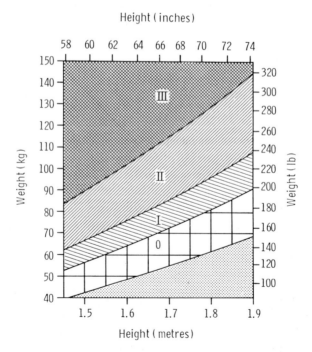

Fig. 1.1 Relation of weight to height defining desirable range (0), and grades I, II and III obesity, marked by boundaries W/H^2 = 25–29.9, 30–40, and over 40 respectively

that he or she is overweight, and indicates the amount of weight which must be lost in order to enter the 'desirable' range of weight for height (i.e. grade 0). It should be noted that there is no allowance for age, sex or frame size. Life insurance tables may distinguish between large and small frames, but all attempts to refine the estimation of fatness from weight and height by adding various body diameters have failed (Himes & Bouchard 1985, Rookus et al 1985). There is no advantage in specifying different weight ranges for people of large, medium or small frame if there is no usefully accurate way in which frame size can be measured.

The 1959 Metropolitan life insurance standards of weights for women were consistently lower than for men of the same height, but the 1979 standards have closed this gap, and the range W/H^2 20–25 quite adequately indicates the desirable range of weight-for-height in both sexes.

A case could be made from mortality data for having a higher range of desirable weight with increasing age. Among Finnish men aged 80 years or more, the highest 5-year survival was among those with a QI over 30 (Mattila et al 1986). Andres et al (1985) have fitted quadratic curves to insurance company data relating mortality to QI, and these authors show that among men the minimum mortality is associated with an index of 21.4 at age 20–29 years, and with succeeding decades this minimum mortality occurs at an index value of 21.6, 22.9, 25.8 and 26.6 at age 60–69 years. For women the QI values for minimum mortality at age 20–29 is 19.5, but this increases to 23.4, 23.2, 25.2 and 27.3 at age 60–69 years. However a striking feature about the curves relating QI to mortality ratios is that they become very much flatter in older age groups. This is illustrated in Figure 1.2, which shows data about mortality in ostensibly well non-smokers from the American Cancer Society study (Lew 1985). In the younger age groups there is a sharp decrease in mortality ratios around or somewhat below average weight, with a high mortality ratio in the most overweight individuals, but in the older age groups relative weight has less and less influence on mortality ratios.

It cannot therefore be concluded that there is no disadvantage to an old person in being overweight, since exercise tolerance and mobility may be greatly impaired by excess weight in an elderly person with degenerative disease of weight-bearing joints. In practice, therefore, the classification given above of grades of obesity serves quite well, at least over the range 20–65 years. (The problem of defining obesity in children is considered in Chapter 17.)

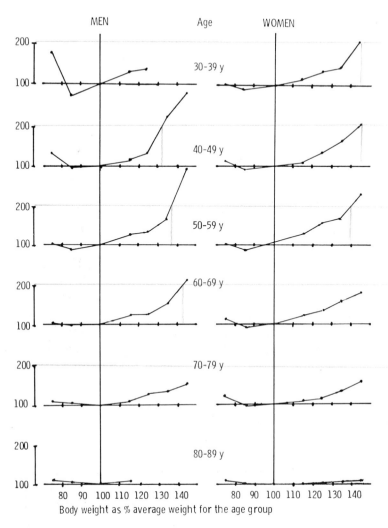

Fig. 1.2 Mortality ratio among ostensibly well non-smoking men and women by age and relative weight. Mortality among individuals of average weight is taken to be 100 at each age range (Data of Lew 1985, from American Cancer Society study)

It has been suggested that the desirable range of weight-for-height for cigarette smokers differs from that for non-smokers, but there is no reasonable basis for this. Smokers tend to be lighter than non-smokers, and have a greater risk of early death, but when the relation of weight-for-height to mortality is examined for smokers and non-smokers separately the curves are virtually identical in shape for both men and women, with the smokers showing a higher mortality at each weight. These data from the American Cancer

Mortality ratio as % average

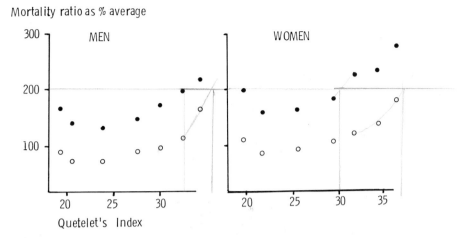

Fig. 1.3 Mortality risk as percentage of average for all ages related to grade of obesity among men and women non-smokers (open circles) and those who smoke 20 or more cigarettes per day (filled circles). (Data of Lew & Garfinkel 1979)

Society study are shown in Figure 1.3. A non-smoker in grade 0 would have to increase weight to grade II obesity in order to experience the same mortality risk as a person in grade 0 who smokes 20 or more cigarettes a day.

1.b PREVALENCE OF OBESITY

The prevalence of obesity (as defined above) is accurately known in the adult population of the UK. Between August and September 1980 a representative sample of households was drawn from the electoral rolls in a manner which reproduced the distribution of social class and type of district (metropolitan or rural) in the country as a whole. This yielded about 5000 households in which all the adults between 16 and 64 years were to be interviewed. Interviews were achieved at 82% of eligible households, and the height and weight of 79% of all eligible adults was measured. The sample of 10021 adults showed only minor differences in age structure from that of the UK population as a whole (Rosenbaum et al 1985).

The distribution of QI in the whole population of men and women is shown in Figure 1.4. A little over half the population is in the grade 0 range, a minority (10% of men and 13% of women) are underweight, and the remaining 40% of men and 32% of women are obese to some degree. However, although there are fewer women

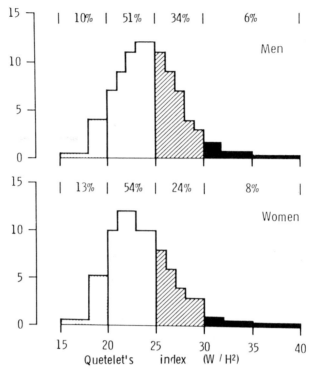

Fig. 1.4 Distribution of Quetelet's index (W/H²) in a representative sample of 10 000 men and women aged 16–64 years in the UK (Data of Rosenbaum et al 1985)

than men over QI 25, there are more women than men in the more serious grade II obesity.

The effect of age on the distributions of QI in this sample is shown in greater detail in Figures 1.5 and 1.6. Figure 1.5 shows that underweight (QI <20) is relatively uncommon among men and women over the age of 40 years, but that about one-third of men and women between 16 and 20 years are in this range. Grade I obesity increases with age in quite a linear manner among women between the age of 16 and 64 years, but among men the increase is rapid up to age 40, and then levels off. The reason for this difference between the sexes is not known.

The evolution of grade II obesity with age is shown in Figure 1.6. Among both men and women the proportion in the range QI 30–35 increases from about 2% at age 16–20 to about 10% at age 60–64. Among men there are relatively few over QI 35, but among women the prevalence increases with age to about 4% at age 60 years. Grade

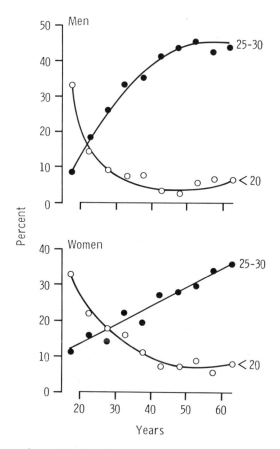

Fig. 1.5 Percentage of men (above) and women (below) in each age group who had a Quetelet index <20 (open circles). Closed circles show percentage with grade I obesity (index 25–29.9) (Data of Rosenbaum et al 1985)

III obesity is relatively rare: in this survey there were less than 0.5% of men in this grade at any age group, but among the women age 40 and more years about 1% were grade III. We can calculate that for the whole population about 0.1% of men and 0.3% of women are in grade III, and these are mainly over 40 years old.

In other countries, surveys have been done using slightly different techniques for selecting the sample to be measured, and often using different criteria of obesity. However, it is possible to judge that the prevalence of obesity in the UK is similar to that in other developed countries. In Table 1.1 the prevalence rates for UK are compared with the results of large surveys in other countries, using as far as possible similar criteria. The data on height and weight from the

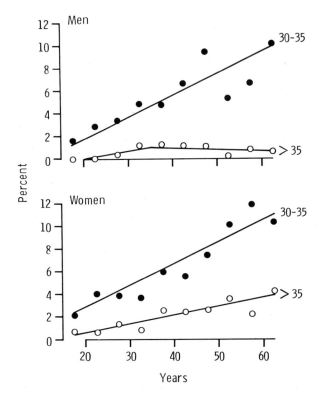

Fig. 1.6 Proportion of men (above) and women (below) in each age group with a Quetelet index of 30–35 (closed circles) or >35 (open circles) (Data of Rosenbaum et al 1985)

Table 1.1 Prevalence rates (%) of obesity among adults in the UK compared with other countries

Country	Age (yr)	Grade I		Grade II		Grade III		Author
		M	F	M	F	M	F	
UK	16–64	34	24	6	8	0.1	0.3	Rosenbaum et al 1985
Netherlands	20–34	20	10	2	2	?	?	Van Sonsbeek 1985
	35–49	37	21	4	5	?	?	
	50–64	46	36	5	10	?	?	
Norway	20–24	17	11	1	2	—	0.1	Waaler 1984
	40–44	41	30	5	5	—	0.5	
	60–64	44	43	8	24	0.1	1.1	
Australia	25–64	34	24	7	7	?	?	Bray 1985a
Canada	20–69	40	28*	9	12*	?	?	Millar 1985
U.S.	20–74	31	24	12	12	?	?	Abraham et al 1983

? Grades II and III not separated.
— prevalence <0.05%.
*criterion for women: grade I >23.8, grade II >28.6.

1981, 1982 and 1983 Continuous Dutch Health Interview Survey have been published so far only in Dutch (Van Sonsbeek 1985). The findings are very similar to the UK survey: the prevalence of obesity increases with increasing age in both sexes, and this increase is more marked among women than among men. The Norwegian data are derived from the National Mass Radiography Service files, which contained height and weight measurements on 1.8 million Norwegians — the total population of Norway is about 4.1 millions (Waaler 1984). Each of the age/sex categories shown in Table 1.1 contains some 70 000 individuals. Again the data show the increase in obesity with increasing age, especially in women. The oldest age group of the Norwegian data (age 60–64) shows a remarkably high prevalance of grade II and III obesity among women. The data from Australia resemble the UK data, but Canada and the USA have somewhat higher rates of obesity. Rookus et al (1986) have commented on the greater prevalence of obesity in the USA compared with the Netherlands. All these surveys report a higher prevalence of obesity among subjects of lower socio-economic status.

Thus the prevalence of obesity seems to be higher in North America than in European countries, with the UK in an intermediate position. Grade I obesity is less common in women than in men, but there are more women in grades II and III obesity, especially over the age of 50 years.

1.c DISEASES RELATED TO OBESITY

A Consensus Conference in 1985 in the USA (National Institutes of Health Consensus Development Panel 1985) concluded:

> The evidence is now overwhelming that obesity, defined as excessive storage of energy in the form of fat, has adverse effects on health and longevity. Obesity is clearly associated with hypertension, hypercholesterolaemia, non-insulin-dependent diabetes mellitus, and excess of certain cancers and other medical problems . . . . Thirty-four million adult Americans have a body mass index greater than 27.8 (men) or 27.3 (women); at this level of obesity, which is very close to a weight increase of 20% above desirable, treatment is strongly advised. When diabetes, hypertension, or a family history for these diseases is present, treatment will lead to benefits even when lesser degrees of obesity are present.

Medical experts have been curiously slow to recognise that obesity impairs health and reduces longevity through an effect on related diseases. Since the first actuarial investigation of mortality in 1903, life insurance companies have been aware that overweight people tended to die young, and hence were less profitable to insure. They were aware that the excess deaths among obese people were mainly 'cardiovascular', which is the commonest cause of death classification among normal-weight people also. Figure 1.7 shows the mortality experience among insured men who were either normal-weight or more than 20% overweight (Preston & Clarke 1966). Data are shown for men aged 35–49 years, and 50–74 years. In both age groups and weight groups cardiovascular and cancer are the commonest causes of death, with the obese men having a somewhat higher mortality rate than the normal-weight men. Accident is an important cause of death in younger men, and again the obese men are worse affected. In this series, suicide and leukaemia were much commoner in the obese group, but quantitatively these were rare causes of death. It is not surprising that from data such as these the manner in which obesity contributed to mortality was not appreciated.

Several factors tended to conceal the medical importance of obesity. The effects of overweight on mortality take years to become evident, but they are clear enough to the insurance companies, which necessarily take a long view. However, after the onset of a disease such as diabetes the patient usually loses weight (Knowler et al

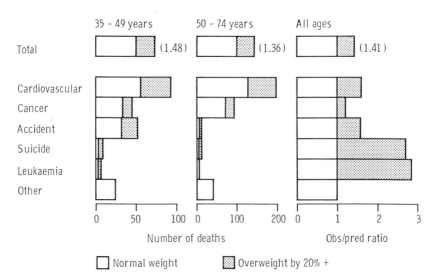

Fig. 1.7 Mortality rate and cause of death among insured men of normal weight or 20% overweight, aged 35–49 years, or 50–74 years at time of insurance (Data of Preston & Clarke 1966)

1981), so the contribution of obesity to the illness is not so obvious. Another confounding factor is cigarette smoking: smokers tend to be lighter than non-smokers and to die younger, so when studied in a population mixed with non-smokers they distort the true relation of weight to mortality which is seen in Figure 1.2. Finally there is the logical problem of interpreting multiple regression analysis, which was well shown in the 7-country study (Keys et al 1984). This survey showed that overweight men were more more likely to have heart attacks, but that when age, smoking, blood pressure and serum cholesterol were taken into account, relative weight did not significantly predict coronary heart disease among men aged 40–59 years. This finding may be interpreted to mean that weight is irrelevant to coronary heart disease, or alternatively that it increases the risk of death from coronary heart disease by contributing to hypertension and hypercholesterolaemia.

We now know that hypertension, hypercholesterolaemia and diabetes mellitus all increase the risk of coronary heart disease, and all these risk factors are associated with obesity. The critical question is: does the obesity cause the hypertension, hypercholesterolaemia and diabetes, or is it just a non-causal association? It might be that people with a certain genetic profile were liable to obesity and various other diseases. If this were so, then preventing or treating the obesity would not necessarily have any beneficial effect on the associated diseases. It has recently been shown by studies on identical twins that if one twin develops non-insulin-dependent diabetes mellitus (NIDDM), the other twin almost always develops the disease also. It has therefore been argued that the aetiology of NIDDM must be primarily genetic, and there is little room for other factors such as obesity in its causation (Leslie & Pyke 1985). However, other workers conclude that obesity plays an important role in precipitating the onset of NIDDM in people who have the genetic disposition to this disease (Baird 1973, Bonham & Brock 1985). It is not known if obesity alone could cause NIDDM in a person with no family history of the disease, and therefore presumably no genetic predisposition to it.

The only way to obtain a definitive answer to this important question is to take normal volunteers without a family history of diabetes or obesity, and overfeed them so they become obese, and see if any or all of them become diabetic. The practical difficulties of such an experiment are obvious, but it was attempted by Sims et al (1973) in Vermont, using volunteers from the State prison. The changes

Table 1.2 Changes in fasting blood concentrations, and insulin responsiveness among 19 male volunteers who over-ate a normal diet and increased body weight by 21 ± 1.0% and increased body fat by 73 ± 4.4% (Data of Sims et al 1973)

	Change	P<
Fasting blood		
cholesterol	increased	0.1
triglycerides	increased	0.01
aminoacids	increased	
glucose	increased	0.05
insulin	increased	0.005
oral glucose tolerance	decreased	0.005
intravenous glucose tolerance	decreased	0.05
Insulin response		
to oral glucose	increased	n.s
to intravenous glucose	increased	0.1
to intravenous arginine	increased	0.01

produced by overfeeding all elements of the diet in 19 volunteers are shown in Table 1.2. The study certainly proves that normal weight people can be made obese by experimental overfeeding, and that they then show biochemical changes in the direction of those found in spontaneous obesity and in non-insulin-dependent diabetes. However, the changes are small and do not take the values outside the normal range, so this degree of experimental obesity does not, on its own, cause diabetes. That would be too much to expect, since spontaneous obesity does not always cause diabetes either. At least we know that obesity (either experimental or spontaneous) causes some degree of insulin resistance, which is the cardinal feature of NIDDM. It is therefore reasonable to conclude, on the available evidence, that obesity plays some part in causing NIDDM in individuals who have a genetic disposition to this disease.

Does obesity cause hypertension? The Vermont study described above was not focused on blood pressure changes, so the evidence to answer this question depends on the observed associations between the two conditions. The prevalence of hypertension among white and black men and women of different weight categories is shown in Table 1.3. The black population has higher blood pressure levels than whites at similar relative weight, but in all groups increasing obesity is associated with increasing prevalence of hypertension (Stamler et al 1978). Obese normotensive subjects (children, adolescent or adult) when followed prospectively are more likely to become hypertensive than normal-weight normotensive subjects (Berchtold et al 1981). There are several mechanisms by which obesity might cause hypertension, but the evidence is inconclusive

Table 1.3 Frequency of hypertension (diastolic >95 mmHg) per 1000 among white and black men and women aged 20–39 and 40–64 years (Data of Stamler et al 1978)

Age	Weight	White men	White women	Black men	Black women
20–39	underweight	38.7	38.6	88.3	88.7
	normal weight	72.4	41.3	122.5	101.9
	overweight	175.9	110.9	259.9	149.1
40–64	underweight	182.4	172.5	300.4	377.2
	normal weight	244.2	221.7	374.7	411.8
	overweight	361.2	352.7	519.0	539.2

(Berchtold & Sims 1981, Dunstan 1985). It may be that the hyperinsulinaemia associated with obesity causes sodium retention by the kidney (DeFronzo 1981), or the increased sympathetic tone associated with overfeeding may be involved. Whatever the mechanism, obese subjects have an increased risk of hypertension, and this is another important cardiovascular risk factor in obesity. Hyperinsulinaemia may itself be an independent risk factor for atherosclerosis (Stout 1982). Cardiovascular disease is particularly associated with fat deposition in the abdominal region (Bjorntorp 1985). The measurement and significance of fat distribution on the body is considered in greater detail in Chapter 3.i.

The idea that obesity is benign unless associated with risk factors such as hypertension and hypercholesterolaemia is challenged by recent results from the Framingham study (Hubert 1984) and other long-term prospective studies. It now appears that obesity is a significant and independent predictor of disease, especially among women. Indeed obesity in women is the next best predictor of cardiovascular disease after age and blood pressure. The Framingham data also show a gradient of cardiovascular risk with adiposity in the subset of men and women who had no major risk factors for cardiovascular disease (Hubert 1984, see Ch. 14). Although obese people have a significantly increased rate of hyperlipidaemia and hypercholesterolaemia compared with normal-weight people, the degree of hyperlipidaemia bears no simple relation to the degree of obesity. Figures 1.8 and 1.9 show the fasting plasma triglyceride and cholesterol concentrations respectively in an unselected series of obese patients admitted to a metabolic ward. The highest values for cholesterol are not seen in the most extremely obese, but among those with moderate obesity. Autopsy analyses of extremely obese patients show that the degree of coronary atherosclerosis is not particularly severe (Warnes & Roberts 1984).

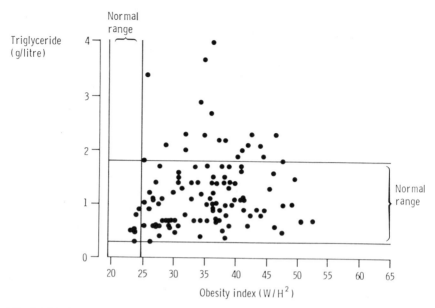

Fig. 1.8 Fasting plasma triglyceride concentration and Quetelet's index in unselected series of obese adults. Horizontal lines mark upper and lower limits of normal range.

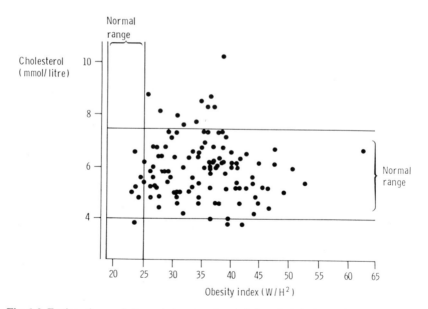

Fig. 1.9 Fasting plasma cholesterol concentration and Quetelet's index in unselected series of obese adults. Horizontal lines mark upper and lower limits of normal range.

Obese people also show an increased mortality and morbidity from disease of the gallbladder (Bray 1985b). Increased secretion of cholesterol into the bile is a characteristic of obese patients: in the study of Reuben et al (1985a) those with and without gallstones had secretion rates of 107 and 81 μmol/h, which was significantly greater (P<0.01) than non-obese patients with and without gallstones (51 and 42 μmol/h). Obese subjects also secreted more cholesterol in relation to bile acid, thus making the bile more liable to form stones. Gallbladder disease was found at operation in about 90% of morbidly obese patients (Amaral & Thompson 1985). Also, a significantly increased prevalence of abnormal liver function tests has been reported among moderately obese people (Nomura et al 1986).

Obesity also has adverse effects on reproductive function (Friedman & Kim 1985). Very thin and very fat women often have problems with menstrual irregularity and ovulatory failure. The syndrome of polycystic disease of the ovaries is associated with obesity, androgen excess and failure of ovulation. Ovarian function may improve dramatically with substantial weight loss. Overweight is also associated with an excess mortality from cancers of the colon, rectum and prostate in men, and the gallbladder, endometrium, cervix, ovary and breast in women (Garfinkel 1985).

Apart from the metabolic penalties associated with overweight, the extra fat also constitutes a physical burden. Diminished exercise tolerance is an objective consequence of quite modest degrees of obesity, and with severe obesity in older patients osteoarthritis in weight-bearing joints is often a major cause of disability. Finally, obesity is associated with social and psychological disadvantages, since our society tends to have a low valuation of obese individuals and, in the case of only slightly overweight people, low self-esteem may be the most crippling penalty of obesity (Wadden & Stunkard 1985).

1.d MORTALITY AND MORBIDITY ASSOCIATED WITH OBESITY AND RELATED DISEASES

Uncomplicated obesity is seldom fatal: some massively obese patients go into respiratory or cardiac failure, and there is no other apparent cause of death, but such cases are rare. Evidence has been presented above that obesity is associated (probably causally) with non-insulin-dependent diabetes and heart disease, but if an obese diabetic dies of a myocardial infarction should the death be ascribed to the obesity or the diabetes? Data of Fuller et al (1980) go some way towards answering this question. They observed the death rate from coronary heart disease in a prospective $7\frac{1}{2}$ year survey of 18 403 civil servants aged 40–64 years, divided according to their response to an oral glucose tolerance test. As might be expected those with impaired glucose tolerance (IGT) had a higher mortality rate than those with normal glucose tolerance (NGT), and those who were overweight (W/H² >27) had a higher mortality than those who were lighter. When the 418 deaths from coronary heart disease are assigned to both weight and glucose tolerance categories the effect on mortality rate is as shown in Figure 1.10.

In the period of study 21.6/1000 normal-weight NGT men died, but among overweight NGT men the mortality rate was modestly increased to 24.5/1000. Among men with IGT the mortality rate was 39.8/1000 for those who were not overweight, but 56.0/1000 for those who were overweight. Thus overweight increased mortality only 10% in NGT men, but by 40% in men with IGT. When calculating mortality attributable to obesity, therefore, we should consider not only that the obese person is more likely to become diabetic or hypertensive, but also that he or she is more likely to die of these conditions. The overall effect on mortality is shown in Figures 1.2 and 1.3. In general a person in grade II obesity (say W/H² 35) has roughly twice the chance of premature death compared with a person of similar age who is in grade O. Among younger people the gradient is steeper, so at age 45 years grade II obesity

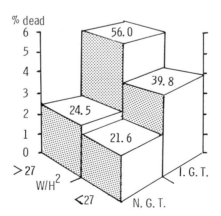

Fig. 1.10 Interaction of obesity and impaired glucose tolerance in causing death from coronary heart disease among 18 403 civil servants aged 40–64 years (Data of Fuller et al 1980)

carries about three times the mortality of grade O, while at age 80 there is virtually no effect of weight on mortality.

The effect of obesity on morbidity is more difficult to measure, and is confounded by the effect of age. In general older people are more overweight, but they also suffer more illness regardless of their weight status. Some studies have compared morbidity in overweight and normal-weight people matched for age, and they all give similar results. The survey of a representative sample of adults in the UK (Knight 1984) showed that complaints of pain in the hips and knees is associated with overweight in both men and women irrespective of age. Among women shortness of breath is associated with over-weight, but among men this is mainly related to age. A survey of overweight in relation to health care in the Netherlands showed that overweight men were more hypertensive, and that among grade II women there was a significantly increased prevalence of hyperten-sion, diabetes, varicose veins, asthma/bronchitis and haemorrhoids. Grade II patients used more medication and more medical care than normal-weight people (Seidell et al 1986b). A survey in a general practice in Somerset found an increased morbidity among patients with $W/H^2 >28$, especially in women. The main diseases causing this morbidity were hypertension, cardiovascular disease and muscu-loskeletal disease (Dawes 1984). Overweight patients were more likely than normal-weight patients to have several complaints at once. There are no objective studies of the morbidity which arises from the social and psychological problems arising from obesity.

In summary, therefore, obesity is associated with serious morbidity and mortality, and the more overweight and the younger the patient the more severe are the health implications. Many of the diseases related to obesity, such as diabetes and osteoathritis of weight-bearing joints, are crippling rather than killing diseases, so the mortality figures tend to underestimate the importance of obesity as a public health problem. Since grade II obesity affects about 7% of adults in the UK, USA, Australia and Canada, and is associated with a two-fold increase in mortality risk, it must rank next to cigarette smoking in importance as a cause of avoidable ill health in these populations.

1.e REVERSIBILITY OF MORTALITY AND MORBIDITY WITH WEIGHT LOSS

From a clinical viewpoint the crucial question is: can the excess mortality and morbidity associated with obesity be reversed by successful treatment? We cannot conduct an experiment to answer this question, since it would involve two large well-matched groups of obese subjects, one of which was reduced to normal weight, while the other group was required to remain obese. The practical and ethical objections to such a study make it impossible that it will ever be done. However there is enough evidence of a less well-controlled nature to make it very probable that most, if not all, the health risks of obesity are reversible by treatment. This does not mean that damage done by hypertension or degenerative disease of weight-bearing joints is reversible, but if weight and body composition are restored to normal then the prognosis of the formerly obese person with these complications is no worse than that of a normal-weight person with similar complications. Thus it is always worth while to treat significant obesity, but in younger people it is particularly worth while, since effective treatment will confer relatively more benefit in later life than it would to an older person with a similar degree of obesity.

The experience of life insurance companies provides evidence that weight loss to normal levels reduces the mortality risk of obese people to normal. Table 1.4 shows the mortality ratio experienced by people who were refused life insurance by the Metropolitan Life insurance company because they were overweight, but who subsequently achieved 'desirable' weight-for-height (Dublin 1953). It may be argued that those overweight clients who were able to lose weight to save on their insurance premiums were a particularly highly motivated and self-selected group, and they may not be typical of all obese people. Nevertheless the data in Table 1.4 show that, at least in this group of obese people, weight loss reverses the increased mortality risk of obesity.

Recent reports from the Framingham study confirm that weight change during adult life affects the risk of cardiovascular disease (Hubert et al 1983). Among both men and women weight gain

Table 1.4 Effect of weight loss on mortality ratios in men and women who were otherwise healthy* (Data of Dublin 1953)

| | 25% overweight | | | 35% overweight | | |
	n	Before	After	n	Before	After
Men	1300	142	113 (129)	400	179	109 (36)
Women	400	142	90 (18)	200	161	135 (15)

* 'n' shows number of individuals who lost weight to normal levels to obtain reduced insurance premium. 'Before' ratios show mortality experience in whole group without weight loss, and 'after' shows observed mortality ratios in those individuals who lost weight. Figures in parentheses show number of deaths on which mortality ratios were calculated.

increases the risk, and weight loss decreases the risk, both in terms of risk factors such as blood pressure and serum cholesterol, and also in observed disease incidence. Studies on morbidly obese patients have shown significant improvement in cardiac function after weight loss (Alpert et al 1985). It is also well documented that hypertensive obese patients show a significant decrease in blood pressure with weight reduction, even before all the excess weight is lost. Eliahou et al (1981) report that two-thirds of their obese hypertensive patients achieved normal pressures by the time they had lost half their excess weight.

The effect of correct dietary treatment on non-insulin-dependent diabetic patients is often dramatic, and probably it is possible to achieve normoglycaemia in virtually all such patients if they adhere to the correct diet. In the treatment of osteoarthitis of the hips and knees weight loss is often more effective in relieving pain and improving mobility than any form of drug treatment (Dixon & Henderson 1973). The effect of weight loss on the social and psychological penalties of obesity is difficult to evaluate objectively, but it is reasonable to suppose that the effect is beneficial.

The liability of obese patients to form gallstones, however, is not diminished during weight reduction: indeed the risk may become greater since the body fat being burned off is a large store of cholesterol, which is then excreted in bile.

2

Definitions and usage

The purpose of this chapter is to list, for convenient reference, the way in which terms and conventions have been used in this book. No special merit is claimed for these definitions over alternative definitions: they are chosen for clarity and convenience when discussing obesity in man.

ENERGY METABOLISM

Two units of energy are in common use. The older unit, still almost exclusively used in the USA, is the *kilogramme calorie (kcal)*. This is the amount of energy required to raise the temperature of 1 kg of water from 3.5°C to 4.5°C. The other unit is the *joule (J)* which is the energy dissipated when one ampere flows through a resistance of one ohm for one second. 1 kcal = 4.183 kJ. The Royal Society Conference of Editors (1968) recommended that SI units (i.e. the joule rather than the calorie) should be used in scientific publications, but progress has been slow in this direction. In this book, energy values are given in kcal with (in parentheses) the value in kilojoules (kJ) if that seems appropriate. A scale is provided in Figure 2.1 to facilitate conversion between kcal and MJ (10^6 joule) over the range encountered in human energy metabolism.

Energy intake normally means metabolisable energy intake, which is less than total energy in the diet as determined by bomb calorimetry. In this book, the metabolisable energy per gram of protein, fat, available carbohydrate and alcohol have been assumed to be 4 kcal, 9 kcal, 4 kcal and 7 kcal respectively. For a fuller discussion of these values see Chapter 4, pages 53–6.

Rate of working may be expressed as kcal/min, or kcal/ 24 h, or as watts (W). A watt is 1 J/s. In direct calorimetry, heat loss is

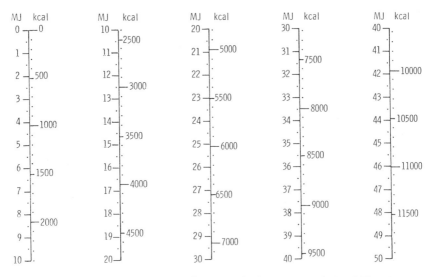

Fig. 2.1 Scale to facilitate conversion of energy units between megajoules (MJ) and kilocalories (kcal)

usually measured in watts, since calibration of the calorimeter is usually achieved with a standard electrical source whose energy output in watts is known. In indirect calorimetry, energy output is often expressed as ml O_2/min, and by assuming an energy equivalent of 4.9 kcal (20.5 kJ)/litre oxygen (see Ch. 5, p. 79–80) these four methods can be related thus: 204 ml O_2/min = 1 kcal/min = 1440 kcal/24 h = 70 W. (Note that for rapid conversion of ml O_2/min to kcal/day, a factor of 7 serves quite well: i.e. 200 ml/min = 1400 kcal/day, 300 ml/min = 2100 kcal/day, etc.)

External work load on a bicycle ergometer is usually expressed in W, or in kiloponds (kp). 1 kp = 50 W. To perform 70 W external work the oxygen uptake of the subject will need to increase by about 1000 ml/min, not the 204 ml/min suggested above. This is because the efficiency of muscular work is such that metabolic rate must increase by some 4 times the extra work load.

Resting metabolic rate is usually expressed as oxygen uptake — the units in which it is measured. The term 'basal metabolic rate' is avoided if possible, since the conditions in which it should be measured — postabsorptive, in a thermoneutral environment, and mentally and physically at rest — are difficult to achieve.

Thermogenesis is used to describe any increase in metabolic rate above resting metabolic rate in response to any stimulus other than physical activity. This is not a generally accepted use of the word, but it is very convenient, because then by definition:

Total energy expenditure =   Resting metabolic rate + Physical activity + Thermogenesis

BODY COMPOSITION

Fat vs adipose tissue, and fat-free mass vs lean body mass

To study body composition in living subjects it is necessary to make simplifying assumptions so the body is made of two components only. These components may be fat and fat-free mass (FFM), or alternatively adipose tissue and lean body mass (LBM), but the two systems cannot be mixed. Fat + LBM do not equal body weight, nor do adipose tissue + FFM. Fat is a pure chemical substance, the glyceryl ester of fatty acids. It contains no water, protein or potassium. The fat-free mass is everything apart from fat in the body. The fat + FFM convention is used in this book, because the exact composition of adipose tissue and lean body mass is so difficult to define.

Obesity in adults is defined operationally by Quetelet's index: values above 25 are considered to indicate obesity. The calculation of Quetelet's index is described in Chapter 1, page 2, and the justification for basing the definition of obesity upon this index is given in Chapter 3, pages 39–44. It is not possible to offer an objective definition of obesity in children for reasons which are given in Chapter 17.

STATISTICAL CONVENTIONS

Data for groups of subjects are normally presented as mean ± standard deviation (SD), and the number of observations is indicated by n. This is more informative than the practice of quoting the mean and standard error of mean (SEM), where $SEM = SD/n^{0.5}$. Approximately 66% of results will be within ± 1 SD of the mean, and about 95% within ± 2 SD.

A difference is described as 'not significant' if statistical tests indicate that this difference might have arisen by chance more than once in 20 trials.

Accuracy and precision

The accuracy of a measurement indicates how close it comes to the correct value, while precision is a measure of repeatability. A precise measurement may not be very accurate if there is a systematic bias which causes the answer to be consistently higher or lower than the true value. Measurements which are not precise are unlikely to be accurate, but the mean of several imprecise measurements may give an accurate answer if the errors are not systematically biased.

Correlation and prediction

The correlation coefficient (r) indicates if two variables x and y are related, but it does not indicate how accurately y can be predicted from x. If x and y are weakly associated, but the data on x and y cover a ten-fold range, the correlation coefficient will be far higher than it would be if the data related to only 10% variations in x and y, but clearly the error in predicting y from x would be similar in the two cases.

'Prediction equations' are often misnamed: an investigator finds an association between x and y, does a regression analysis, and presents the regression equation as a prediction equation. It may or may not have useful predictive power, but this can only be discovered when the equation is used to predict values of y from values of x, using data which were not used in the original regression analysis.

CONTROL AND REGULATION

A quantity which is regulated is maintained at a constant value ('kept regular'). To achieve this state, other variables must be controlled. For example a thermostat *controls* the output of a heating device so the temperature of a room is *regulated*.

3

Measurement of energy stores

Body weight is easy to measure to one hundredth of one per cent with a simple beam balance, but the weight of the body bears no simple relationship to the size of the energy stores, nor is a change in energy stores necessarily reflected in a change in weight. Under carefully controlled conditions, in a subject who is close to energy balance, it is possible to obtain the relationship between change in weight and change in energy balance, as shown in Figure 3.1. These data were obtained by feeding the subject meals which differed in energy content by several hundred kilocalories, and measuring body weight twice a day for 10 days. The slope of the regression line indicates that under these conditions body weight changes by 1 gram

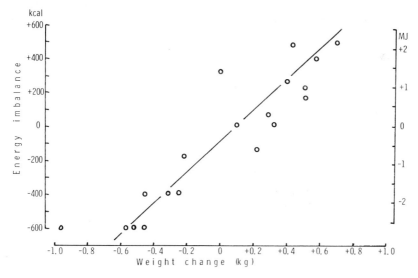

Fig. 3.1 Relation of weight change to small degrees of energy imbalance in normal subject. The regression line has slope indicating change of weight of 1 g/kcal energy imbalance: this corresponds to a glycogen:water mixture with 1 g glycogen binding 3 g water

for each kilocalorie of energy inbalance. In this case it is reasonable to suppose that the small imbalances between intake and output are being met from the glycogen stores of the body. Since each gram of glycogen binds about 3 g water (Olsson and Saltin 1970) the glycogen/water mixture has an energy value of about 1 kcal/g. However, when large imbalances occur the excess or deficit is balanced by changes in the store of adipose tissue, which has a much higher energy density. Therefore, it is necessary to know the nature of the energy store which is being changed before weight change can be interpreted in terms of energy balance. To do this we must measure the energy stores in the body.

Our understanding of the composition of the human body is based on chemical analyses of 6 cadavers which were performed between 1945 and 1956. Mitchell et al (1945) analysed the body of a 35-year-old white male who died suddenly of a heart attack. Widdowson et al (1951) analysed 2 adults and 1 child; the adults were a man of 25 who died of uraemia and a woman of 42 who drowned herself. Forbes et al (1953) analysed a man of 46 who died of a fractured skull, and Forbes et al (1956) reported two more analyses: one a Negro male with bacterial endocarditis who died aged 48, and the other a man of 60 who was found dead, presumably of a heart attack. Further data on the electrolyte composition of the last two bodies was published by Forbes & Lewis (1956). The composition of individual organs has been extensively investigated by Dickerson & Widdowson (1960) and Widdowson & Dickerson (1960).

It is obviously not practicable to measure the energy stores of a patient by direct chemical analysis, so various indirect methods have been developed, which are discussed later in this chapter. These all to a greater or lesser degree rest on the assumption that the body consists of two components: fat, and fat-free tissue of a fairly constant composition. The limitations of this approach are indicated in Table 3.1, which shows the water, protein and potassium concentration of the fat-free bodies which were analysed by the investigators mentioned above. It can be seen that each kilogram of fat-free tissue contains about 725 g water, 205 g protein and 69 mmol potassium, but that there is considerable variation between the individual bodies. In the lower part of Table 3.1 the composition of various organs is shown, and it is obvious that fat-free skin, for example, has a very different water and potassium content from, say, brain or muscle.

The body composition of a hypothetical normal adult male

Table 3.1 Contribution of water and protein to fat-free weight of 6 adult bodies, and in some organs (for sources of these data see text)

Age yrs	Water g/kg	Protein g/kg	Remainder g/kg	Potassium mmol/kg	K : N ratio mmol/g
Fat-free whole bodies					
25	728	195	77	71.5	2.29
35	775	165	60	—	—
42	733	192	75	73.0	2.38
46	674	234	92	66.5	1.78
48	730	206	64	—	—
60	704	238	58	66.6	1.75
Mean	725	205	71	69.0	2.05
Selected organs					
Skin	694	300	6	23.7	0.45
Heart	827	143	30	66.5	2.90
Liver	711	176	113	75.0	2.66
Kidneys	810	153	37	57.0	2.33
Brain	774	107	119	84.6	4.96
Muscle	792	192	16	91.2	2.99

is shown diagrammatically in Figure 3.2. The components of body weight which contribute to the energy stores are fat, protein and glycogen; water and mineral are irrelevant in this matter, and the component of body weight marked 'other' in Figure 3.2 is composed of material such as nucleotides and hormones which can also be neglected for purposes of calculating energy stores. The factors 4 kcal (17 kJ) per gram for protein and glycogen, and 9 kcal (37 kJ) per gram for fat enable us to convert the body composition shown in Figure 3.2 into energy equivalent: this calculation is set out in Table 3.2. A further complication, when trying to relate body weight to energy stores, is that body weight includes the weight of gut contents and of urine in the bladder, although physiologically this is not material within the body.

Weight change would accurately reflect change in energy stores if, when body weight changed by 5% (for example), all the components of body weight changed in similar proportion. However this is not so. During a period of total starvation body weight decreases rapidly at first, and then more slowly. The weight curve can be well described by two exponential functions (Forbes & Drenick 1979). There are at least four factors influencing this changing rate of weight loss: first, starvation is associated with ketosis, and consequent osmotic diuresis; second, during the early stages of starvation the glycogen stores become depleted, and so the water normally bound to glycogen is lost at this stage; third, there is an early loss

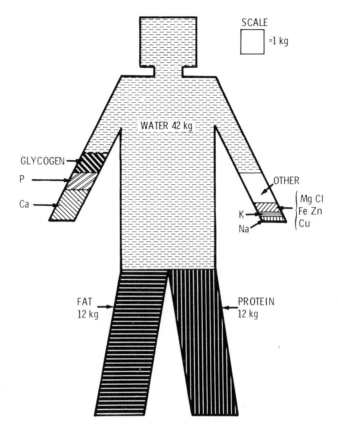

Fig. 3.2 Diagrammatic representation of body composition of normal adult male weighing 70 kg. Contributions of components to body weight represented by their area in diagram: only fat, protein and glycogen contribute to energy stores of the body.

Table 3.2 Energy stores in body of normal adult male (values are approximate)

Component	Weight kg	Energy equivalent Mcal	MJ
Water	42.0	0	0
Protein	12.0	48	200
Fat	12.0	108	450
Glycogen	0.5	2	8
Mineral and other	3.5	0	0
Total	70.0	158	658

of lean tissue, which decreases with time; fourth, there is a decrease in metabolic rate, so the energy deficit in the starving subject becomes less. With so many factors involved it is difficult to assign correct values for the relative importance of each one.

In practice, if we want to estimate the fat content of a living person we have to assume that the body consists of fat and fat-free tissue of constant composition, although, as the above discussion shows, we know this assumption is not correct. Various methods for estimating fat-free mass are described below and, although the assumptions about fat-free mass on which they depend are not necessarily correct, different methods involve different assumptions. It will be shown that if a battery of methods (such as density, water and potassium) are used on a group of subjects the combination of tests provides quite a good estimate of fat-free mass.

Before discussing individual methods in detail three general points should be made about comparisons between methods for the measurement of body fat. First, it is very difficult to validate any method objectively, since there is no 'gold standard' of absolute accuracy with which the method under test can be compared. If there were we would not need so many methods. It is a rather fruitless process to show that method A correlates better with method B than method C: method C might still be best, and methods A and B may merely share similar errors. Techniques for validation are discussed further in section 3.e.

Second, body weight can be measured easily and accurately, but body fat cannot. Methods such as total body water and total body potassium estimate fat-free mass, and fat is obtained by subtracting fat-free mass from weight, so 1 kg error in the estimation of fat-free mass causes 1 kg error in the estimation of fat. If the error is expressed as percentage of fat content this 1 kg will be a large percentage error in a thin person, but a small percentage error in a fat person. The point is of importance, since methods such as density and skinfolds measure percentage fat, not weight of fat. Probably the most valid way to compare two methods is to compare the accuracy with which they can measure the weight of fat in the subject, not % fat.

Third, it is necessary to give a warning about 'prediction equations'. Since almost everyone now has access to computers which perform regression analyses, many people are delighted to find that their data on human body composition, obtained by some of the laborious methods described below, could have been 'predicted' by a regression equation involving a few simple anthropometric measurements. Since they wish to share their fortunate discovery with others, they send off a paper about it to a journal, pointing out that their prediction equation fits the data very well, indeed far better than other people's equations. Of course it does: the computer made the equation fit the *retrospective* data as well as possible. However, to find out if the equation has any *predictive* power it is necessary to apply it to data which were not used to derive the equation. When this harsh test is used many 'prediction' equations are found to have very little ability to predict anything.

3.a MEASUREMENT OF BODY DENSITY

The measurement of body density as an index of obesity was pioneered by Behnke et al (1942) and developed by many investigators (Goldman & Buskirk 1961; Siri 1961; Durnin & Rahaman 1967). The density of tissues has been measured (Allen et al 1959) and the validity of the method for estimating the fat content of sheep has been confirmed by chemical analysis of their homogenised bodies (Beeston 1965). Human fat at body temperature has a density of 0.900 g/cm^3 , and a reasonable approximation for the density of the fat-free body of white people is 1.100 g/cm^3 (Keys & Brozek 1953). Black people have more bone mineral than whites of the same height, so the density of fat-free mass in blacks has been calculated to be about 1.113 g/cm^3 (Schutte et al 1984). Therefore a white person in whom half the body weight was fat would have an average density of 1.000. Obviously any mixture of fat and lean will result in an average density somewhere between 1.10 and 0.90. Making the assumptions stated above, it is possible to calculate percentage of fat from average body density. It may be that in individuals who are very fat or very severely malnourished the hydration of the fat-free body is altered (Streat et al 1985), but this causes only a small error in the estimation of body fat from density.

The practical problem is to make a very accurate estimate of the volume of the tissues of a human subject in a manner acceptable to patients. Few patients are able and willing to immerse themselves totally but gently in water so the volume of water displaced can be accurately measured, either by displacement or from the apparent weight loss of the submerged subject. These measurements cannot be made unless the water around the subject is at rest, and in practice this means that the subject must submerge calmly and remain still under water for about 30 s. This is quite possible if you understand what is needed and have confidence in the competence of the investigator, but it is not easy to induce this state of mind in all patients. A major technical advance was that of Irsigler et al (1975), who combined the good qualities of the usual water immersion plethysmograph with the acceptability of the gaseous system of Siri (1961): their subjects were immersed in water up to the neck, but their head was in a clear plastic cover. The volume of the air space around the subject's head was estimated by noting the pressure change produced by withdrawing a known volume of water from the plethysmograph. However, this system still has snags which affect both its acceptability and the reproducibility of the results. The general principle has been adopted, but the apparatus has been considerably modified by Diethelm et al (1977), and the construction of the modified apparatus is shown in Figure 3.3.

The subject stands in a vertical cylindrical water tank (17) with his head in a clear plastic cover which is sealed to the tank with metal rings and a silicone rubber gasket (5). The tank is lagged (15) and the temperature of the water is recorded with an electronic thermometer (13). Pressure changes in the air space are produced by a motor driven pump (12) and alternate between positive and negative. The pump is also connected to a reference chamber (2), and electronic pressure tranducers (1) compare the pressure cycles in the

1. Pressure transducers
2. Reference chamber
3. Perspex hood
4. Rubber balloon
5. Silicone rubber gasket·
6. Side arm for observation of
   water level and addition or
   subtraction of water
7. Taps
8. Air leak
9. Electronic circuitry
10. Power supply
11. Motor
12. Pump
13. Electronic thermometer
14. Recorder
15. Insulation
16. Steel pipe
17. Water
18. Aluminium rings
19. Intercom

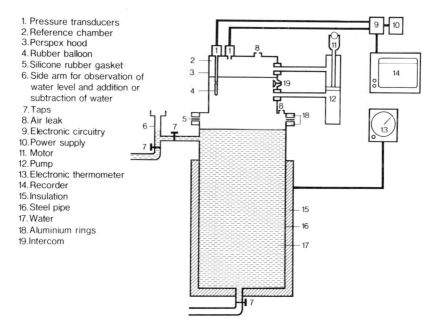

Fig. 3.3 Plethysmograph for measuring volume (and hence density) of human subject without requiring subject to immerse totally in water. For description of apparatus see text

space around the head of the subject with those produced in the reference chamber. Both the air space around the subject and the reference chamber are connected to the outside air by a small leak (8) to prevent drift in the baseline pressure between the two chambers due to any change in barometric pressure or change in volume, temperature or humidity in the air around the subject. The output of the transducers is fed to a unit which compares the signal from the two chambers (9), compares the difference with a reference voltage from a power unit (10) and displays the answer on a recorder (14). The system is made more acceptable to patients because it is recessed into the floor and hence is easy to enter, there is a flow of air continuously around the subject's head and a microphone loud-speaker (19) allows the subject and operator to communicate at all times. The stability and reproducibility of the system are greatly increased by using a balanced alternating system, in which unwanted changes in pressure are allowed for by comparison with the reference chamber.

The measurement procedure is described in detail elsewhere (Garrow et al 1979). Briefly, the plethysmograph is filled with water and adjusted so the signals from the two transducers (1) are equal and opposite: the output to the recorder is then zero. Water is then removed from the tank in 4 steps of 1 litre quantities to produce a calibration curve. The water is returned to the tank and the recorder zero is checked. The patient is now weighed on a beam balance, and a weight of water equal to the weight of the patient is removed from the tank. The patient is lowered into the tank, the lid is replaced, and the pump is switched on. If the density of the patient is equal to that of water the recorder will again read zero, since the volume of the patient will have exactly replaced the volume of water removed. If the density of the patient is greater than that of water the recorder will deflect, and the deflection of the recorder is read against the calibration curve to show the difference between the volume of the patient and that of an equal weight of water (x litres). The density of water at 34°C is 0.993 g/cm^3, so the volume (V litres) of a subject of weight (W kg) is

$$\frac{W}{0.993} - x$$

and density (d) is W/V. Percentage body fat (F%) is given by

$$F\% = \frac{495}{d} - 450$$

Replicate measurements on subjects of different fatness show that the reproducibility of measurements by this technique is better than 0.5 kg fat (Garrow et al 1979). However in this context reproducibility is not the same as accuracy, a point which is considered further in section 3.e.

Durnin and Satwanti (1982) have investigated the effect of variations in experimental technique on the estimate of density by underwater weighing. They conclude that ideally the subject should be measured in the fasting state and under conditions of maximal expiration to reduce errors arising from gas in the body. Theoretically with the non-immersion technique this should not cause significant errors anyway.

3.b MEASUREMENT OF TOTAL BODY WATER

The volume of water in the cooling system of a car can be measured by the dilution principle: if 1 litre antifreeze is added to the radiator, and after thorough mixing of the water in the cooling system the concentration of antifreeze is found to be 5%, the total volume of water must be 20 litres. Even if there is a slow leak in the system this will not introduce much error in the estimate of volume at the time the antifreeze was added, since any leakage after complete mixing was achieved will not affect the final concentration, because the same proportion of water and antifreeze will be lost in any given time period.

Body water in living man can be measured by a similar principle by giving a dose of water labelled with either tritium (the radioactive isotope of hydrogen) or deuterium (the stable heavy isotope of hydrogen) or ^{18}O (a stable heavy isotope of oxygen). The concentration of tritium in body water after equilibrium is reached is measured in a scintillation counter, but if either stable isotope is used it is necessary to use an isotope ratio mass spectrometer to measure the enrichment of isotope in the equilibrium sample (Halliday & Miller 1977, Schoeller et al 1985). To obtain a measurable concentration after mixing with body water it is necessary to give a dose of about 100 microcuries (3.7 MBq) of ^3H_2O or about 1 g of D_2O or $H_2^{18}O$. (The use of doubly-labelled water ($D_2^{18}O$) to measure energy expenditure is discussed in Chapter 5.b.)

The dose of labelled water may conveniently be given orally diluted in 100 ml of tap water. The weight of water given is measured by weighing the container before and after the subject has taken the dose through a drinking straw. It is necessary to allow about 3 h to achieve isotopic equilibrium, and during this period no food or drink may be taken by the subject, otherwise the recently ingested water will dilute the plasma water and cause a falsely low reading which will result in too large an apparent total body water and too low an estimate of total body fat. The loss of isotope in urine during the equilibration period of 3 h does not contribute a significant error ($<$ 1%) so it is not necessary to measure this loss. An error of about 2% occurs because the labelled hydrogen exchanges with labile organic hydrogen atoms as well as water hydrogen (Culebras et al 1977), but this small overestimate of water can be ignored.

Having obtained an estimate of total body water (TBW,kg) Fat-free mass (FFM, kg) can be obtained thus:

$$FFM = \frac{TBW}{0.73}$$

on the assumption that FFM is 73% water (Pace & Rathbun 1945). The fat content (F,kg) of a person of body weight W,kg) is then: F = W − FFM.

In fact the water content of FFM may not be 73% as is shown in Table 3.1, and also when this method is compared with other methods for measuring body composition such as neutron activation (Streat et al 1985) or total body potassium (Dempsey et al 1984) or density (Garrow et al 1979). However, measurement of total body water is a useful member of a battery of tests with which the energy stores of the body can be measured.

3.c MEASUREMENT OF TOTAL BODY POTASSIUM

All potassium, including that in the human body, is labelled with the natural radioactive isotope ^{40}K, so each gramme of potassium emits about 3 gamma rays of high energy (1.46 MeV) each second. These rays can be detected by suitable apparatus (Burch & Spiers 1953, Boddy et al 1976, Smith et al 1979) and thus the total body potassium can be estimated.

Figure 3.4 shows the general construction of a whole body counter designed to measure ^{40}K. Since the radiation coming from the body is very weak it is necessary to enclose the apparatus and subject in a massive shield made (usually) of steel and lead to reduce interference from cosmic radiation and other extraneous sources of radio-

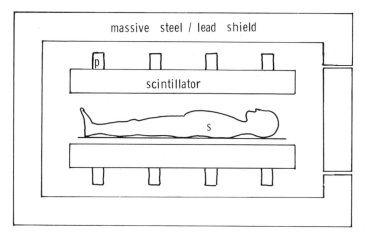

Fig. 3.4 Diagram of one type of whole body counter designed to measure ^{40}K. Subject (S) lies between tanks of scintillation liquid. Gamma rays emerging from subject pass through scintillator and cause flashes of light which are detected by a series of photomultipliers (p). To reduce background count rate from cosmic rays and other local radioactivity the whole instrument is enclosed in a massive shield

activity. The steel itself must be free from radioactivity; pre-war battleship steel is a suitable material. Within the shielded volume the subject (S) lies with detectors arrayed around him to try to catch as much as possible of the radiation. Ideally the detectors should totally enclose the subject, but this causes problems in getting the subject in and out of the counter so a usual compromise is to have detectors above and below the couch on which the subject lies. In Figure 3.4 the detectors shown are tanks containing liquid scintillator, with photomultipliers (p) detecting the burst of photons emitted when a gamma ray passes through the scintillator. An alternative design is to use crystal detectors made from NaI which has a greater capacity to absorb the energy from gamma rays, and therefore produces a burst of photons which is more closely proportional to the energy of the gamma ray. This sharp photopeak makes it easier to distinguish counts attributable to the potassium radiation from other radioactive events, and is particularly valuable if it it required to measure ^{40}K in a subject who already contains traces of other radioactive isotopes. The disadvantage of NaI crystals is that they are much more expensive than an equivalent volume of liquid scintillator.

Whatever the design of the counter it is necessary to have an expert operator who makes careful calibrations to check the effect of different sizes and shapes of subjects on the ^{40}K count obtained.

All the radiation does not escape from the body, and the larger the subject the more of the radiation will be absorbed in the tissues and never emerge through the skin. All of the radiation which emerges is not counted: the proportion which is captured will depend on the geometrical relation of the subject to the counters. Thus each counter needs calibration with a range of phantoms which mimic the range of body size of subjects who will be measured, so appropriate corrections can be made to derive the total body potassium from the observed count rate. Typically the counting time for an average subject is about 1000 s, and the coefficient of variation is about 3%. Longer counting times will give greater precision, but ultimately accuracy is limited by the stability of the electronics and the validity of the calibration equations.

Having obtained an estimate of total body potassium (TBK,mmol) the FFM (kg) can be calculated for women from

$$FFM = \frac{TBK}{60}$$

and for men from

$$FFM = \frac{TBK}{66}$$

on the assumption that fat-free tissue contains 60 mmol K/kg or 66 mmol K/kg for women and men respectively. (1 g K = 25.6 mmol).

It is clear from Table 3.1 that the 5 cadavers for whom we have analyses did not have the concentration of potassium in fat-free tissues which are used in the equations above, and that the variation in potassium content is very large from one tissue to another. Also there is some evidence that the potassium concentration in the lean tissues of obese people is lower than normal (Colt et al 1981). However, provided total body potassium is measured in an adequate counter which has been well calibrated, this measurement is useful in assessing body fat stores.

3.d MEASUREMENT OF BODY COMPOSITION BY NEUTRON ACTIVATION

The technique for measuring total body potassium described in the previous section depends on the fortunate accident that potassium has a natural isotope with a high-energy gamma emission. If a human subject is irradiated with neutrons of appropriate energy many other elements become transiently radioactive: O, H, N, Ca, P, Na, Cl and Mg. The facilities for this investigation have been available for some time at the Brookhaven National Laboratory in the US (Cohn et al 1982) and in Leeds at the UK (Bogle et al 1985), but are not generally available elsewhere. The accuracy with which total body nitrogen can be measured is about 3% (Cohn et al 1974) so estimates of fat-free mass from neutron activation measurements of total body nitrogen are less accurate than by other methods previously mentioned. Recently an improved model has been proposed which uses a combination of estimates of N, Ca, Cl by neutron activation, K by ^{40}K counting, and total body water by tritium dilution (Cohn et al 1984). The estimated errors in measurement of total body fat are 2.7% or 5.1% depending on the model used.

It is suggested that this technique provides estimates of total body fat which are not vulnerable to the changes in hydration and electrolyte balance which so often occur in the ill patient on whom body composition measurements are required. At present there is no evidence on which to judge if this claim is true or not.

3.e MEASUREMENT OF BODY FAT BY SKINFOLD THICKNESS

Many authors have pointed out that most of the fat stored in the body lies immediately under the skin (Edwards 1950) and that the thickness of a fold of skin picked up at strategic sites indicates the amount of subcutaneous fat (Montoye et al 1965, Seltzer & Mayer 1965). Various sites for measurement have been suggested: Hermansen & Von Dobeln (1971) used 11 sites, Strakova & Markova (1971) 15 sites, and Seltzer & Mayer (1965) relied only on a single skinfold over the triceps. However, probably the best established system is that using four sites: biceps, triceps, subscapular and supra-iliac. These were proposed by Durnin & Rahaman (1967) and developed by Durnin et al (1971), Durnin & Womersley (1974) and Womersley & Durnin (1977) to include standards based on 245 men and 324 women covering the age range from 17 to 72 years. Fat-free mass (calculated from skinfolds) agrees well with total body nitrogen (measured by neutron activation analysis). Hill et al (1978) found a coefficient of variation of 8.5% between the two measurements.

However, measurement of skinfolds requires skill and training. Ruiz et al (1971) showed that it was important that the triceps skinfold was measured at exactly the correct site, otherwise false results were obtained. In very fat people it is impossible to obtain a true fold of skin and subcutaneous fat, and if you do so it will not fit between the jaws of the standard caliper. Attempts have been made to measure the thickness of the subcutaneous fat layer by X-rays (Garn 1961, Tanner 1965) or by ultrasound (Booth et al 1966, Hawes et al 1972, Haymes et al 1976, Weits et al 1986), but these techniques are less convenient than skinfold caliper measurements with little compensating advantage. A theoretical limitation to the skinfold measurement is that it assumes a constant relationship between subcutaneous and deep fat stores, which is not confirmed by measurement at post-mortem examinations (Alexander 1964), but the tables of Durnin & Womersley (1974) give different standards for percentage body fat according to age and sex, which to some extent compensates for age- and sex-related changes in the distribution of fat in the body. Jones et al (1976) found differences between the proportion of fat which was subcutaneous in Europeans, Gurkhas, Rajputs and South Indians, so there are also probably ethnic differences which should be considered when converting from skinfold thickness measurements to estimates of body fat.

Despite these reservations skinfolds are certainly the most convenient method for estimating fat in people of reasonably normal build, provided that the measurements are made by a trained observer, and an error of about 3% of body weight (i.e. 2 kg of fat in an average subject) is acceptable. This is probably the error in skilled hands (Womersley & Durnin 1977).

In unskilled hands, and with fatter subjects, the error will be much greater, but this does not prevent some authors from applying the method in circumstances which are quite inappropriate. Grimes & Franzini (1977), for example, suggest that skinfolds should be used to 'measure change in behavioural weight control studies', and explain, with diagrams, how to take measurements at the sites used by Durnin & Rahaman (1967). They note the 'lack of normative data for extremely or morbidly obese patients' but solve this difficulty with a stroke of the pen: since the standards of Durnin and Rahaman stop at a total skinfold reading of 95 mm, they simply extend the line to 150 mm. These investigators would do better to use ordinary bathroom scales, which would be a much more reliable measure of change in behavioural weight control studies.

If skinfolds are to be used to estimate body fat the procedure of Durnin & Womersley (1974) should be used. The Harpenden caliper is used (Holtain Ltd, Bryberian, Crymmych, Pembrokeshire) which is designed so the surface of the jaws applied to the skin surface remain parallel and exert a constant pressure. The skinfold is picked up between forefinger and thumb of the left hand, the caliper is applied so it closes under the spring pressure, and the reading is taken on the micrometer dial as soon as the rapid phase of compression is over (after about 5 s). The sites of measurement are biceps, triceps, subscapular and supra-iliac. The position of the first two sites is on the anterior and posterior mid line respectively of the upper arm, at the mid-point between the acromion and olecranon processes when the elbow is flexed at 90 degrees. The skinfold is oriented in the long axis of the limb. The subscapular site is at the lower angle of the scapula at 45 degrees to the vertical, and the supra-iliac site is a horizontal skinfold just above the iliac creast in the mid-axillary line. To make the measurement it is necessary to have the subject stripped to the waist or, with female subjects, wearing only a brassiere above the waist. Three measurements should be made at each site, and if the span of readings is greater than 2 mm more readings should be taken until a set of three consecutive readings agreeing to 2 mm is obtained. The average of the three readings is taken at each site, and the sum of these values is entered into the table given by Durnin and Womersley (1974) in the column appropriate to the age and sex of the subject. The percentage body fat related to the sum of 4 skinfolds is given in Table 3.3.

3.f MEASUREMENT OF FATNESS BY QUETELET'S INDEX

The origin of Quetelet's Index (W/H^2), where W is body weight in kg, and H is height in m) has already been mentioned in Chapter 1.a. It is identical to the 'body mass index' of Keys et al (1972b), but the term Quetelet's index (QI) is preferred because Quetelet had priority by 103 years.

The use of QI as a measure of fatness has been analysed by Garrow & Webster (1985a). There are two ways in which fatness can be expressed: either fat as percentage of body weight, or else fat in absolute amount (kg). If (as will shortly be shown to be the case) a person becomes obese by adding tissue with a constant ratio of fat

Table 3.3. Percentage body fat in men and women related to sum of 4 skinfolds (biceps, triceps, subscapular and supra-iliac). (Data of Durnin and Womersley 1974).

Skinfold (mm)	Men				Women			
Age(y): 17–29	30–39	40–49	50+	16–29	30–39	40–49	50+
20	8.1	12.2	12.2	12.6	14.1	17.0	19.8	21.4
30	12.9	16.2	17.7	18.6	19.5	21.8	24.5	26.6
40	16.4	19.2	21.4	22.9	23.4	25.5	28.2	30.3
50	19.0	21.5	24.6	26.5	26.5	28.2	31.0	33.4
60	21.2	23.5	27.1	29.2	29.1	30.6	33.2	35.7
70	23.1	25.1	29.3	31.6	31.2	32.5	35.0	37.7
80	24.8	26.6	31.2	33.8	33.1	34.3	36.7	39.6
90	26.2	27.8	33.0	35.8	34.8	35.8	38.3	41.2
100	27.6	29.0	34.4	37.4	36.4	37.2	39.7	42.6
110	28.8	30.1	35.8	39.0	37.8	38.6	41.0	42.9
120	30.0	31.1	37.0	40.4	39.0	39.6	42.0	45.1
130	31.0	31.9	38.2	41.8	40.2	40.6	43.0	46.2
140	32.0	32.7	39.2	43.0	41.3	41.6	44.0	47.2
150	32.9	33.5	40.2	44.1	42.3	42.6	45.0	48.2
160	33.7	34.3	41.2	45.1	43.3	43.6	45.8	49.2
170	34.5	34.8	42.0	46.1	44.1	44.4	46.6	50.0

to FFM, that person's percentage of fat will not increase linearly with equal increments in weight. Indeed, since the composition of weight gained is about 75% fat and 25% fat-free tissue (Webster et al 1984) the percentage of fat in the body will approach the asymptote of 75% at infinite weight, but can never be greater than 75%. However, if fatness is expressed in absolute terms it will increase indefinitely in a linear manner with successive additions of tissue which has a constant proportion of fat.

The data on which the argument rests are shown in Figure 3.5. Among 104 women aged 14 to 60 years, who ranged from very thin to very fat, the relation of fat to body weight was well described by a straight line, with a slope of 1.27 and a correlation coefficient of 0.960 (Webster et al 1984). To some extent this close association might be due to the fact that the women varied also in height, and even if they all had the same percentage of fat the taller women would tend to be heavier and have more fat than the shorter women. To correct for differences in stature both axes may be divided by H^2: this yields the result shown in Figure 3.6. The intercept of the regression line has changed but the slope (1.28) and the correlation coefficient (0.955) is hardly changed. The estimates of fat used to construct Figures 3.5 and 3.6 were the average values derived from measurements of density, water and potassium in each of these 104 women, using the calculations explained in sections 3.a, 3.b and 3.c above. If, instead of using this average figure, we take the values for

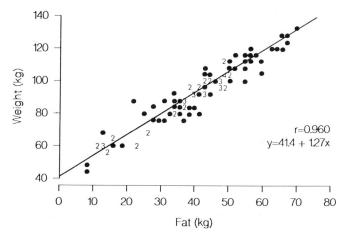

Fig. 3.5 Relation of body weight to total body fat in series of 104 women. Body fat was calculated from mean of estimates by density, water and potassium in each woman (Data of Webster et al 1984)

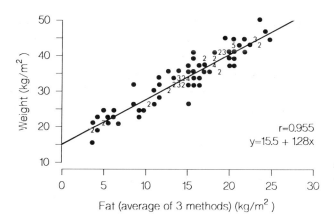

Fig. 3.6 Data shown in Figure 3.5 corrected for differences in stature by dividing both variables by H^2. The y axis now becomes Quetelet's index

fat derived from density alone, or water alone, or potassium alone, the results are shown in Figures 3.7, 3.8 and 3.9 respectively. When the estimates of body fat are based on a single method of measurement the errors are greater, and hence the correlation coefficient with weight is slightly reduced, but the slope of the line is still close to 1.27. In the case of men similar data are obtained (Garrow & Webster 1985a).

The data in Figures 3.5 and 3.6 suggest that as women (of a given height) increase in weight they gain 1 kg fat for every 1.27 kg weight

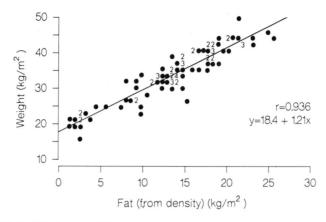

Fig. 3.7 Relationship shown in Figure 3.6, but based on fat estimated by density alone

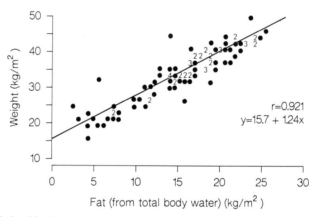

Fig. 3.8 Relationship shown in Figure 3.6, but based on fat estimated by water alone

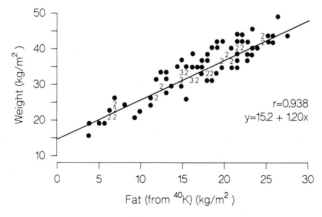

Fig. 3.9 Relationship shown in Figure 3.6, but based on fat estimated by potassium alone

gained: in other words 1/1.27, or 78.7%, of the excess weight is fat. However if we regress fat on weight, instead of weight on fat, we obtain the formula:

$$F/H^2 = 0.713W/H^2 - 9.74$$

for women and

$$F/H^2 = 0.715W/H^2 - 12.1$$

for men which implies that 71.3% (or 71.5%) of the excess weight is fat (Garrow & Webster 1985a). If the correlation coefficient between W/H^2 and F/H^2 had been 1.00 the slope would have been identical whichever way the regression had been performed, but since the association is not perfect we have to accept that the true figure for the proportion of fat in excess weight is about 74 ± 4% which can conveniently be rounded to 75%.

If it is true that throughout the range of fatness excess weight is about 75% fat and 25% non-fat, then it must be possible to calculate body fat using QI. In fact this has been done for the 104 women and 24 men studied by Garrow & Webster (1985a), and the estimate of body fat was compared with that obtained from the average of density, water and potassium measurements, which was assumed to be the 'true' value. Among women the standard deviation from this 'true' value of fat estimated by density, water, potassium and QI was 3.4, 3.3, 3.5 and 4.2 kg respectively. Among men the standard deviations were 5.8, 3.8, 4.1 and 5.8 kg respectively.

Evidently QI is not quite as accurate a method for estimating body fat as the more complex laboratory techniques described in sections 3.a, 3,b and 3.c, but these techniques are also liable to significant error, which can be measured only if a still more accurate method for measuring body composition is available for comparison. There is no perfectly accurate method applicable to living subjects, but under very carefully controlled conditions in a metabolic ward it is possible to estimate *change* in fat stores with considerable accuracy from measurements of energy balance or nitrogen balance. Measurements of body fat by density, water and potassium have been made on a series of 19 obese women, and repeated after a few weeks. The change in fat stores during the interval was estimated by energy balance and nitrogen balance, and the change estimated in this way (2.77 ± 0.71 kg fat) was assumed to be the 'true' change. By comparing the change in fat stores indicated by the change in density, water and potassium with the 'true' value for each subject, the errors of the various methods can be estimated: they are calculated to be 2.2, 2.3 and 3.5 kg of fat by density, water and potassium respectively (Garrow et al 1979).

3.g OTHER TECHNIQUES FOR ESTIMATING BODY COMPOSITION

Since body density or total body potassium is rather difficult to measure there have been innumerable papers in which it is claimed that by making some simpler anthropometric measurements the value of density or total body potassium can be predicted. For example Burkinshaw et al (1971) predict total body potassium from weight and the width of muscle and of fat measured on a radiograph of the thigh. Ellis et al (1974) multiply the square root of weight by the square of height and then use a constant related to age. Turner & Cohn (1975) have another formula using weight, height and age. Pollock et al (1975) predict body density from skinfolds at thigh and suprailiac sites, plus knee diameter and wrist girth. Shizgal (1976) predicts total body potassium from a measurement of body water and exchangeable sodium. And so on. These techniques will not be reviewed in any detail because, although the proffered formula can be shown to have a highly significant correlation with potassium or density as the case may be, there is no evidence that these formulae predict the proportions of fat and lean in the body any more accurately than QI, used as described in the preceding section.

Other methods have a sound theoretical basis, and deserve some comment. It is an attractive idea to establish an equilibrium between a fat-soluble gas inhaled by the subject and total body fat, and thus to calculate body fat by observing the amount of gas absorbed (Hytten et al 1966, Lesser et al 1971). Unfortunately the equilibration time is impossibly long, so the method is impractical.

Creatinine excretion has been used as a measure of muscle mass, since creatine and phosphocreatine in muscle is non-enzymically dehydrated to form creatinine, which is excreted in the urine (Forbes & Bruining 1976, Heymsfield et al 1983). However muscle mass is only about half the total fat-free mass, so it is not possible to calculate body fat from creatinine excretion. The creatinine excretion of 42 obese women related to QI is shown in Figure 3.10: although total fat-free mass increases linearly with QI (see Fig. 3.6) creatinine excretion does not. This suggests that muscle does not contribute a large part of the extra fat-free mass in obese subjects (Webster & Garrow 1985).

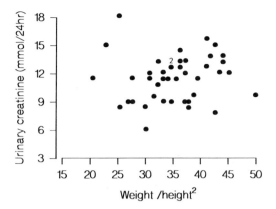

Fig. 3.10 Relation of 24 h urinary creatinine excretion to Quetelet's index in 42 obese women

A recently described technique for estimating fatness is infrared interactance (Conway et al 1984). Light in the wavelength range 700–1100 nm is shone onto the skin surface at selected sites, and the spectrum of wavelengths reflected is analysed by computer. Fat and lean tissue have different interactive spectra, and so the lean:fat ratio at the test sites can be calculated. So far there is no information by which the reliability of this technique can be compared with other techniques.

Body imaging techniques have developed greatly in recent years. A very simple system for estimating the amount of fat, muscle and bone in a segment of limb is shown in Figure 3.11. A source of gamma rays of suitable energy (such as the radioisotope americium) is mounted in a shielded enclosure on one side of the limb, and a detector consisting of a NaI crystal viewed by a photomultiplier is mounted in a similarly shielded enclosure on the other side of the limb. The radiation detected depends on the attentuation of the beam by the tissues of the limb in the path of the beam: bone mineral, muscle and fat have characteristic attenuation coefficients. If both source and detector are scanned across the long axis of the limb the proportion of bone, muscle and fat can be calculated.

A similar principle is used in computer-assisted tomography (CAT-scanning), but in this case the source of radiation and the detectors are rotated around the subject, thus generating a large number of scans at different angles. The computer resolves this information into an image by calculating the attenuation attributable to each small part of the cross-sectional area (called a pixel) and plotting the answer as a shade of grey appropriate to this attenuation.

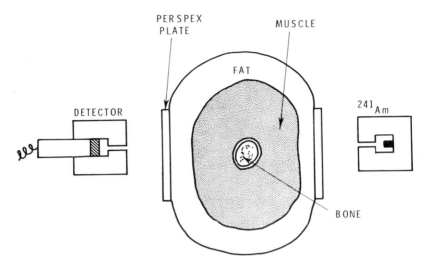

Fig. 3.11 Simple system for estimating proportion of fat, muscle and bone in cross-section of limb from attenuation of mono-energetic gamma beam scanned across it. In computer-assisted tomography the source and detector rotate around subject, and an image is constructed by the computer from multiple scans in different planes

CAT-scanning is very useful in indicating the distribution of fat in the human body, which is further considered in the next section, but it is not a particularly convenient or accurate method for estimating total body fat, and it involves some dose of ionising radiation to the subject. It is also a very expensive procedure.

Finally, two methods have been developed which depend on the difference in electrical conductivity of lean tissue (which is virtually an electrolyte solution, and hence a good conductor) and fat, which is a non-conductor. In the total body electrical conductivity (TOBEC) system the subject lies within a solenoid coil through which radiofrequency pulses are fed at a frequency of 5 MHz (Segal et al 1985b). This generates an alternating magnetic field within the coil which induces a response in the subject depending on the conductivity of the tissues, and the strength of the evoked field is measured by a secondary coil. The advantage of this system is that it makes the measurement very quickly: the device was originally designed to measure the fat content of processed meat travelling on a conveyor belt. The disadvantage is that the evoked field depends on the shape of the subject as well as on the fat content, since a short stout person would trap more of the magnetic radiation than a tall slim person of similar body weight and composition.

The other device which measures electrical conductivity uses a pair of electrodes attached to the left hand and left foot of the subject (Lukaski et al 1985). A current of 800 μA at a frequency of 50 MHz is passed between the outer electrodes, and the voltage drop is measured at the proximal electrodes, from which the resistance of the tissues is calculated. Both these methods show highly significant correlations with other methods for measuring body composition, but we do not yet know if they can provide an estimate of body fat any more accurate than that provided by QI.

3.h BODY SHAPE AND FAT DISTRIBUTION

After puberty the fat distribution of males and females shows characteristic differences: women tend to store fat around breast, hip and thigh regions, whereas men tend to accumulate fat in and on the abdomen. However some women have a relatively central, or android, fat distribution, while some men have a relatively peripheral or gynaecoid fat distribution. Vague (1953) was the first to draw attention to the clinical implications of these differences: he showed that an android fat distribution was more strongly associated with atherosclerosis, diabetes and gout than a similar amount of fat in a gynaecoid distribution. His method for classifying fat distribution was rather complex, and did not attract much international attention for another two decades. The metabolic consequences of different fat distributions will be discussed elsewhere, but the techniques for measuring and classifying fat distribution can conveniently be described here.

The outline front and side views of three women with roughly similar degrees of fatness are shown in Figure 3.12. These outlines are obtained from projections of somatotype photographs, which are taken in a standard format (Stalley & Garrow 1975). This technique was developed to follow changes in fat distribution with weight loss, and it has the merit that photographs taken many months apart can be superimposed to demonstrate change in shape. To derive a classification of obesity the ratio of waist diameter to thigh diameter on the side view is used. Alternatively the circumference of waist and thigh can be measured with a tape measure, which yields a ratio which correlates well with the diameters measured on somatotype photographs (Ashwell et al 1982). The technique using a tape measure is more convenient, but when obese subjects have a pendulous abdomen it is difficult to find landmarks which permit replicable

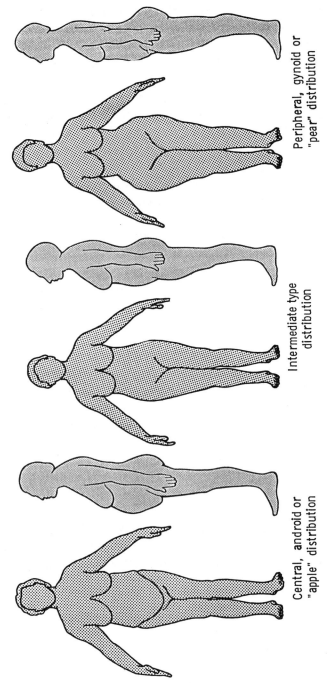

Central, android or
"apple" distribution

Intermediate type
distribution

Peripheral, gynoid or
"pear" distribution

Fig. 3.12 Outline of three obese women with approximately the same Queteler's index, but differing in pattern of fat distribution

measurements of waist diameter: with weight loss the circumference at the level of the umbilicus may no longer be the true waist circumference.

Kalkoff et al (1983) and Larsson et al (1984) have used the waist: hip ratio to classify fat distribution: waist circumference is measured at the level of the umbilicus and hip circumference at the level of the iliac crest with the subject standing. An average value for waist:hip ratio in men is about 0.93, with a range from 0.75 to 1.10. Among women an average value is about 0.83 with a range from 0.70 to 1.00, so the ranges for the two sexes show considerable overlap. The femoral fat depots in women probably have a special importance as an energy reserve to support pregnancy and lactation (Rebuffe-Scrive et al 1985).

Since interest is now focused particularly on abdominal fat the new techniques of CAT-scanning have been used to determine the proportion of abdominal fat which is subcutaneous or within the peritoneal cavity (Borkan et al 1982, Tokunaga et al 1983, Grauer et al 1984, Ashwell et al 1985, Kvist et al 1986). These studies suggest that the metabolic complications of obesity may be specifically related to the amount of intra-abdominal fat rather than subcutaneous fat in the abdominal wall.

Ashwell et al (1987) have recently reported the effect of weight loss on the waist:hip and waist:thigh ratio in 58 obese women. After reducing weight from an average of 94.7 kg to 83.0 kg the waist:hip ratio was unchanged (0.826 vs. 0.829) but the waist:thigh ratio decreased significantly (P<0.01) from 1.208 to 1.176. It appears, therefore, that whatever the prognostic significance of waist:hip circumference ratios the ratio is unlikely to change much with weight loss. There is other evidence that the pattern of fat distribution is genetically determined: Borjeson (1976) showed that identical twins showed much less difference in the pattern of skinfold thickness than dizygotic twins. However, this is not to say that the total quantity of fat is genetically determined: the influence of heredity and environment in the aetiology of obesity is discussed in section 6.d.

3.i MEASUREMENT OF FAT CELL SIZE AND NUMBER

Hirsch & Gallian (1968) demonstrated that it is easy and relatively painless to obtain a sample of subcutaneous adipose tissue by percutaneous needle biopsy. If the tissue is treated with osmium tetroxide the fat in the cells is fixed within the fat cell, and these particles of fixed fat can be separated and counted, so the number of fat cells in a given weight of adipose tissue can be measured. If this sample of adipose tissue is taken to be typical of all the adipose tissue in the body the average weight of fat per cell can be calculated, and if total body fat is measured then the total number of fat cells in the body can be calculated. This calculation depends on various assumptions which are not necessarily true. First, the osmium tetroxide method counted cells which contain a certain amount of fat, but cells with very little fat were not detected, so the estimate of cell number in a biopsy was too low. Second, it is now known that fat cell size varies considerably from one site to another, so a single biopsy does not yield a reliable sample of total body adipose tissue (Ashwell et al 1976).

Despite these limitations there was considerable interest in measurements of fat cell number because there was evidence that fat cell number was constant in adults, and that people who had become obese in childhood had more fat cells that those who had become obese later in life. These observations gave rise to the hypotheses 'that obesity may be accompanied by an excessive number of adipocytes, possibly brought about by excess feeding in infancy and childhood, and that the excessive number of adipocytes remains constant and in some way causes a drive for maintaining the obese state' (Hirsch 1975), and that 'when the fat cell size in different regions of an individual is known, as well as the total fat cell number, the success of an energy-reduced dietary regimen might be approximately predicted both in terms of remaining total body fat and regional fat depot decrease' (Bjorntorp et al 1975). These were plausible hypotheses with important implications: if fat cell number is set during childhood, and subsequently determines the ability of the obese person to lose fat, then clearly preventive measures should be directed towards stopping an undue increase in fat cell number in early life.

However, intensive work on fat cells over the past ten years has shown that, during adult life, cells which are histologically indistinguishable from fibroblasts can become adipocytes, and fat cells can lose their fat and become indistinguishable from fibroblasts, so we can no longer believe in the constancy of fat cell number in adult life. It is of little significance to calculate the fat cell number in an adult at any particular time, since more cells will be recruited for this purpose if there is a need to store more fat. It appears that increase in fat storage over a short time (weeks or months) is achieved mainly by increasing the amount of fat stored in existing fat cells, but if fat cells reach a particular size then gradually recruitment of more storage cells is initiated.

Probably the most valuable advance from the study of adipose tissue biopsies has concerned the function rather than the morphology of fat cells from different adipose tissue depots. In vitro measurement of rates of lipolysis in biopsies of adipose tissue have shown similar basal rates in femoral and abdominal adipose tissue in non-pregnant women. However, lipolysis increases in the femoral fat during lactation. In non-pregnant women noradrenalin has less lipolytic effect on femoral fat than abdominal fat, but lipolysis in femoral fat increases during pregnancy (Rebuffe-Scrive et al 1985). This implies that the femoral fat depot is conserved in the non-pregnant woman, but made available as an energy source in the later stages of pregnancy and lactation.

The discussion of adipose tissue so far has concerned white adipose tissue, which is the predominant energy storage tissue in adult man. However there has been much interest in brown adipose tissue, which has powerful heat-generating capacity, and which is required to maintain the body temperature of small mammals when the ambient temperature is low (Himms-Hagen 1984). The histological appearance of a typical white and brown adipose tissue cell is shown in Figure 3.13. The white fat cell has a thin rind of cytoplasm surrounding a large fat globule. The nucleus is displaced to

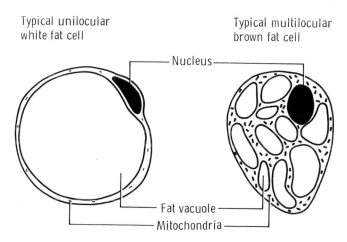

Typical unilocular white fat cell

Typical multilocular brown fat cell

Nucleus

Fat vacuole

Mitochondria

Fig. 3.13 Diagram to illustrate chief morphological differences between white and brown fat cells

the edge which gives the cells a signet-ring appearance in a stained section. There are very few mitochondria in the cytoplasm of a white fat cell, which is metabolically relatively inactive. The brown fat cell, by contrast, has small fat droplets in a cytoplasm rich in mitochondria. These mitochondria are the site of heat production.

The interest in brown fat in connection with obesity arises from the demonstration that in certain strains of obese rodent there is a defect in thermogenesis in brown fat, so in a cold environment the animal becomes hypothermic and dies. It has further been demonstrated that during overfeeding the thermogenic activity of brown fat is activated, energy expenditure increases, and thus the animal does not become as obese as it would have done without the protective action of the brown fat (Stock & Rothwell 1982). It is tempting to suggest that some obese human subjects, who seem to have quite a modest energy intake, have become obese because they lack an analogous thermogenic mechanism (James & Trayhurn 1981, Jung & James 1986). This possibility is considered in section 6.b., but we should note that estimates of the activity of brown fat in human adults indicate that it could not account for more than 2% of energy expenditure (Cunningham et al 1985, Astrup 1986). Therefore, if human obesity is due to a defect in thermogenesis it is unlikely that this defect is related to brown fat.

4

Measurement of energy intake

The energy stores in the body are derived exclusively from the energy-yielding constituents of food and drink, namely carbohydrate, fat, protein and alcohol. It is not difficult to measure how much of these nutrients is present in a given amount (usually 100 g) of an item of food. However, the measurement of habitual energy intake in man with useful accuracy is one of the most difficult enterprises a nutritionist can attempt. There are three problems. First, analysis of food yields an estimate of gross energy, but only part of this (called 'metabolisable energy') is available to the person eating the food. Second, if an accurate method is used to record the energy intake of a subject over a given period, it is very likely that the intake over that period has been affected by the monitoring procedure, so what is measured is not in fact habitual intake. Third, spontaneous intake fluctuates widely from day to day, and week to week, so even if the habitual intake were known over a period of several days there would still be considerable uncertainty about extrapolating this value to give an estimate of habitual intake over a period of, say, 1 year. These problems will be discussed in turn.

The gross energy content of a food is determined by bomb calorimetry: a dry sample of the food is ignited in a crucible in a pressure container with pure oxygen at high pressure. Under these conditions combustion is complete, and the gross energy content of the food is indicated by the amount of heat generated. For fat, alcohol and simple carbohydrates the gross energy and metabolisable energy is virtually identical, since when these foods are eaten by man they are virtually totally absorbed from the gut, and completely combusted to yield carbon dioxide and water — the same end products as those formed in the bomb calorimeter, with the same energy yield, namely 9 kcal/g for fat, 7 kcal/g for alcohol and 3.75 kcal/g for monosaccharides. With protein the oxidation of nitrogenous compounds in man does not go to oxides of nitrogen as it does in the bomb calorimeter, but stops at urea. Therefore,the gross energy of protein is about 5.25 kcal/g, but of this 1.25 kcal/g is lost as urinary urea, so the metabolisable energy is 4 kcal/g.

The chief difficulty in calculating the metabolisable energy in human diets concerns the complex carbohydrates — starch, and 'dietary fibre' — about the definition of which the experts still dispute. If starch such as cornflour is cooked it is as readily digested and absorbed as glucose. This can be demonstrated by giving an oral dose of 50 g cooked cornflour which is enriched with ^{13}C. The timecourse of evolution of carbon dioxide labelled with ^{13}C after such a meal in normal fasted subjects is shown in Figure 4.1. Within

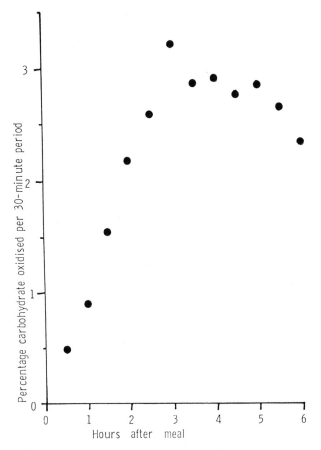

Fig. 4.1 Evolution of labelled carbon dioxide after oral meal of cooked starch enriched with labelled carbon. About 25% of the carbohydrate is oxidised 6 h after ingestion, and remainder is stored (Data of Garrow et al 1983)

30 min expired CO_2 is significantly labelled, indicating that some of the starch has already been absorbed and oxidised. Peak labelling of expired CO_2 occurs about 3 h after the meal, and by 6 h about 25% of the ingested starch has been oxidised and the remainder has been stored. The results for a glucose meal are very similar (Garrow et al 1983).

The gross energy of starch is 4.2 kcal/g, and for purposes of food tables a value of 4 kcal/g can conveniently be used for 'available' carbohydrate to account for both starch and monosaccharides (Paul & Southgate 1978). To validate this procedure it is necessary to feed diets of different composition, and to make very accurate measurements of gross energy intake and of energy losses in urine and faeces. This was done by Southgate & Durnin (1970) who found satisfactory agreement between the metabolisable energy as calculated and as measured by the difference between gross energy and energy losses in excreta. However, this has been disputed by Goranzon et al (1983) who measured the energy losses in excreta with diets high and low in protein and fibre, and compared the results with the metabolisable energy calculated by various methods. On average the errors were less than 5% for most diets, but with the high fibre diet there was a 13% difference between the observed metabolic energy and that calculated by the method of Paul and Southgate. There are at least two reasons why it is difficult to calculate the metabolisable energy of a high fibre diet: one is that the presence of a large amount of fibre in the lumen of the gut decreases the absorption of other nutrients, in particular fat, so faecal fat excretion on high-fibre diets is higher than would be expected for the fat content of the diet (Goranzon et al 1983).

The other problem concerns the availability or otherwise of dietary carbohydrate. If certain chemical species, like cellulose and lignin, were simply excreted unchanged in the faeces, while all other carbohydrates were absorbed, the calculation of metabolisable energy would be simple. However, recent work has shown that certain forms of starch are not digested by intestinal amylase, so they pass to the large bowel and serve as an energy source for the anaerobic metabolism of colonic bacteria. The starch in leguminous seeds is protected by a relatively resistant cell wall, and the digestion of these starches depends on the way the food was processed and cooked to expose the starch granules to the action of digestive enzymes (Wursch et al 1986).

Another interesting example is provided by the studies of

ileostomy effluent by Englyst & Cummings (1986). Patients with an ileostomy were fed bananas of varying ripeness: with the least ripe banana very little of the banana starch was hydrolysed and absorbed in the small bowel, so this starch made up the great majority of 'non-available' carbohydrate passing to the colon, but when fully ripe bananas were fed the carbohydrate was mainly in the form of sugars which were readily absorbed. Thus a week of ripening changes most of the carbohydrate in a banana from non-available to available. For this reason it is impossible for food tables to give a very accurate indication of the energy value of high-fibre foods. (The question of carbohydrate digestion is also of importance in diabetic diets, which are discussed in Chapter 13).

It should be stressed here that the total energy losses in faeces is normally only about 5% of intake. The suggestion is sometimes made that the difference between lean and obese people who apparently eat the same diet is due to the greater efficiency with which obese people extract energy from the diet (Macnair 1979). This cannot be so, since many studies have shown that both lean and obese people absorb about 95% of the energy which they ingest.

4.a ENERGY INTAKE UNDER EXPERIMENTAL CONDITIONS

To measure daily energy intake it is necessary to know the weight and energy concentration of each item of food consumed. For the reasons given in the previous section high-fibre foods should be avoided if high accuracy is required, and if the diet consists solely of one item of food both analysis and calculation are greatly simplified. Furthermore, if the diet consists of a homogeneous liquid, such as milk, it is very easy to take a representative sample for analysis, and if all the diet provided is not consumed the composition of that which is left will be identical to that which was consumed. Liquid formula diets also lend themselves to use in feeding machines (Campbell et al 1971, Pudel & Oetting 1977). These can be constructed so the subject does not know what quantity he is taking, or even so the subject is deliberately given misleading information about his intake. Snack vending machines can be adapted so as to provide the subject with items of solid food in discrete quantities of which the composition is accurately known (Durrant & Wloch 1978).

The features of liquid dispensed diets which make it convenient for the experimenter — that it is uniform and homogeneous — also make it monotonous and unacceptable for the subject. The penalty which the experimenter pays for ease of analysis is that the subjects will probably reject the diet after a few days, or relieve the tedium by surreptitiously eating more interesting fare, unless restrained by efficient policing or unusual loyalty to the investigator. In our experience, 3 weeks' incarceration in a metabolic ward on a formula diet is about as much as most patients will tolerate in the service of research (Garrow et al 1978). Certainly energy intake on a liquid formula gives little information about what the subject would have eaten if normal food had been avaliable.

For these reasons enlightened self-interest, as much as humane considerations, stimulates investigators to provide varied diets for metabolic studies, although this involves much more analytical work and some loss in accuracy of measurement. It is possible to measure energy intake with an accuracy of about $\pm 2\%$ if the diet is carefully prepared in a diet kitchen from items of food which have been bought in bulk and of which a sample of each batch has been analysed, and provided the subjects are under continuous surveillance in a closed metabolic ward. I have no faith in estimates of food intake (or collection of excreta) when the subjects are allowed to roam freely, since there is a very good chance that some mistake will occur and thus invalidate any calculation of energy balance.

Examples of excellent energy balance technique are given in the studies reviewed by Porikos & Pi-Sunyer (1984): in some of these studies patients were confined to a metabolic ward for up to 62 days and provided with varied palatable meals every item of which had been weighed and analysed before the meal was served, and every item of plate waste was weighed back. These studies demand a high degree of dedication both for subjects and investigators. It is tempting to take short-cuts like using food-table values for the composition of food, assuming that all the food offered is eaten so plate waste is not analysed, and trusting that the subjects will eat only the food provided on the protocol. These short-cuts save time, but they introduce errors of unknown magnitude. Balance studies are always demanding, but if they are not done properly they might as well not be done at all.

4.b ENERGY INTAKE UNDER NATURAL CONDITIONS

In most clinical applications it would be interesting to know what people habitually ate in their normal life, rather than the diet which was imposed by experimental conditions. The obvious way in which such information could be collected is to ask subjects to weigh and record the food they eat over a typical period of, say, a week. Shorter periods of recording are of little value, since intake usually differs considerably between working days during the week and leisure time at the weekend. The pioneering studies of Widdowson (1936) which were the first to show the large variation in intake between individuals, used the 7-day weighed diet inventory method. In their review of methods for measuring energy intake Stern et al (1984) conclude that this technique, although very tedious, is the most accurate available. The same truth can be expressed by saying that other methods are still less accurate.

An insight into the validity of weighed dietary intakes, particularly in connection with the differences between the intakes of obese and lean subjects, can be obtained from the study of Prentice et al (1986). They obtained weighed intake records from a group of lean women for a period of 7 days, and for two periods of 7 days from a group of obese women. They concurrently measured total energy expenditure using the doubly-labelled water technique. The relevant data from non-pregnant women who made acceptable records are shown in Figure 4.2. Although it is not to be expected that the intake and output of each individual would be accurately matched over a 7-day period, the average of the groups should be roughly equal, or if not the discrepancy should be indicated by a change in body weight over the period of the study.

The results from the lean and obese women are strikingly different. Data from the 11 lean women show an average recorded intake of 7.85 MJ/day, and an average observed energy expenditure of 7.99 MJ/day. This is very satisfactory agreement. The change in body composition of these women over the monitored period suggested that they were in negative energy balance by about 0.3 MJ/day, so if the recorded intake is 'corrected' for this imbalance the agreement with observed output is still good. The results from the obese group are less reassuring. On average their recorded intake was 6.73 MJ/day, and observed output was 10.22 MJ/day. Changes in body composition indicate a negative energy balance of 1.75 MJ/day, but even with this addition the reported intake falls short of observed output by nearly 2 MJ/day. These results indicate that the recorded intake of the lean women may well have been correct, and only 0.3 MJ/day (3.8%) less than their habitual intake. The recorded intake of the obese group is most implausible:

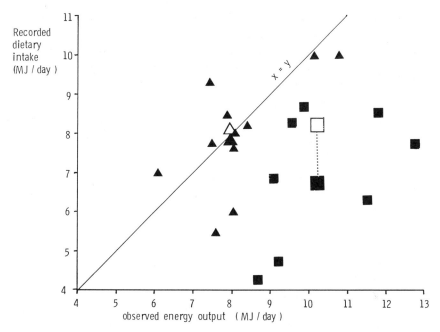

Fig. 4.2 Relation of recorded daily energy intake to observed daily energy expenditure in lean women (triangles) and obese women (squares). Open symbols indicate mean value for each group adjusted for observed change in body composition during period of study. Average reported energy intake matches observed energy output well in lean women, who showed little change in body composition. In the obese group, reported intake was lower than for the lean women, but observed output was higher. Even when reported intake of the obese group is corrected for changes in body composition there is still a deficit in average reported intake compared with output. This suggests that the obese group systematically under-reported their actual intake, although this was already less than their habitual intake (Data of Prentice et al 1986)

certainly what they recorded was less that the intake required to maintain weight by about 1.75 MJ/day, because the measurement of body composition indicated a deficit of about that amount. This is not surprising since it is well known that the act of weighing the diet results in a decrease in food intake in most people, although the decrease indicated here of about 25% is unusually large. What is more disturbing is that the intake 'corrected' for energy imbalance is still about 2 MJ short of expenditure. By far the most likely explanation for this discrepancy is that the group of obese women were, on average, making a weighed record of food intake which was about 2 MJ/day less than the food they were actually eating.

Since weighing and recording the diet tends to inhibit food intake an alternative way of assessing food intake in natural conditions is to take a diet history of what was eaten in the past. This escapes the danger of influencing food intake, but involves even bigger errors for other reasons. The best that can be expected of a dietary history is that the investigator obtains a true account of what the subject believes he or she ate, but even under favourable conditions this may differ considerably from what was actually eaten.

Any illusions about the validity of dietary recall methods should have been shattered by the report of Acheson et al (1980). The subjects were members of the British Antarctic Survey who lived for a year at the base of Haley Bay. Every item of food had to be brought to the base by relief ship once a year, so it was very easy to check food consumption among 12 members of the expedition. For a total of 1085 man-days the subjects kept weighed rcords of all items of food and drink, and on 86 occasions they were asked to recall what they had just recorded for the previous 24 h. This task is obviously much easier than that of a person who is asked to recall intake which he had not recorded, but even with this advantage the recalled intake ranged from 33–132% of the recorded intake. When the subjects were given a blank sheet of paper on which to recall their intake they underestimated on average by 33.6%, while if they were given a printed dietary questionnaire they underestimated by 21% on average.

The only reasonable conclusion from this report is that it is a waste of time for both investigators and subjects to use dietary recall data, because the results are so unreliable that it would be easier, and just as accurate, to make a guess at energy intake based on the published average values for energy requirements.

A good example of misplaced faith in dietary recall data is provided by Braitman et al (1985). They observed that analyses of dietary surveys had failed to show that obese people were eating more than lean people, and considered the possibility that this failure was due to the small databases which had been used. With the massive HANES database of 24-hour dietary recall data on 6219 adults obtained by a skilled dietitian or nutritionist in a 20-minute interview they were still unable to show that obese people ate more than lean, so they suggest that the cause of obesity must lie somewhere other than with overeating. This conclusion will be discussed elsewhere, but it is appropriate here to indicate the frailty of the reasoning which led to it. The HANES data on dietary intake are certainly no more reliable than the weighed 7-day records illustrated in Figure 4.2, and if Prentice et al (1986) had obtained diet records from 19 million people, rather than 19 people, they would still have failed to show that obese people eat more than lean. To paraphrase the late Henry Ford: 'Twenty-four hour diet histories are bunk', and an investigator with a large database of bunk is no better placed to investigate small differences in energy intake than an investigator with a small database of bunk.

If 24-hour diet histories are useless, how long a period must be reviewed to obtain a useful measure of intake, and how can this estimate be validated? These important questions have been addressed by many workers, most recently by Van Staveren et al (1985) and Bingham & Cummins (1985). Urinary nitrogen excretion in adults over a period of several weeks closely resembles nitrogen intake, so if nitrogen excretion is measured this can be compared with the protein intake estimated by dietary recall. It seems that if dietary histories are to provide useful quatitative information they need to relate to intake over a period of at least 1 month.

An alternative approach has been used by Obarzanek & Levitsky (1985). They asked 8 subjects who were 'conscientious and trained to keep accurate food records' to weigh and record all they ate and drank for 4 days (Monday to Thursday) on one week, and the next week over the same 4 days they ate all their food in the research unit, where it was weighed by the staff. The day-to-day variation in energy intake during the 4-day periods was about 16% of average at home and 10% of average in the laboratory: both these estimates of day-to-day variability are rather smaller than those found in studies which were not limited to weekday records (Acheson et al 1980). The home and laboratory data were analysed by analysis of variance and intraclass correlation coefficient. The paired differences were not significantly different from zero, and the intraclass correlation coefficient was highly significant ($p < 0.005$). The authors conclude 'that food consumed in a laboratory setting is a reasonable approximation of caloric intake as measured under free-living conditions'.

One would like to believe this conclusion, but Figure 4.3 shows a plot for each subject of his or her 4-day average intake at home and in the laboratory. For two of the subjects the agreement is very good (mean difference 67 kcal and 71 kcal respectively), but the largest difference is 628 kcal, and the mean difference is 382 kcal, or about 15% of mean intake. So with well-trained subjects during weekdays this is the average error of a prediction based on 4 days, eating in the laboratory, but it is safe to assume that with less well-trained subjects, or at weekends, the error would be considerably greater. When this technique is compared with the technique of dietary

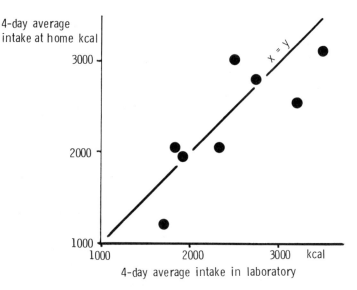

Fig. 4.3 Relation of average daily energy intake of 4 men and 4 women based on 4-day recordings at home or in the laboratory (Data of Obarzanek & Levitsky 1985)

history in one of its forms (Stern et al 1984) it is doubtful if any accuracy gained by getting subjects to eat in the laboratory justifies the much greater inconvenience to both subjects and investigators.

The paper of Krantzler et al (1982) contains the surprising statement: 'Results of this study demonstrate that it is feasible to collect accurate data on food intake using the telephone.' The study involved students from a single dormitory complex at University of California, Davis, who were observed eating in the dormitory dining hall. At the beginning of each meal the participants were given a printed form listing all the foods available at the meal, on which they marked their selection. After 18–46 h they were asked by telephone to recall what they had eaten — not the quantity, but the menu items they had selected. The average under-reporting (ie foods observed to have been eaten, but not recalled) was 13–31%, and the average over-reporting (foods recalled, but not observed to have been eaten) was 10–18%. The average agreement between what was observed and reported was highest for breakfast (83%) and lowest for 24-hour recall of lunch and dinner (both 65%). I think this study is a striking demonstration of the fact that intelligent sujects, under favourable conditions, often cannot recall what kind of food they ate the previous day, and still less what quantity of this food they ate.

No one need be surprised that the very poor techniques available to the researcher who wishes to measure habitual energy intake have failed so far to show any consistent difference between the intake of lean and obese subjects. Fortunately more reliable information about habitual energy intake can be derived from measurements of energy expenditure (discussed in the next chapter) and application of the principles of energy balance.

4.c ASSESSING HUNGER, APPETITE AND RESTRAINT

Although habitual energy intake is almost impossible to measure, for reasons given above, it is not difficult to devise experiments to investigate the regulation of energy intake. For example two groups of subjects, one lean and the other obese, may be presented with a meal shortly after ingesting a milk shake which has either a high-energy or low-energy content. If the lean group eat less of the meal when preceded by a high-energy milk shake than when it is preceded by a low-energy milk shake, while this difference is not seen with the obese group, the study would support the hypothesis that lean people have better physiological regulation of energy intake than obese people. However, eating in human subjects is a very complex process, and the simple experimental design outlined above probably would not yield a clear difference between the lean and obese groups, and even if it did this result would be open to several interpretations.

The amount a person eats at a given time is a result of several conflicting factors, among which we may identify at least three: hunger, appetite and restraint. Hunger is a drive to eat which can be reliably caused in any normal animal or human subject by an energy deficit, and which is removed when this energy deficit is abolished by refeeding. Appetite is a drive to eat a food which is palatable in that particular situation: for example a person who has eaten a large meal may still have an appetite for strawberries, but a fruit-picker who has eaten strawberries all day probably would not have such an appetite. Finally, a person who experiences hunger or appetite for a food may not eat it as a result of restraint, arising from a belief that for some reason (such as politeness, or the need to avoid obesity) it would be wrong to eat that food. This factor of restraint makes it particularly difficult to study eating behaviour in obese subjects, since as soon as they are aware that their food intake is observed they are liable to be inhibited in food intake. Psychologists have shown great ingenuity in overcoming this problem by devising experiments in which the subjects are deprived of food for several hours while completing meaningless questionnaires, and then covertly observed as snack foods are made available to them as they complete a last irrelevant task. A masterly review of the many studies of human eating behaviour published up to 1979 was made by Spitzer & Rodin (1981) who comment: 'Collectively the studies continue to be impressive in their demonstration of the lack of clear overweight–normal differences in eating behaviour'.

It would be impractical and unnecessary to attempt to review here the huge literature on the regulation of food intake in man, which was the topic of a supplement to the *American Journal of Clinical Nutrition*, vol. 42, no. 5, 1985. Only those findings which are relevant to an understanding of the aetiology and treatment of human obesity will be discussed. The first point to note is formulae which predict reasonably well the intake of rats on laboratory chow will not work with human subjects offered a varied palatable chow. For example Russek (1976) proposed a mathematical model based on the concentration of glucose, insulin, adrenalin and glucagon in the blood, liver glygogen, the rate of glucose utilisation by the lateral hypothalamus, body weight and osmolarity, and air temperature. Perhaps in man also these factors could be shown to affect food intake if everything else was held constant, and only a monotonous diet like laboratory chow was available to the experimental subject. However these are not the conditions which apply to obese patients. Hypothalamic damage is a rare but well-documented cause of obesity in man (Bray & Gallagher 1975), but food intake in intact man is dominated by cognitive factors which do not apply to the chow-fed rat.

A method to evaluate restraint in eating was proposed by Herman & Mack (1975). The subject is asked the following 5 questions. How often are you dieting? What is your maximum weight gain in a week? Do you eat sensibly before others and make up for it alone? Do you give much time and thought to food? Do you have feelings of guilt after overeating? The more strongly positive the response the higher the restraint score. However, Spitzer & Rodin (1981) point out that the questions do not necessarily reflect the extent to which the respondent consciously restricts food intake, nor does the restraint score reliably predict the amount eaten in test situations. This is unfortunate, because we need a good method for measuring restraint. If a group of normal-weight subjects contains some individuals who are effortlessly lean, and others who would be obese if they did not constantly restrain their intake, this will not make a suitable control group with which to compare the eating behaviour of obese subjects.

Two facts of great importance have been established by studies on eating behaviour. First, that habit plays an important part in regulating intake. If the energy content of the diet is covertly decreased, by substituting the non-nutritive sweetener aspartame for sucrose, there is some increase in the weight of food consumed, but not enough to compensate for the decrease in energy concentration (Porikos et al 1977, 1982). If, in another type of experiment, energy expenditure is increased by increasing exercise, then voluntary food intake increases very little, and fails to match the increased energy requirements (Woo et al 1982a,1982b, McGowan et al 1986). The practical implication of these observations is that it is probably useful to use low-energy foods, and increased exercise, to help to generate a negative energy balance in obese patients, since there is no immediate physiological drive to replace the energy thus removed (Porikos & Pi-Sunyer 1984).

The other important fact about human food intake is that it is greatly influenced by palatability, which is itself dependent on variety in the diet. Rolls et al (1984) have done a series of experiments showing that appetite for a particular food decreases as that food is ingested, but appetite for a different type of food is not affected. Thus when subjects were offered a meal of four separate courses — sausages, bread and butter, chocolate dessert, and then banana — they ate 60% more calories than when the meal consisted of one food type only. The practical implication of this finding is that it may be easier for an obese person to keep to a low energy diet which is relatively monotonous, and hence does not stimulate appetite, than a more varied and palatable diet.

'Satiety' is one of the terms which has not so far been defined in this discussion on the regulation of food intake. It is a sensation intermediate between the relief of hunger and the nausea which ultimately limits overeating, and is difficult to define either operationally or in the abstract. It would be helpful to identify foods which had a high satiating capacity relative to their energy content, since these foods would presumably enhance the acceptability of a low energy diet. Kissileff (1982) reports that a quadratic curve describes the cumulative intake of a single-course liquid meal, but this approach is difficult to apply to calculate the satiating efficiency of more normal meals consisting of several different foods (Kissileff et al 1984).

For many years there have been two great mysteries concerning the control of food intake in man:

a. How does the signal for satiety work in time to stop the meal? Whatever the signal may be — a change in blood glucose, a change in body temperature, even the taste of food — it cannot be generated until the food has at least entered the mouth, and once in the mouth it is likely to be eaten rather than spat out. It is difficult to believe that a person who needs, say, 500 kcal (2 MJ) at a particular meal would rely on a satiety signal generated half-way through the meal to terminate it at 500 kcal, because there is no certainty that, having set up conditions which would produce satiety some time later, the second half of the meal would actually be eaten. Therefore if we believe that the signal comes from the last mouthful actually eaten, how can this operate in time to stop the next mouthful when there is probably less than a minute for the last mouthful to be analysed by the control system, whatever that may be?
b. Since the control system seems to work well in the long term, how is it possible to fool it so easily in the short term with changes in the energy density of food?

Both these problems may be explained on the hypothesis that satiety is a conditioned reaction: that it arises, not from the properties of the meal which we are currently eating, but from our experience of similar meals which we have eaten in the past. If our past experience is that about 500 kcal is a comfortable and satisfying amount to eat at a particular meal we will experience satiety when we think that we have eaten about 500 kcal. If some scientist has adulterated the food, so that when we think we have had 500 kcal we have in fact had more or less, this will not affect satiety until the experiment has gone on long enough for us to acquire a new set of experience about the consequences of eating the adulterated food.

The history of this important idea is given by Booth (1977). It is important from a clinical viewpoint, because it offers hope that a satiety mechanism may be susceptible to retraining. A convincing demonstration of the acquired sensory control of satiation in man was given by Booth et al (1976). They recruited university staff and students to take 100 ml of a starch drink before a sandwich lunch, with a flavoured yoghurt as dessert. Every day the lemon-flavoured starch drink looked and tasted the same, but on some days the drinks contained 5 g starch and the yoghurt was one flavour, and on other days the drink contained 65 g starch and the yoghurt was a second flavour. In time subjects came to eat less on the days when the meal started with the higher starch preload, than when it started with the smaller starch preload. So far the experiment has told us nothing about the mechanism by which this adjustment was made.

The second phase of the experiment was to change all the starch drinks to an intermediate value (35 g starch) and observe the effect of the flavour of the yoghurt dessert on the amount eaten at the meal. At first, when subjects were offered the flavour of yoghurt which had previously been associated with the large starch preload they ate less yoghurt than when offered the flavour previously associated with the small preload. When the experiment was repeated with the 35 g preload several times the difference disappeared. This is as convincing evidence as possible that the subjects had come to associate a flavour with a particular state of satiety under conditions when this association was appropriate, and had continued to make the association even when there was no reason for it.

Blundell & Hill (1986) have reported a decrease in satiety in volunteers after taking drinks sweetened with aspartame. They found that the sweet taste of aspartame decreased the pleasantness of sweet taste (as glucose does) but (unlike glucose) aspartame was followed by an increased motivation to eat. They ascribe these paradoxical results to the dissociation of the sweet taste from the satiating effect of glucose.

The idea that habit, experience and teaching are important influences in regulating food intake is one supported by much animal experimentation. The phenomenon of 'bait shyness' is well known: if an animal has been injured by eating poisoned food neither that animal, nor other members of the same colony, will eat food of the same flavour, even if unpoisoned food is offered. It is obvious that this learned aversion to certain types of food is necessary for survival of the species, and it is not difficult to accept that similar types of conditioning are powerful factors in determining the amount, as well as the type, of food eaten. The system breaks down when conditions change, and experience is no longer a reliable guide. In the case of human obesity it is striking that migrants from a less affluent to a more affluent culture may experience a very high incidence of obesity. Presumably it takes time to learn the appropriate intake of new and palatable foods.

Can the composition of diets be manipulated to increase satiety without increasing the energy content? One method which has been proposed is to increase the fibre content of the diet, although the difficulties in measuring the energy content of a high-fibre diet have been mentioned above. Heaton (1973) has suggested that the fibre content of the diet is an important factor in regulating energy intake, and Hunt et al (1978) suggest that the lower the energy density of the diet the slower the absorption of energy, since gastric emptying is slower. Grimes & Goddard (1977) have shown that gastric emptying is slower after eating wholemeal bread than after eating white bread. It might be expected, therefore, that volunteers given substantial amounts of wholemeal bread would have a lower spontaneous energy intake thereafter than when they were given white bread, but Bryson et al (1979) failed to observe this effect.

Krotkiewski (1984) found that 10 g guar gum daily reduced hunger ratings in obese subjects more than a similar weight of bran. Porikos & Hagamen (1986) found that obese subjects ate less after a meal which supplied 5.2 g crude fibre than one which supplied 0.2 g crude fibre, but the intake of normal-weight subjects was unaffected by the fibre load.

An interesting attempt to find out what in fact happens to spontaneous intake when the fat: carbohydrate ratio was altered was reported by van Stratum et al (1978). A formula diet, providing 4.18 kJ (1 kcal) per g, was prepared in two recipes: formula A provided 20% of the energy as fat and 61% as carbohydrate, while formula B had the proportions reversed. In both formulae, protein provided 19% of the energy. Over a period of 4 weeks 22 Trappist nuns derived most of their energy from one or other formula, with a balanced crossover design. If either fat or carbohydrate was much more satiating there should have been a significantly lower intake of one or other formula, but this was not found. There were large variations between individuals, but no general pattern emerges. It should be noted that the test foods were made up as drinks, and the formulae were adjusted to give equal energy density, so the results do not necessarily reflect behaviour when eating normal food.

A final question to consider in this section is: does stress induce eating? It is common for obese patients to say that they eat when under stress, but usually this means that they have been trying more or less successfully to limit their energy intake when some emotional crisis occurs and they lose control of their diet. The point is debated by Robbins & Fray (1980) and Herman & Polivy (1980). Certainly all stressful situations do not induce eating, nor does eating always relieve stress, which it would need to do in order to reinforce this behaviour. The point is not very important therapeutically, since the therapist has no power to protect the patient from stress. A more useful approach is to recognise the situations in which collapse of a dieting effort is likely to occur and to provide all possible support for the dieter at that time — especially to try to arrange that food is not freely available to the dieter at a vulnerable period.

5

Measurement of energy expenditure

The measurement of energy expenditure is a much simpler task than the measurement of energy intake, provided that the appropriate apparatus is available. The immediate energy source for metabolic work in the tissues is a phosphate bond in adenosine triphosphate (ATP) or some other high-energy phosphate compound, which must be resynthesised if metabolism is to continue. The oxidation of 1 mol (180 g) glucose involves the uptake of 6 mol (134.4 litres) of oxygen, and the production of 6 mol (134.4 litres) of carbon dioxide and 6 mol (108 g) water, with the liberation of 2.78 MJ (665 kcal). Of this energy less than half (about 44%) is recovered in high-energy phosphate bonds which can be used to drive further metabolic work, and the remainder is degraded to heat. However, as soon as the newly synthesised high-energy phosphate bonds are hydrolysed (which in practice will be in a few seconds) this energy also is degraded to heat, so for the purpose of measuring energy expenditure fuelled by the oxidation of 1 mol of glucose we have the option of observing the liberation of 2.78 MJ heat (direct calorimetry), or the uptake of 6 mol oxygen (indirect calorimetry).

In practice the situation is not quite so simple as indicated above, because the fuel may not be glucose, but fatty acid, alcohol, or the deaminated carbon skeleton of aminoacids. Furthermore the dietary fuel may not be directly oxidised, but may take a circuitous path through various storage compounds before being oxidised, and this will affect the yield of ATP from a given weight of dietary fuel. For example the direct oxidation of 1 mol of glucose would yield 38 mol ATP, but if the glucose was first stored as glycogen and then oxidised the yield would be 37 mol ATP, and if it was converted to palmitic acid, stored as triglyceride and then oxidised, the overall yield would be 33.7 mol ATP. The theoretical yield on direct oxidation of 100 g dietary fat is 51 mol ATP, but if the fatty acids were broken down into acetoacetate and then oxidised the net yield would be only 49 mol ATP (Davidson et al 1979).

The classical teaching was that the generation of ATP took place by three sequential phosphorylation steps, and that 3 mol ATP were generated per mol oxygen consumed, given a P:O ratio 3.0, but a more modern view is that this is not necessarily so (Flatt 1985). Under some conditions P:O ratios ranging from 2.4 to 3.5 have been found. There can also be a dissociation, at least temporarily, between heat production and oxygen utilisation: for example at the very start of vigorous exercise the heat production exceeds the rate of fuel oxidation, because initially pre-formed ATP in muscle is used, and there is a delay of a minute or two before the flow of substrate utilization matches the energy expenditure (Flatt 1985). Not all substrate oxidation is linked to ATP production, because some energy is used in substrate cycling, for example between fructose 6-phosphate and fructose 1,6-biphosphate in muscle (Challis et al 1985). An extreme case of metabolic inefficiency is seen in brown adipose tissue which has the capacity to use fuel and generate heat without any net gain in ATP.

Fortunately the direct calorimetrist can afford to ignore the metabolic processes which use the energy generated by the oxidation of fuels, since whatever the metabolic route taken by dietary fuel, or fuel derived from tissue stores, the total heat generated by the oxidation of 1 g carbohydrate or 1 g protein is about 4 kcal (17 kJ), 1 g alcohol is about 7 kcal (29 kJ), and 1 g fat is about 9 kcal (38 kJ). When we talk about measuring energy expenditure in man we really mean the rate of fuel consumption. The situation is analogous to rating the energy output of an automobile engine by measuring the weight of petrol consumed per hour. For a given weight of fuel the power output will vary according to the tuning of the engine, but the heat generated by the complete combustion of the fuel will not be affected.

The indirect calorimetrist has some problems, since to interpret gaseous exchange in terms of energy production it is necessary to know what fuel is being burned, but in practice the difficulties are not very great. Before we consider techniques for direct and indirect calorimetry it may be noted that the two techniques give very similar answers for energy expenditure, by which we mean the rate at which fuel is being used. It is possible that two individuals may have similar rates of fuel use (and hence similar rates of heat production and oxygen uptake) but be forming high-energy phosphate bonds at different rates, since one is using a more efficient route for oxidative phosphorylation than the other. To detect this difference it would be necessary to make both subjects perform a similar amount of additional metabolic work, which would cause a smaller increase in metabolic rate in the subject with the more efficient metabolism. One way to apply this test is to observe the metabolic cost of a standard work load on a bicycle ergometer after steady-state conditions have been achieved: the muscle would then need to restore the high-energy phosphate lost from the phosphocreatine, which is the immediate energy source for muscular work. In fact the metabolic efficiency of muscular work is remarkably constant at about 27% in different individuals, and in the same person whether overfed or underfed, which suggests that the overall cost of ATP synthesis does not differ greatly from one person to another (Flatt 1985).

5.a MEASUREMENT OF ENERGY EXPENDITURE IN EXPERIMENTAL CONDITIONS

Direct calorimetry

'Every year I have the pleasure of describing Atwater's beautiful experiments to a new class of medical students . . . it is possible to make measurements on a human subject over a period of several days with the precision customary in the physical sciences'. (Passmore 1967). It is possible indeed, but only with skill, vigilance and dedication.

The Atwater calorimeter was developed and perfected over a period of 12 years, and a description of the final instrument is given in great detail by Atwater & Benedict (1899). It was situated in a basement room in the Orange Judd Hall of the Wesleyan University, at Middletown, Connecticut: a holy place to any student of energy balance in man. The calorimeter chamber was essentially a box 2.15 m long, 1.22 m wide and 1.93 m high, made from sheets of 24-gauge copper soldered together. The subject entered through an aperture 49 cm wide and 70 cm high, which was then sealed with a sheet of plate glass bedded in melted beeswax. The chamber was furnished with a table and a bed, both of which could be folded away when not in use, a chair, a telephone, and a bicycle ergometer. There was no source of light inside the chamber, but the aperture faced an outside window of the building.

Completely surrounding the copper chamber and separated from it by an air space of 7.6 cm was another box made of sheet zinc. Surrounding the zinc box were two further concentric coverings of wood, again with an air space of about 7 cm between them. To detect differences in temperature between the copper and zinc shells there were 304 pairs of thermocouples bridging the air gap at selected points over the entire surface of the chamber, and provision was made for heating or cooling the air outside the zinc shell to ensure that the two metal shells could be held at the same temperature at all times, whatever the change in heat production within the copper chamber. Thus escape of heat through the walls of the chamber was prevented.

In order to remove heat from the chamber as fast as it was produced by the subject, water was circulated through cooling pipes inside the chamber. The temperature of the ingoing and outgoing water was read from specially calibrated mercury thermometers to 0.01°C, and the flow rate of water was monitored by an ingenious system which weighed the outcoming water in pans which held about 10 kg water. As one pan became full the flow was switched to another, and the weight of the pan was determined to 2 g. When the subject was asleep at night 10 kg of water, entering at about 5°C and leaving at about 15°C, would suffice to keep the calorimeter at 20°C for 2 or 3 h. When the subject was hard at work 10 kg water might last only 7 min.

Throughout the experiments, which lasted from 1 to 13 days, a team of observers kept records of the temperature of the various layers of the calorimeter wall, and of the cooling water, and of the air which was pumped through the calorimeter at 75 l/min, and that of the subject (by rectal thermometer) every 4 min. After each reading, the flow rate of the cooling water, and the temperature of the air outside the zinc shell, was adjusted so as to maintain a constant temperature in the calorimeter chamber and a zero temperature gradient across the walls. Each experimental day was divided into four 6-hour periods, starting at 07.00 h. Thus at 07.00, 13,00, 19.00 and 01.00 h there was a stocktaking of the total amount of heat removed by the cooling water, and by the water vapour in the expired air. Carbon dioxide production was calculated by the change in weight of soda lime absorbers, the composition of the gas in the calorimeter was analysed, and the subject, his clothing and bedding were weighed to correct for changes in humidity.

If the experimental procedure was exacting, the calculations were no less laborious. Corrections had to be made for the thermal mass of the calorimeter walls (60 kcal/°C); for the thermal mass and temperature of all food entering, or excreta leaving, the calorimeter; for changes in atmospheric pressure (since with a volume of about 5000 litres a change of 1 mm Hg in barometric pressure represents a change of over 6 litres in effective gas volume); and many other minor factors. In the circumstances it is understandable that by 1905, after 12 years of development, these indefatigable workers had completed only 22 experiments on 5 human subjects. This section is concerned with direct calorimetry, so it is this aspect of the work which is here described, but simultaneously Atwater and Benedict were doing complete metabolic balance studies, including complete measurements of gas exchange.

The precision of the results was indeed awe inspiring. There were two standard calibration checks for the calorimeter; the electrical check and the alcohol lamp check. A known amount of heat was generated inside the calorimeter by these means. For a known dissipation of heat from an electric fire 99.72% was recovered, and the recoveries of the products of combustion of a known amount of ethyl alcohol were for heat 99.8%, for carbon dioxide produced 100.1%, for water produced 100.6% and for oxygen consumed 101.0%.

With a human subject as the source of heat the results were less precise, but still magnificent by modern standards. Atwater & Benedict (1899) report the results of their first experiments on man. In each case the subject was Mr E. Osterberg, a man of 31 years 'in excellent health and accustomed, as laboratory janitor and chemical assistant, to moderate muscular labour'. The first four experiments were primarily concerned with calibration or were 'so vitiated by accident as not to be completed'. The results of experiments 5–10 are shown in Table 5.1.

The authors comment on the unsatisfactory discrepancy between predicted and observed heat production in experiment 5, an error of 4.1%. This they ascribe principally to the diet which was more varied than that of some of the later experiments. Mr Osterberg's tolerance seems to have been as excellent as his health, because he ate the experimental diet for 8 days before entering the calorimeter, instead of the normal 4 days, as unexpected circumstances delayed the start of the experiment proper, and he then went on for his further 4 days in the calorimeter. The agreement between predicted and observed heat production becomes greater as the diet is made

Table 5.1. Energy balance in man by direct calorimetry (Data of Atwater & Benedict 1899) Values are average kcal/day, based on 4-day experiments

| | Experiment no. | | | | | |
	5	6	7	8	9	10
Heat determined	2397	2829	2434	2361	2277	2268
Protein change	−24	+40	−69	0	−21	−40
Fat change	−93	−455	−135	+266	+171	+199
Energy store change	−117	−415	−204	+266	+150	+159
Alcohol eliminated	0	0	21	0	0	8
Difference between heat estimated and heat observed	−4.1%	−2.7%	−1.6%	−3.2%	+1.4%	+0.7%

more uniform and easy to sample, and as the team of operators become more expert at maintaining precise temperature control. The results of experiments 9 and 10 have not been surpassed by any investigator in this century.

With modern electronic techniques it is possible to operate a heat-sink calorimeter like that of Atwater and Benedict with much less trouble. Jacobsen et al (1985) describe a large heat-sink calorimeter with a PDP 11/24 computer which controls the calorimeter and processes data from it, and other designs of smaller direct heat-sink calorimeters have been published by Dauncey et al (1978), Tschegg et al (1979) and Snellen et al (1983). Other types of direct calorimeter are a chamber constructed of a gradient layer which generates a voltage proportional to the heat flow across it (Benzinger et al 1958, Spinnler et al 1973) or a water-cooled garment (Webb et al 1972), but for economy and convenience the heat-sink direct calorimeter has much to commend it.

The design of a rather simple direct calorimeter constructed at the Clinical Research Centre, Harrow, UK. is shown in Fig 5.1. Its advantages are that it was relatively inexpensive to construct, it is acceptable to most patients for measurement periods of 26 h, and it gives an estimate of 24-hour energy expenditure which is reproducible within about 2% under fairly standard conditions. Its main disadvantage is that it does not permit separate measurement of heat loss by evaporative, convective and radiative routes, but registers the sum of total heat loss, which, for energy balance studies, is what we require. The chamber is similar in size to that of Atwater & Benedict (1899), and 6 m³ in volume, with walls of expanded polystyrene 20 cm thick, lined inside and outside with aluminium (P). Air is circulated by a fan (F) at 3 m³/min in a duct along the rear wall under the bed. The end walls of the chamber have false walls of

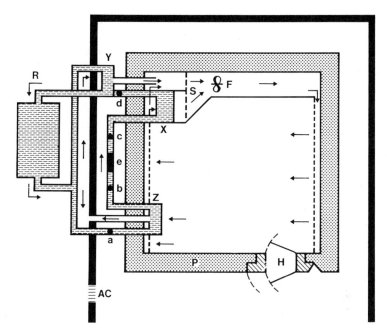

Fig. 5.1 Heat-sink direct calorimeter built at the Clinical Research Centre in 1976 (Webster et al 1986). See text for description

perforated hardboard, so the circulating air emerges from the perforations in the right-hand wall, and passes in a laminar flow fashion across the chamber to enter the perforations in the left-hand wall. During the passage across the chamber it picks up heat from the subject. This heat is removed by a heat exchanger in the duct under the bed. The proportion of the air flow which goes through the heat exchanger is controlled by a semicircular shutter (S) driven by a servo motor. The servo motor is in turn controlled by thermistors which monitor heat flow across the walls of the chamber, and the whole system is adjusted for zero heat flow across the walls. Thus the amount of heat lost by the subject equals the amount of heat gained by the heat exchanger (X).

The heat exchanger is supplied with cold water from a refrigerated reservoir (R) in an adjacent room. This water passes in series through a reference heater (e), at which point exactly 100 W is injected into the water, and then to the main heat exchanger. The temperature rise across the heat exchanger is in the same proportion to the temperature rise across the reference heater as the heat loss of the subject is to 100 W. In order to supply the subject with fresh air, 50 l/min of air is admitted to the chamber through a subsidiary heat exchanger (Y) and an equal amount of chamber air is removed through a twin heat exchanger (Z). Entry to the chamber is by a door containing a window and pass-through hatch (H), and the room housing the chamber is maintained at a constant temperature by an air conditioning unit (AC). Thus it is possible to observe the heat loss of a subject throughout the 24 h, eating, sleeping, watching television, or (if desired) riding a bicycle ergometer. It is not necessary to make any assumptions about the energy equivalence of respiratory gases (see below) and the apparatus can easily be calibrated by either an electrical heat source or a butane lamp with known energy output.

Ideally the direct calorimetrist wishes to measure the heat produced by the subject, but what the calorimeter measures is the heat lost by the subject, which is the same as heat production provided the store of heat in the body does not change. It is difficult to measure the heat stored in a person: as a first approximation the body may be considered to be composed thermally of a warmer core and a cooler shell, and the temperature of these two components can be measured. However under conditions of thermal stress the relative mass of core and shell components may change, so it is virtually impossible to measure changes in heat storage (Livingstone 1967). It is therefore best to make measurements by direct calorimetry over relatively long periods (such as 24 h) so small changes in heat storage will cause only a small percentage error in the answer. Furthermore if a 24-hour period of measurement is used the subject will start and end the period of measurement at the same point in the diurnal cycle of body temperature, so there is less risk that there will be significant changes in heat storage.

Indirect calorimetry

Atwater & Benedict (1905) described how, by analysing the air coming from a calorimeter chamber, the energy expenditure of the occupant could be calculated, and they were able to demonstrate close agreement between this 'indirect' calorimetry and the heat loss measured by direct calorimetry. With indirect calorimetry a change in energy expenditure is reflected almost immediately by a change in the rate of oxygen utilisation, since the oxygen stored in the body is too little to support aerobic metabolism for as much as a minute.

Table 5.2. Gas exchange and energy yield from 1 g foodstuffs, based on analyses of Zuntz (1897)

Food	Gas exchange			Energy yield		Energy/1 O_2	
	ml O_2	ml CO_2	RQ	kcal	kJ	kcal	kJ
Glucose	747	747	1.00	3.75	15.7	5.1	21.3
Starch	829	829	1.00	4.2	17.6	5.1	21.3
Fat	2019	1427	0.71	9.4	39.6	4.7	19.6
Protein	966	781	0.81	4.4	18.4	4.6	19.2
Alcohol	1461	973	0.66	7.0	29.3	4.8	20.1

In this respect indirect calorimetry has the advantage of a shorter response time than direct calorimetry. However, a disadvantage of indirect calorimetry is that the energy value of oxygen varies according to the fuel which it is oxidising.

Table 5.2 shows the amount of oxygen required to oxidise 1 g of various fuels, the respiratory quotient (RQ) — the ratio of carbon dioxide produced to oxygen consumed — and the yield of energy. In classical energy physiology an attempt is made to calculate the metabolic mixture (protein, fat and carbohydrate) which is supplying fuel under given conditions. Theoretically this can be done by calculating the oxidation of protein from the rate of urea excretion, and thus calculating a 'non-protein RQ' which indicates the mixture of carbohydrate and fat being oxidised. This is a tedious exercise which is anyway of doubtful validity, since it assumes that the urea which is excreted, and the carbon dioxide which is exhaled, relates to the same batch of fuel as that which the oxygen oxidised. This is improbable, since both the urea and bicarbonate pools in the body are relatively large and the rate of excretion of these compounds does not necessarily match the rate of production, at least over short periods of an hour or so.

Weir (1949) made a valuable contribution when he showed that the rate of energy production (E watts) can be calculated with little error from the volume of expired air (V l/min) and the difference between the oxygen concentration of inspired and expired air (d %) by the formula

$$E = 3.43 \, Vd$$

This appears to be same as saying that 1 litre oxygen is equivalent to 20.5 kJ, whatever the substrate oxidised, and regardless of the RQ. However, as McLean (1985) has pointed, out Weir's formula works well because it involves two roughly equal and opposite errors, which virtually cancel out. As the RQ decreases from 1.00 to 0.70

the energy equivalence of oxygen decreases by about 6%, but the volume of expired air also decreases relative to the volume of inspired air. If oxygen uptake is calculated by multiplying the concentration difference between inspired and expired air by the minute-volume of expired air (not the minute-volume of inspired air) the calculated oxygen uptake is too high, and at an RQ of 0.7 the error is roughly 6%, which cancels the error arising from the too-low energy equivalence of 1 litre oxygen at an RQ of 0.7. The net effect is that provided flow rate of expired air is measured the energy equivalence of 1 litre oxygen can be assumed to be 20.5 kJ (4.9 kcal) without significant error. The measured volume of gases must be corrected to STPD values (i.e. standard temperature 0°C, and pressure 760 mmHg, dry) before being used in any calculation.

For indirect calorimetry it is necessary to ensure that a true sample of expired air is analysed, and if the subject is confined in a respiration chamber with a suitable ventilating system this is easily arranged. For measurements of energy expenditure extending over several days is it necessary to provide quite a large and comfortably furnished chamber, such as the one in Lausanne (Jequier & Schutz 1983). However for shorter periods of measurement some enclosure around the head will suffice. For measurements of resting metabolic rate it is not satisfactory to use a mouthpiece or tightly fitting face mask to collect expired air, since these are quite uncomfortable after about an hour, so the subject is not at truly rest. It is not a solution to use shorter sampling periods of about 10–15 min to avoid this discomfort, since in short sampling periods the subject does not settle to a true resting state. The most convenient arrangement is to use some form of canopy or ventilated hood over the subject's head though which air is drawn at about 20–30 l/min.

Many such devices have been described (Benedict 1930, Ashworth & Wolff 1969, Garrow & Hawes 1972, Kinney 1980, Head et al 1984, Weissman et al 1985). The essential components are a comfortable enclosure over the subject's head to collect expired air, a quiet and reliable pump which will suck air through the system at a rate of about 20 l/min for resting subjects, but up to 50 l/min for exercising subjects, a meter which will indicate the rate of air flow with an accuracy of about 1%, a small pump which will take a sample of the air stream, dry it and pass it to the gas analyser, and a gas analyser which will measure the difference in oxygen concentration between room air and the air coming from the ventilated hood (typically about 1% difference) also with an accuracy of 1%. It is convenient if an analyser for carbon dioxide is also included, an automatic system for switching the analysers between inspired and expired air to correct for drift in the analysers, and a recorder or printer to display the output. The system chosen will depend on the money and other equipment available to the investigator. Whatever system is used the accuracy of the results will probably depend on the effectiveness of the calibration procedure.

Modern physical gas analysers are deceptively easy to use: gone is the mystique of the Haldane volumetric apparatus from which only experienced technicians could coax a probable answer. If the results are computerised and output in digital form to four significant figures it seems impertinent to doubt their accuracy. However, an elementary understanding of the way the analysers work may save the novice from some pitfalls. The oxygen analyser depends upon the fact that oxygen is paramagnetic — its presence between the poles of a magnet weakens the magnetic field, and the more oxygen present the weaker the field becomes. In paramagnetic oxygen analysers the test gas is admitted to a chamber between the poles of a magnet through which a galvanometer suspension passes, which also carries a small coil. The more oxygen present in the sample gas the greater the current which must be passed through the coil to cause a given deflection on the galvanometer. It is therefore understandable that if the sample gas is passes at too high a rate through the analyser cell it will become unstable, because the turbulence in the sample cell physically shakes the suspension. Also it should be remembered that although the output of the analyser is calibrated to display percentage oxygen, in fact it measures the amount of oxygen in the magnetic field, so it is important when calibrating to ensure that known and unknown gases are admitted to the analyser at the same pressure. Finally, paramagnetic analysers work much better if the air is dried before being admitted to the analyser cell.

Many carbon dioxide analysers work on the infrared absorption characteristics of carbon dioxide. Radiation of the appropriate wavelength is shone through the sample cell, and the more carbon dioxide present the more energy is absorbed and degraded to heat. This heating effect is detected and displayed in term of percentage carbon dioxide. Infrared analysers are remarkably sensitive, robust and generally trouble-free instruments, but again the calibrating and unknown gases must be measured at the same pressure. Infrared analysers must be left switched on: they rely on detecting small temperature changes, and take many hours after first switching on to achieve internal temperature stability.

Any measurement of metabolic rate takes at least 1 h — measurements over shorter periods are liable to too great error from the unsettled state at the beginning of the recording. In a laboratory which makes many measurements of metabolic rate — especially resting metabolic rate before breakfast in the morning — it is convenient to be able to measure two patients simultaneously. It saves operator time, and the patients do not have to wait for the apparatus to become available if another patient is being measured.

We have recently described a system for measuring two patients simultaneously, with control and data acquisition by microcomputer (Garrow & Webster 1986a). The layout is shown in Figure 5.2. One pump, set of gas analysers, computer and printer serves both patients,thus saving money on the more expensive components of the system. Each patient has a loosely fitting face mask (which is adapted to permit sampling of breath for isotope tracer studies) and a rotameter which displays the ventilation rate for that mask. The air stream from each patient in turn, and from room air, is sampled and analysed by the operation of solenoid valves (A, B and C, Fig. 5.2) which open sequentially at intervals controlled by the microcom-

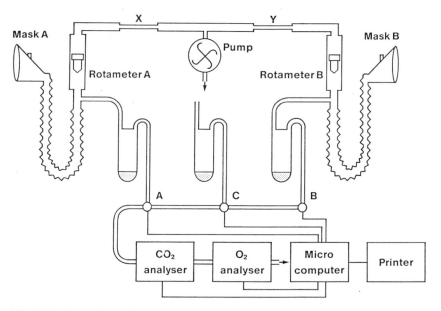

Fig. 5.2 Indirect calorimeter controlled by a microcomputer which will measure two subjects simultaneously (Garrow & Webster 1986a)

puter. Under typical conditions there is a period of 2 min after the opening of a valve during which the tubing is purged of the previous sample, then for 3 min the gas analysers are read and the output is stored by the computer, and then that valve closes and the next is opened. The complete cycle of both patients and room air is therefore completed each 15 min, the calculation of oxygen uptake, carbon dioxide production and RQ for each patient is made by the computer, and the result is displayed on the printer.

The two-channel design saves time in measuring patients, but it also confers advantages in calibration and fault-finding. Calibration is achieved by using a butane lamp in a box as a phantom patient. The RQ of butane is 0.61, and the oxygen consumed in oxidising 1 g butane is 2.51 litres. Both the patient A and B tubes are connected to the box, so the composition of gas in each channel is the same. If the RQ displayed on the printout is not 0.61, but is equal for both 'patients' then it is likely that one of the gas analysers is not correctly calibrated. If the readings for the two patients are not equal this cannot be the fault of the analysers, but indicates that there is a leak on one side, or that the purge time is insufficient. If the RQ is correct and equal both sides, but the printout does not agree with the theoretical oxygen consumption calculated from the weight of butane burned, then the measurement of flow rate should be checked. Thus a simple calibration procedure, which should be done at least once a week, checks all the likely sources of error in the system.

For workers in industrial situations, or in the field where it is not possible to use laboratory apparatus, a very satisfactory estimate of energy expenditure can be obtained with a portable battery-operated indirect calorimeter, the 'Oxylog' (Humphrey & Wolff 1977). This uses a tight-fitting face mask connected by corrugated tubing to the analyser pack which measures the ventilation rate and the oxygen concentration, and displays oxygen consumption, or other variables, on a digital meter.

5.b MEASUREMENT OF ENERGY EXPENDITURE UNDER NATURAL CONDITIONS

Schutz (1981) made an excellent review of techniques available at that time for measuring energy expenditure in free-living man. Most of the methods are not very accurate, but probably the best were the

activity diary or the heart rate method. The activity diary uses measured or estimated energy costs for each activity, and requires the
subject (or a constant observer of the subject) to record the activity
for each minute of the 24 h. I have tried keeping such a record, and
I know of no more irritating procedure. The weaknesses of the
method are therefore that the diary may not be a faithful record of
exactly how subjects spend their time, that the process of keeping
the record may well have deflected the subject from their normal
pattern of activity, and that the energy cost of given activities varies
from time to time according to how they are done, so a single value
cannot always be correct.

The rival to activity diaries was heart rate recording. During any
increase in energy expenditure there is an increased requirement for
oxygen transport to the tissues which requires an increased cardiac
output. As part of this increased cardiac output there is an increase
in heart rate (the other part is achieved by an increased stroke
volume of the heart). Therefore there is quite a good relationship
between heart rate and oxygen consumption in subjects at varying
levels of exercise, and it is possible with modern ambulatory monitoring devices to record heart rate throughout the 24 h with little
disturbance to the subject. Unfortunately there are other factors
apart from oxygen demand which affect heart rate: for example
anxiety and posture. In subjects who are sedentary most of the time
the variations in heart rate due to these factors make estimates of
energy expenditure very uncertain, while in very active subjects,
such as long-distance cyclists, the heart rate method may give a
useful indication of energy expenditure.

Recently, however, these rather unsatisfactory methods have been
overtaken by the development of the doubly-labelled water technique, which is based on the observation of Lifson & McClintock
(1966) that isotopes of hydrogen and oxygen in body water are lost
at different rates, and that the difference in disappearance rate of
the two isotopes is a function of carbon dioxide production. The
reason for this is illustrated in Figure 5.3. where the situation at time
zero is that body water is labelled with both deuterium (the heavy
isotope of hydrogen) and ^{18}O (the heavy isotope of oxygen) to an
extent which is arbitrarily designated as 100% (the true level of
labelling is about 0.02% or less).

Suppose total body water is 40 litres, and water intake is 2 l/day,
then the deuterium label will be eliminated at the rate of 5% per day
in an exponential fashion, which is a linear decline when plotted on

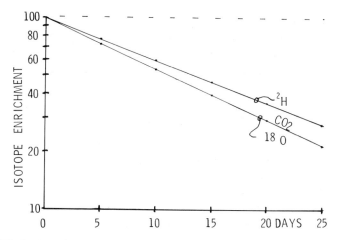

Fig. 5.3 Elimination of isotopes of hydrogen and oxygen from body water. Vertical scale is logarithmic. Increased rate of loss of oxygen compared with hydrogen indicates rate of production of carbon dioxide, and hence energy expenditure

log-linear paper. The oxygen label will also be lost in the course of water turnover, but the oxygen has an additional route of excretion in expired CO_2, since the oxygen in carbon dioxide is in isotopic equilibrium with the oxygen in body water. If we assume that the subject exhales 200 ml/min of carbon dioxide, that is 288 l/day, or 12.8 mol/day. One mol carbon dioxide contains 32 g oxygen, so the oxygen eliminated as carbon dioxide is 411 g/day in the above example. This is contained in 463 g water, so the loss of oxygen in carbon dioxide is equivalent to the excretion of another 463 g water/day, or 1.16% of body water. Thus while the deuterium label decreases at 5% per day the oxygen label will decrease at 6.16% per day, and the difference of 1.16% is a measure of carbon dioxide production.

Obviously this technique depends on the ability to measure very accurately differences in the rate of loss of the stable isotopes in water, and this depends on the competence of the investigator and the isotope mass spectrometer he uses. At present the doubly-labelled water is very expensive. However in expert hands the method gives good results (Schoeller et al 1985, Coward et al 1985, Westerterp et al 1985). The application of the technique will be discussed later.

There are, of course, prediction equations based on weight, height, age and sex from which resting metabolic rate can be esti-mated. Warwick et al (1978) demonstrated that individuals of the same age and sex, and almost identical weight and body composition could have resting metabolic rates (and total energy expenditures) which differed by as much as 40%. Thus the formulae of Harris and Benedict, and later similar prediction equations, are better than nothing, but cannot be considered to be accurate methods for estimating energy expenditure. A recent comparison of measured basal energy expenditure and that calculated from the Harris–Benedict formulae was reported by Daly et al (1985) using data from two centres on 127 normal subjects. Both sets of data showed a significant correlation between measured resting metabolism and the Harris–Benedict prediction ($r = 0.83$ and $r = 0.82$ respectively), but both centres found that the prediction formulae overestimates energy expenditure: by $10.4 \pm 11.7\%$ at one centre, and by $12.3 \pm 10.6\%$ at the other.

5.c MEASUREMENT OF RESTING METABOLIC RATE

The difference between resting metabolic rate (RMR) and basal metabolic rate (BMR) is somewhat academic. The earliest clinical application of indirect calorimetry was to investigate thyroid disease. At the Mayo Clinic, USA, in the 1920s a group under Boothby performed a vast number of determinations of what they termed 'basal metabolic rate'. The BMR is defined as the energy output of an individual under standardised resting conditions: bodily and mentally at rest, 12–18 h after a meal, and in a neutral thermal environment. Strictly speaking it is also necessary to define the conditions with respect to circadian rhythms, which persist throughout the day, however rigorously the environment may be controlled (Aschoff & Pohl 1970). Thus oxygen consumption falls in the early hours of the morning, whether or not the subject is asleep. In women this circadian rhythm persists, but the oxygen uptake is consistently lower post-menstrually than it is premenstrually. Cyclical variations in body temperature are well known, and in the rabbit these may persist even after ovariectomy (Kihlstrom & Lundberg 1971). There are similar circadian rhythms in human urinary aminoacid excretion (Tewksbury & Lohrenz 1970) and in the plasma-free aminoacids (Feigin et al 1971) which persist regardless of diet or exercise.

In practice it is far more difficult to achieve the conditions of 'basal metabolism' than it is to define them. Given a suitably co-operative subject it is easy to arrange for measurement to be done in a neutral thermal environment 12–18 h after a meal; the problems arise when you try to measure the subject's oxygen consumption under conditions of mental and physical rest. For indirect calorimetry it is essential that all the expired gases are collected; if any is lost the measurement is invalid. Therefore, the subject must wear some form of mask or mouthpiece which seals perfectly to his face, and only well-trained subjects can approximate to mental and physical rest in these circumstances. Even quite minor disturbances in the room may cause a transient change of 10% in the oxygen uptake of a trained subject at rest.

It is understandable that the early investigators should have chosen to measure 'basal' metabolic rate in order to obtain readings which were as reproducible as possible, but it is evident that even so they had difficulty in obtaining technically satisfactory measurements. Boothby & Sandiford (1929) report that at the Mayo Clinic up to December 1926 measurements of BMR had been performed on more than 60 000 individuals, but when they came to report their normal values they used only '6888 subjects (1822 male and 5066 female), who on careful physical examination revealed no abnormality which would influence their rate of heat production' and who also had technically satisfactory recordings. The later definitive 'standard for basal metabolism, with a nomogram for clinical application' (Boothby et al 1936) was based on an even more selected sample of the total available measurements. One of the tenets of the Mayo Clinic, which has been rather uncritically accepted up to the recent times, is that it is appropriate to express basal metabolism in relation to the subject's surface area. This quaint idea has an interesting history.

It was observed that when physiological measurements of many kinds (such as glomerular filtration rate) were made on individuals of different size, the larger individuals gave higher values. Thus, if the observer was asked if a given patient had a high or low glomerular filtration rate, he had to make some correction for body size. Simply to divide by body weight was not satisfactory, since in general, people who weigh 120 kg do not have double the glomerular filtration rate of those who weigh 60 kg. McIntosh et al (1929) thought it reasonable to correct renal clearance rates by dividing by the weight of the kidneys, but this cannot be determined in living human subjects: however, further research revealed that kidney weight was quite well correlated with body surface area on the evidence of post-mortem data. Thus it came about that renal clearance rates were quoted relative to surface area, and since medico-actuarial tables of the time stated that the average area of normal young men was 1.73 m^2, nephrologists 'corrected' renal clearance measurements to a value of 1.73 m^2. All this was empirical and perfectly sensible within its limitations. However, the limitations were soon exceeded, and physiologists noted with delight that the basal metabolic rates of mice and elephants, and of species of intermediate size, were fairly similar when related to their surface area. The temptation to elevate this observation to the status of a physiological law was irresistible: it was pointed out that surface area determined rate of heat loss, and basal metabolism the rate of heat production, so it was inevitable that the two were inextricably linked.

It is clear to anyone who has given the matter thought that, in the human species at least, the BMR is not determined by the rate of heat loss. If this were so the BMR would be higher if the subject is lying spread-eagled, and thus presenting the maximum area for heat loss, than if he curled up in as small a volume as possible, but this is not so. The conditions for measurement of BMR specifically require a neutral thermal environment, so even if there were a heat loss effect (as of course there is when the range of shivering thermogenesis is reached) it would not be detected by the test.

It is astonishing, therefore, that BMR is still often reported in relation to surface area or, more obscurely, as a percentage of 'normal' values which have themselves been derived using surface area as a parameter. It would be understandable if in practice it worked well, but it does not. The traditional Du Bois formula for calculating surface area gives an answer which is about 6.6% too low, and has a coefficient of variation of 11% (Van Graan & Wyndham, 1964). In practice body weight is as good a reference standard as calculated surface area (Durnin 1959).

The case for abandoning the 'BMR' and substituting 'resting metabolism' is well made by Durnin & Passmore (1967). The 12–18-hour period of fasting is inconvenient for the subject, and if the measurement of metabolic rate is made 2–4 h after a light breakfast, as much is gained by making the test less trying as is lost by abandoning the true fasting state. The problem of correction for body size remains, but, before deciding how to correct for body size, it is important to be clear why we should correct for body size. Usually we should not do so; certainly in the study of energy balance it is nonsense to measure the energy cost of every other activity in kcal/min, and that of basal metabolism in kcal.m^2/min. The problem of correcting for body size arises only when it is necessary to say if a given RMR is 'normal' or not, or when the metabolic rates of subjects of very different build are being compared. Durnin & Passmore (1967) give a very useful table of normal values for resting oxygen consumption adults of average build, and this is a better reference standard than tables based on 'surface area', for reasons given above. When the problem arises of defining the 'normal' RMR of a grossly obese person weighing, for example, 150 kg, it is as well to recognise that there is no such thing as a normal value for an abnormal person. It may be informative to compare the observed metabolic rate of such a patient with the normal rate for a person of the same height and normal build, but anyone who gives values for the metabolic rate of obese patients as 'percent normal for surface area' is not thinking about what he is doing.

5.d MEASUREMENT OF THERMOGENESIS

'Thermogenesis' means heat production, so etymologically the word should be used to describe all energy expenditure, since all energy expenditure eventually produces heat. Resting metabolism and physical activity are two special and easily defined causes of heat production, but there are other thermogenic stimuli which are less clearly defined: response to food, exposure to cold, increased sympathetic tone due to anxiety or the action of a drug such as caffeine, smoking, fidgeting and so on. The most convenient convention is to say 'diet-induced thermogenesis' or 'cold-induced thermogenesis' to describe the effect of a specific stimulus in raising metabolic rate above the resting level, and to reserve the term 'thermogenesis' for the effect of all thermogenic stimuli, known and unknown, other than resting metabolism and physical exercise. The partition of total energy expenditure according to this convention is shown below:

TOTAL ENERGY EXPENDITURE =

Resting metabolic rate +	Activity + Thermogenesis	
(postabsorptive, resting, thermoneutral, but awake)	(muscle action doing external work or moving the body)	(response to food, cold, anxiety, drugs, isometric exercise, and all other unknown stimuli)

The simplest approach to the study of thermogenesis is to measure metabolic rate in the resting state before and again after a stimulus such as food. The increase in metabolic rate may then reasonably be called diet-induced thermogenesis. However, this approach implies two assumptions, neither of which is quite true: first, that food was the only stimulus given, and second, that metabolic rate would have continued at pre-meal levels if the food had not been given. Several publications report thermogenesis after a meal, but the metabolic rate after the meal never falls to baseline levels, and at least part of the 'response' is simply the diurnal variation in metabolic rate which is seem in all normal subjects. The average values for hourly heat loss from 5 subjects measured in a direct calorimeter is shown in Figure 5.4: between 0200 h and 0700 h the rate of heat loss is about 60 W, but during the morning it increases to reach about 90 W, where it remains until the subject goes to bed. Obviously a test meal given at 0700 h would be followed by a much larger increase in metabolic rate than the same meal given at 1400 h, even if the true thermic response to the meal is the same. The moral, of course, is that when the thermogenic response to anything is measured it is necessary to perform a proper control experiment on the same subject over the same period of time: thus the response to a meal should be compared with the response to a sham meal given under identical conditions.

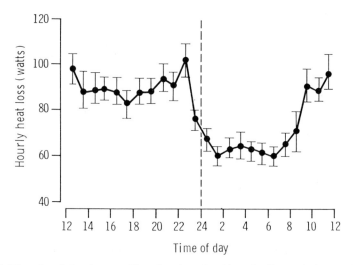

Fig. 5.4 Diurnal variation in rate of heat loss from 5 subjects in direct calorimeter. Vertical bars are s.e.m.

The other approach to the measurement of thermogenesis is to measure total daily energy expenditure under standard conditions in a calorimeter, and then to subtract the energy which can be accounted for by basal metabolism or by physical activity. The remainder is thermogenesis. Figure 5.5 shows a plot of this sort from the data of Jequier & Schutz (1981). This method has the advantage that it is not necessary to specify what thermogenic stimuli are being measured: the list on page 89 includes 'unknown stimuli' which obviously cannot be specified. It also overcomes the difficulty which is experienced with the ventilated hood system of knowing how long the measurement period should be to capture the whole response to a particular stimulus — after a large protein meal the metabolic rate remains elevated for many hours, but if the subject is kept under the ventilated hood too long he usually becomes restless and so base-line resting conditions will never be achieved.

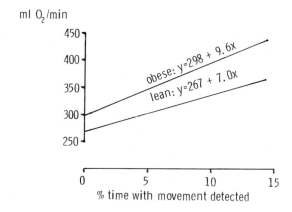

Fig. 5.5 Plot of energy expenditure against physical activity between 0800 h and 2300 h in lean and obese subjects in respiration chamber. Intercept at zero activity is RMR plus thermogenesis: by subtracting RMR (separately measured) total thermogenesis can be estimated (Data of Jequier and Schutz 1981)

Diet-induced thermogenesis

Figure 5.6 shows the time-course of metabolic rate in lean and obese subjects for 150 min after ingesting a meal of 75 g glucose, measured with a ventilated hood system. Before the meal the obese subjects

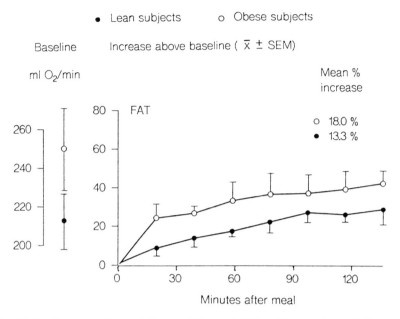

Fig. 5.6 Baseline metabolic rate before meal (mean + SD) and increase in metabolic rate after 75 g glucose. Open circles obese subjects, closed circles lean subjects (Data of Nair et al 1983)

had a significant higher resting metabolic rate than the lean subjects. The metabolic rate in both groups is significantly greater than the baseline at each time-point from 15 min to 150 min. Figures 5.7 and 5.8 show the results obtained on the same group of lean and obese subjects when an isoenergetic meal of protein or fat was given in place of the glucose. With protein the increase in metabolic rate is larger and more prolonged than after the glucose meal. With fat the response is small, and shows a slow rate of rise, which is partly explained by the slow rate of absorption of ingested fat from the gut. In neither case is there any indication that the response of the obese subjects is less than that of the lean subjects. Figure 5.9 shows the result of a control experiment in which water was given instead of the meal. The metabolic rate does not change significantly from the baseline level.

Other studies on the dietary-induced thermogenesis of lean and obese subjects have been reviewed by James (1985). The results may be summarised thus: some investigators find that the response (as an absolute increment of oxygen uptake, or as a proportion of the energy content of the meal) is smaller in the obese subjects, and some find no significant difference between lean and obese subjects.

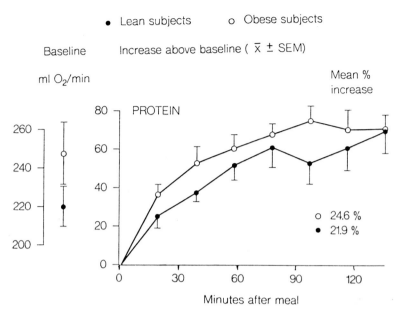

Fig. 5.7 Data shown as in Figure 5.6, but with isoenergetic protein meal

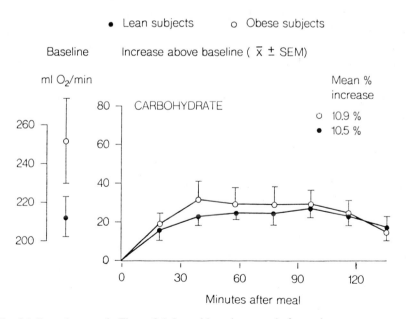

Fig. 5.8 Data shown as in Figure 5.6, but with an isoenergetic fat meal

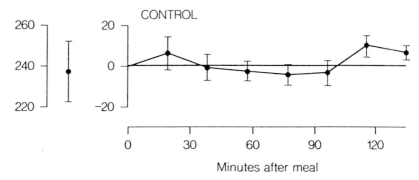

Fig. 5.9 Control experiment in which water was given instead of a meal

All find a higher baseline metabolic rate in the obese group. The response to protein is greater and more sustained than to isoenergetic meals of carbohydrate or fat (Zed & James 1986a, 1986b). The average response to mixed meals is an increase in metabolic rate equivalent to about 10% of the energy content of the meal. We may conclude, therefore, that in a person in energy balance, dietary-induced thermogenesis accounts for about 10% of total energy expenditure, which makes it, next to physical activity, the most important thermogenic stimulus in ordinary circumstances.

Cold-induced thermogenesis

When normal subjects are exposed to severe cold, metabolic rate increases to defend body temperature. In such circumstances obese subjects benefit from the insulation provided by the layer of subcutaneous fat, and do not need to generate so much heat at first, but eventually the maximal cold-induced thermogenesis of lean and obese subjects is similar. This point is illustrated by Figure 5.10, from a study by Wyndham et al (1968). Conversely obese subjects are able to do more muscular work when immersed in cool water, because they can maintain normal core temperatures better than lean people (Sheldahl et al 1982). However such studies belong to the

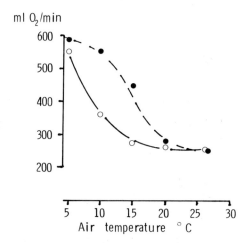

Fig. 5.10 Metabolic response after lightly clad subjects were exposed to cold for 2 h. Open circles fat subject (W/H² = 31.6), closed circles normal subject (W/H² = 22.5) (Data of Wyndham et al 1968)

realm of temperature physiology rather than energy balance. No normal person would endure the severe discomfort of these cold exposure experiments as part of their daily life. The question which concerns us is: does the difference in cold responsiveness of lean and obese subject make any practical difference to total energy expenditure?

It appears that, in general, lean and obese subjects do not differ in their preferred ambient temperature. Fanger (1970) tested subjects seated in light clothing for 3 h at various environmental temperatures, and at the end of the test the subjects rated the conditions on a 7-point scale: −3 for much too cold, 0 for comfortable, and +3 for much too hot. The results are shown in Figure 5.11. At 25°C there were 6% of subjects dissatisfied, half of them because it was too hot and the other half because it was too cold. As the test temperature went down the proportion complaining of cold increased to 78% at 20°C. When it was raised, 79% complained that it was too hot at 32°C. When the subjects were analysed by weight-for-height there was no significant difference in the preference of the fatter subjects compared with the thinner ones.

It also seems that people who describe themselves as 'warm-preferring' do not choose different ambient temperatures from those saying they are 'cool-preferring'. Blaza (1980) tested 6 women and 1 man in a direct calorimeter which was fitted with a control knob which the occupant could set to show if the temperature was too

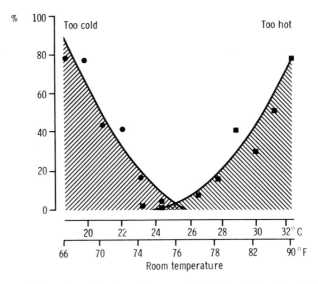

Fig. 5.11 Range of thermal comfort for subjects seated in light clothing for 3 h (Data of Fanger et al 1970)

warm or too cool. When the subject signalled that the it was too warm the temperature of the chamber was reduced at the rate of 2°C/h until a 'too cold' response was elicited, at which time the temperature was increased by 2°C/h until a 'too warm' signal caused it to be reduced again. In this way each subject indicated an acceptable range of temperatures, which are shown in Figure 5.12. There was no correlation between these ranges and the stated temperature preference or the degree of obesity of the subject: the mean thermal comfort zone for 5 obese subjects was 23.2–26.4°C, and for 5 lean subjects it was 23.3–26.2°C (Blaza and Garrow 1983). In the cool temperature (23.3°C) the lean subjects showed an increase in 24-hour energy expenditure of 7.8% above control values, which agrees well with the data of Dauncey (1981) who observed an increase of 7.0% in the metabolism of lean subjects at 22°C compared with control values at 28°C. In the study of Blaza and Garrow (1983) the obese subjects showed no cold-induced thermogenesis at the lower end of the comfort zone chosen by the subject herself in the manner described above. This suggests that cold-induced thermogenesis may have a greater influence on lean people than obese people, but the effect, and the numbers studied, are too small for a statistically significant result.

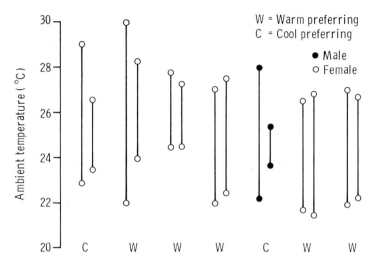

Fig. 5.12 Range of thermal comfort chosen by individuals who described themselves as 'warm-preferring' or 'cold-preferring'. No significant relationship between stated preference and comfort zone chosen under experimental conditions (Data of Blaza 1980)

Thermogenesis induced by anxiety, smoking and caffeine

Benedict & Benedict (1933) tried to measure the energy cost of mental work by studying the oxygen uptake of mathematicians either in a state of mental vacuity, or paying attention, or solving mathematical problems. They failed to find any significant difference between the metabolic rate in these three mental states. Landis (1925) subjected himself and colleagues to severe stress, including sleep deprivation, fasting and gastric intubation, but obtained very variable readings from which it was not possible to assess the effect of anxiety on metabolic rate. Blaza & Garrow (1980) studied a graduate student in a direct calorimeter while she was reading her thesis in preparation for her oral examination, and again after she had passed the examination. Total heat loss was 16% higher on the first measurement compared with the second. To produce anxiety in a controlled manner they studied normal subjects at rest, and when undergoing a protocol involving mental arithmetic and electric shocks. This caused a marked increase in heart rate and cortisol excretion, but the increase in heat loss was only 4%.

The main effect of cigarette smoking on energy balance is through reduction in energy intake. However, Hofstetter et al (1986) showed that smoking 24 cigarettes per day increased total energy output by

11%, and Dallosso & James (1984) found that resting metabolic rate decreased by 4% in smokers who gave up smoking. A decrease in resting metabolic rate on stopping smoking was not found by Robinson & York (1986), perhaps because their ex-smokers increased food intake. However they report a higher thermic effect after a standard meal in smokers than non-smokers.

Caffeine in a dose of 200 mg orally or intravenously increases metabolic rate by about 5–10% over a period of 1 h (Jung et al 1981). The response is similar in lean and obese subjects.

The thermogenic response to cold, anxiety, smoking and caffeine is not likely to be important in regulation of body weight, but since all these stimuli cause measurable thermogenic responses it is necessary to control for these factors when studying thermogenesis.

5.e MEASUREMENT OF PHYSICAL ACTIVITY

Physical activity is the most powerful thermogenic stimulus: highly trained althletes can work for short periods at a rate of 400 W, with a rate of oxygen uptake approaching 6 l/min, which is 15 times the resting energy expenditure. Male students of physical education have an average maximum oxygen uptake around 4 l/min, female students of physical education around 3 l/min, the average fit amateur 2.5 l/min, and the average obese patient perhaps 1 l/min, or three times resting metabolism. It is quite easy to measure the energy cost of exercise on a treadmill or bicycle ergometer using adaptations of the techniques of direct or indirect calorimetry which were described for measuring resting metabolism.

The contribution of inactivity to the aetiology of obesity is discussed in the next chapter; here we are concerned with the problem of estimating the level of physical activity undertaken by a subject, and the effect this activity has on energy expenditure. We encounter the same problem which limits the accuracy with which energy intake can be measured: the more closely the subject is monitored the less likely it is that the observed level of physical activity is the habitual level. If the subject is shut in a chamber, or instrumented with recording devices by which movement can be measured, this may well cause him to be more, or less, active than usual.

Just as it is possible to obtain an idea of energy intake by a dietary questionnaire, so physical activity can be assessed by an activity questionnaire. Subjects are asked about their pattern of physical activity, and this is assigned to light (2.0–4.0 kcal/min), moderate (4.5–5.5 kcal/min) or heavy (>6.0 kcal/min) (Folsom et al 1985). On this basis the average leisure-time physical activity in the Minnesota Heart Study was for men about 200 kcal/day and for women about 100 kcal/day. Alternatively the energy cost of physical activity may be calculated in METs, i.e. multiples of the individual's RMR (Blair et al 1985). Unfortunately, as with dietary questionnaires, it is very difficult to validate this method for estimating physical activity.

Since in affluent societies most people do not undertake strenuous physical activity, it is interesting to know if differences in energy expenditure between individuals can be accounted for by minor movements, fidgeting, or even muscle tension caused by stressful mental work. New light on this subject comes from recent work by Ravussin et al (1987). They recorded 24-hour energy expenditure of 134 non-diabetic subjects in a respiration chamber which was also fitted with a radar device to detect movement. The most powerful determinant of energy expenditure was (as expected) the fat-free mass of the subjects, but on multiple linear regression the minor activity detected by radar also made a highly significant contribution.

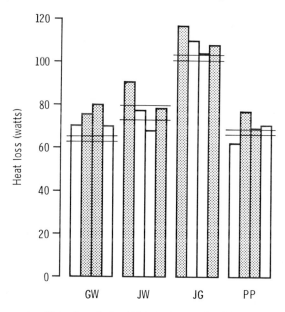

Fig. 5.13 Average rate of heat loss during 7.5 h in 4 normal subjects who either relaxed in a direct calorimeter (open columns) or undertook tiring clerical work (stippled columns). Each subject was tested twice in each condition. Average heat loss was 10% higher on working days than on resting days (Data of Webster et al 1986)

It accounted for an average of 308 kcal/day, or 13% of the total energy expenditure. It is not clear if the fidgeting actually caused the extra energy expenditure, or served as a marker of some other metabolic activity. To distinguish between these two possibilities it would be necessary to ask fidgeters to remain still, and non-fidgeters to fidget, and see if the energy expenditures were then reversed.

Clerical work is tiring, and it is easy to believe that this is associated with muscle tension. To test this theory Webster et al (1986) compared the energy expenditure of normal subjects who either relaxed in a calorimeter chamber, or spent 7.5 h making notes from tape recordings. The results are shown in Figure 5.13. The average heat loss was 10% higher on the working days than the resting days. This was not an effect of stress or anxiety (which is discussed in the previous section) since heart rate and urinary cortisol excretion were not significantly different between the working and control days.

6

Aetiology of obesity in man

6.a INVIOLABILITY OF THERMODYNAMICS

When we consider the aetiology of obesity it is instructive to consider a person (man or woman) for whom the upper limit of the desirable range of weight-for-height (i.e. $W/H^2 = 25$) would be at a weight of 70 kg. If he or she weighs 90 kg ($W/H^2 = 37$) the 20 kg excess weight will contain 75% fat, or 15 kg, which is an excess fat store of 135 Mcal. (We can for simplicity ignore the small contribution to the energy store made by the 5 kg excess FFM.) Fundamentally the aetiology of this obesity is that energy intake has exceeded energy expenditure by 135 Mcal, since unless this was so it would not have been possible to deposit 135 Mcal as excess fat.

From a practical viewpoint the patient wants to know how this energy imbalance of 135 Mcal has arisen: does the abnormality lie in energy intake, or expenditure, or is there some other subtle factor at work involving the psyche, or genes, or hormones, or the activity of some perhaps as-yet-undiscovered enzyme system? Fortunately the aetiological factors, whether psychological, genetic, endocrine or whatever, must ultimately act on energy intake or output or some combination of these. This is an important fact which is sometimes overlooked even by workers in the field. Suppose, for example, a drug was discovered which affected neither energy intake nor expenditure, but which altered the metabolism so that a larger (or smaller) proportion of the fuel used in metabolic processes came from the fat stores of the body. Would this affect the fat stores of a person taking the drug? After the first dose of the drug more (or less) of the fat stores of the body would be mobilised as fuel instead of some of the energy from the diet, but conversely some of the energy from the diet which formerly would have been used as fuel is now being displaced by fat drawn from the fat stores. At the end of the day this dietary energy which is not used as fuel will be deposited as fat in the fat stores, so if there is no change in total energy intake or output there can be no change in total fat stores.

The search for aetiological factors in obesity can therefore be narrowed to factors affecting energy intake or output. Do obese people have a higher energy intake or a lower energy output than lean people?

For reasons explained in Chapter 4 it is fruitless to investigate the aetiology of obesity by comparing the estimated energy intake of lean and obese people, although many workers have wasted time trying to do this. The methods available for measuring habitual energy intake are too imprecise for the task, and the harder we try to make them more accurate the less likely it is that the energy intake being measured is habitual energy intake. We will therefore concentrate on the evidence about the relative energy output of lean and obese people.

There is consensus that, on average, obese people have a higher resting metabolic rate than lean people. The sort of evidence on which this statement is made is illustrated in Figures 6.1 and 6.2. Figure 6.1 shows the distribution of age and W/H^2 among a series of patients admitted to the metabolic unit at the Clinical Research Centre: these two variables are unrelated in this series, and there are

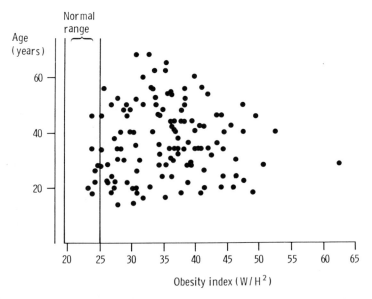

Fig. 6.1 Distribution of age and Quetelet's index in series of 128 subjects studied on a metabolic ward at the Clinical Research Centre, London

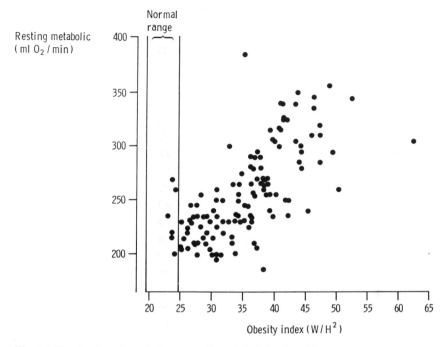

Fig. 6.2 Distribution of metabolic rate vs Quetelet's index in subjects shown in Figure 6.1

subjects throughout the range of adult ages from 16 to 64 years, and of W/H² from normal to extreme obesity. The RMR among these patients, measured fasting, in the morning before getting out of bed, is shown in Figure 6.2. It is obvious on inspection (and confirmed by statistical testing) that there is a very significant positive association between increasing obesity and increasing metabolic rate, although there is considerable scatter in the data points, so some obese patients have a lower metabolic rate than some individuals in the normal range.

These data were further analysed by Dore et al (1982) to examine the relation of metabolic rate to age, height, weight, total body potassium (as a measure of FFM) and surface area. On step-up multiple regression the correlation coefficients were: with weight alone r = 0.798, with weight and potassium r = 0.817, and with weight, potassium and age r = 0.830. Addition of height and surface area did not significantly contribute to the regression. The best subset of variables was therefore weight, potassium and age, and the best-fit equation was

$$RMR = 99.8 + 1.155W + 0.02227TBK - 0.4563A$$

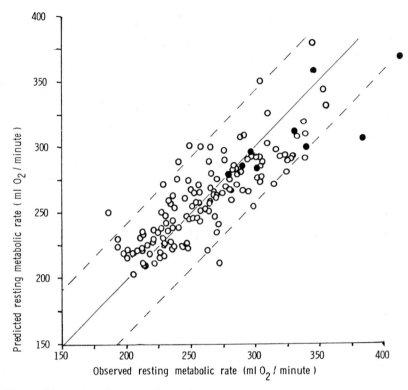

Fig. 6.3 Observed resting metabolic rate in 140 women (open circles) and 9 men (filled circles) compared with metabolic rate predicted by the formula of Dore et al (1982)

where RMR is resting metabolic rate (ml O_2/min), W is body weight (kg), TBK is total body potassium (mmol) and A is age (years). A plot is shown in Figure 6.3 of the observed RMR among 140 women (open circles) and 9 men (filled circles) against the metabolic rate predicted from the above formula. When weight, FFM and age are taken into account about 69% of the variation of RMR in this series is explained.

It has been suggested that obesity may have been due to a low metabolic rate initially, but as weight and FFM are gained the RMR increases, and thus the origins of the obesity are obscured. It is not possible to test this hypothesis by examining people who are going to become obese before they become obese, since there is no way in which such people can be identified. However the form of the regression equation above suggests that both weight and FFM contribute positively to RMR. If fat people had a lower RMR per kg FFM than lean people then the weight factor in the regression equation should be preceded by a minus rather than a plus sign.

This point was further investigated by Garrow & Webster (1985b) using data from the subjects shown in Figure 3.5, in whom body fat had been measured by three independent methods. The RMR of these subjects was 'corrected' for differences in FFM to give a value which would have been obtained if all the subjects had a FFM of 50 kg. A plot of this adjusted RMR against percentage body fat is shown in Figure 6.4. There is a significantly ($p<0.05$) positive relationship, indicating that the most obese patients have a slightly *higher* metabolic rate in relation to FFM than the least obese subjects.

The data discussed so far relate to the RMR of obese patients before they start on a reducing diet. It is possible that obese subjects might respond to dietary restriction by a greater decrease than lean subjects, but the evidence is against this. Figure 6.5 shows the change in RMR among the lean and obese subjects studied by Blaza (1980) when both groups were on a diet supplying 800 kcal (3.4 MJ) per day. There is a somewhat more rapid decrease in metabolic rate in the lean group than in the obese group. The effect of this diet for 3 weeks in a larger series of patients is shown in Figure 6.6. The

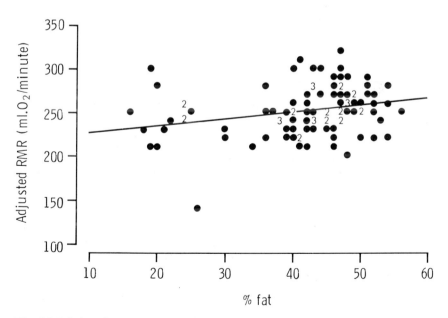

Fig. 6.4 Relation of percentage body fat to resting metabolic rate adjusted for differences in fat-free mass (Data of Garrow & Webster 1985b)

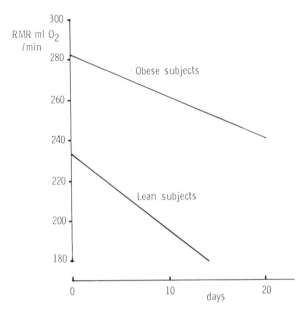

Fig. 6.5 Change in resting metabolic rate with time in lean and obese subjects on 3.4 MJ (800 kcal) diet (Data of Blaza 1980)

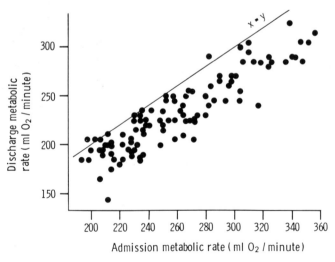

Fig. 6.6 Relation of resting metabolic rate in 104 obese women at start and end of 3 weeks on diet supplying 3.4 MJ (800 kcal)

average decrease is about 14%, and it occurs roughly equally among those with high or low initial metabolic rate. There is therefore strong evidence that obese people have a higher RMR than lean people, and this situation is not altered by dieting, at least in the short term.

It is still possible that obese subjects might have a lower total energy expenditure than lean subjects, but only if their thermogenesis, or energy expended in physical activity, is greatly reduced. There is already a hint that this is not so from the data cited in Chapter 5 to illustrate techniques for the measurement of energy expenditure. The plot of energy expenditure in lean and obese subjects in a respiration chamber (Figure 5.5) shows a higher expenditure by the obese group at every level of physical activity, and the data on dietary thermogenesis (Figures 5.6–5.8) show a higher baseline for the obese subjects compared with lean subjects, and a similar response to the meals.

The conclusion that the total energy expenditure of obese subjects is greater than that of lean subjects is supported by results from both Lausanne and Cambridge, using different techniques. The measured 24-hour energy expenditure among lean, moderately obese and obese subjects in a respiration chamber is shown in Table 6.1. Another set of data on 24-hour energy expenditure among lean and obese women, measured by the doubly-labelled water technique, is shown in Table 6.2. Finally data on the 24-hour energy expenditure of 21 normal women and 20 obese women are shown in Table 6.3. The three sets of results are strikingly similar. All the studies show that the total energy expenditure of the obese group is higher than that

Table 6.1. Energy expenditure of lean, moderately obese and obese subjects measured in respiration chamber. Values for 24h, RMR (i.e. awake, fasting, in morning), and for sleeping metabolism (MJ/day) are given; values for RMR and sleep as percentage 24-hour rate are given (in parentheses) (Data of Ravussin et al 1982)

	Total	RMR	Sleep
Lean			
MJ	8.44 (100)	6.12 (73)	5.67 (67)
kcal	2020	1460	1360
Moderately obese			
MJ	9.60 (100)	6.65 (69)	6.05 (63)
kcal	2300	1590	1450
Obese			
MJ	10.04 (100)	7.59 (76)	6.22 (62)
kcal	2400	1820	1490
Obese/lean	1.19	1.24	1.10

Table 6.2. Total 24-hour energy expenditure and RMR (MJ/day) in lean and obese women, measured by doubly-labelled water. RMR is shown as percentage 24-hour rate (in parentheses) (Data of Prentice et al 1986)

	Total	RMR
Lean		
MJ	7.99 (100)	5.65 (71)
kcal	1910	1350
Obese		
MJ	10.22 (100)	6.71 (66)
kcal	2450	1600
Obese/lean	1.28	1.19

Table 6.3. Total 24-hour energy expenditure and RMR in lean and obese women. RMR as percentage total is given (in parentheses) (Data of Schutz & Jequier 1986)

	Total	RMR
Lean		
MJ	7.36 (100)	5.43 (74)
kcal	1760	1310
Obese		
MJ	9.20 (100)	6.77 (74)
kcal	2140	1620
Obese/lean	1.21	1.23

of the lean group, by a factor of 1.19, 1.28 and 1.21 in the three series. Resting metabolic rate is higher in the obese groups than in the lean groups by factors of 1.24, 1.19 and 1.23 respectively. In the report of Ravussin et al (1982) the energy expenditure during sleep of the obese group is higher than that of the lean group by a factor of 1.10, and in that study the values for energy expenditure for the 'moderately obese' group are intermediate between the values for lean and obese subjects. All three studies show that RMR accounts for 66–76% of total energy expenditure, and the proportion accounted for by resting metabolism is not significantly different between lean and obese subjects.

Taken as a whole the data reviewed above show convincingly that obese people (on average) have a higher energy expenditure than lean people, and thermodynamic considerations demand that they must therefore have a higher energy intake to maintain their body weight.

6.b LESSONS FROM ANIMAL MODELS

Medical research would not have progressed far without the use of animal models. Frequently physiological mechanisms in man are too complex to be easily understood, and an animal model may provide valuable insights which can then be checked, at least partly, in man. For example our understanding of neuromuscular function owes a great deal to the leg muscles of the frog. This splendidly co-operative material can be removed with innervation intact, and it has tendons at each end between which tension can be measured. It is well adapted to the needs of a frog when jumping. However man does not jump like a frog: indeed this function is quite unlike that of any muscle group in man, so obviously there is need for caution when generalising the behaviour of frog sartorius muscle to typical human muscle.

In the field of energy balance the favourite animal model has been the laboratory rat or mouse, which is good at regulating energy balance when fed on laboratory chow. It has to be, because (relative to man) its energy stores are small. Normal man has energy stores equivalent to about 70 days' energy turnover, but the rat has higher energy requirements per unit body weight, and smaller energy stores. What insights have small laboratory rodents provided about the aetiology of human obesity? In my opinion they have contributed to advances, but in other instances also have retarded progress, because fundamental differences between the model and the human situation have been ignored.

Around 1970 it was standard teaching that energy balance was regulated by adjustment of food intake, because that is how rats did it. There was debate about the nature of the sensor — glucostatic, thermostatic or lipostatic — which informed the rat about the state of its energy stores so it could adjust energy intake accordingly. Centres in the hypothalamus were identified which processed this information. Then it was shown that the rat (if it was given the opportunity) responded to changes of variety and palatability in the diet by altering food intake, just as human subjects do, so the hypothalamic nuclei were demoted in importance.

The next advance was the adipocyte hypothesis: that fat cell number was somehow fixed, and in adult life fat cells tended to fill with fat, so fat cell number determined body fat. The model here (unfortunately, in retrospect) was the epidydimal fat pad in the rat, which we now know has specialised functions and behaves somewhat autonomously in respect to energy balance. Also it has been shown that under suitable conditions human subcutaneous fat cells can replicate to store additional fat, so fat cell number is not fixed in adult man.

The latest insight has concerned genetic obesity in certain

laboratory rodents, which is associated with a malfunction or absence of brown adipose tissue (BAT). Attention is now focused on adaptive changes in energy output. This is not the place to discuss adaptive thermogenesis in animals and the role of BAT: interested readers will find reviews written from opposing viewpoints by Rothwell & Stock (1983) and Hervey & Tobin (1983). The important point concerning the aetiology of human obesity is the extent to which adaptive thermogenesis regulates energy balance in man, whether this thermogenesis is due to the action of BAT or any other tissue. Evidence on this point has recently been reviewed by Astrup (1986) whose conclusions are summarised in Figure 6.7. In cold-acclimated rats it is possible to increase metabolic rate three-fold by an infusion of noradrenaline. In warm-acclimated rats the increase for the same stimulus is about 75% above baseline, in normal rats it is about 50% above baseline, and in man it is about 25% above baseline. The hatched part of each column in Figure 6.7 indicates the proportion of the thermogenic response which Astrup attributes to the action of BAT.

Other workers might disagree with this estimate of BAT activity, but it cannot be denied that there is a striking difference in total thermogenic response between man and the rats. This could be predicted on theoretical grounds in view of the difference in volume/surface ratios betweem man and a rat. Large mammals, such as man, generate enough heat as a by-product of metabolism to

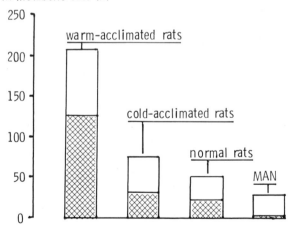

Fig. 6.7 Increase in metabolic rate induced by noradrenaline in rats and man. Cross-hatched section represents proportion of thermogenic response attributed by Astrup (1986) to activity of brown adipose tissue

maintain normal body temperature in normal ambient temperature, so man normally has no energy requirements for thermoregulation. However, small mammals such as a rat have a sigificant energy requirement specifically to maintain body temperature, and must have the capacity to increase this component of energy expenditure if placed in a cold environment.

In summary, therefore, animal models are valuable when they provide a system which is more accessible to investigation than the analogous system in man. Their virtue is that they are relatively simple, and genetically homogeneous, and they can be studied under carefully standardised conditions. However, this simplicity and uniformity also carries a danger, because the more complicated system in man often works in a manner which is quantitatively different. Man does not need leg muscles like a frog because he does not jump like a frog: he does not need BAT like a mouse because he does not have the thermoregulatory problems which a mouse has, and he does not regulate intake like a caged rat on laboratory chow because he usually has access to a varied palatable diet. Finally, the human species shows a genetic heterogeneity which would be unacceptable in the product of a reputable breeder of laboratory animals. Not only do people differ metabolically from rats, they also differ quite a lot from other people.

6.c 'SET POINTS' FOR BODY WEIGHT

The presence of excessive fat stores might indicate that the system which should regulate energy balance is not working correctly. Alternatively it might mean that regulation is taking place about a 'set point' which is too high. To distinguish between these two views it is necessary to establish the characteristics of set-point and non-set-point regulatory systems. A hydraulic analogy of several possible systems is shown in Figure 6.8. A reservoir of water provides a gravity feed to 4 cylinders, each of which has a different control device. Cylinder 'a' has water dripping in at the rate of 1 l/day, and when the amount stored is 50 litres the outlet also drips at the rate of 1 l/day, so the level remains constant. If the input pressure was increased, so the filling rate would increase, the amount stored would also increase until the outlet dripping rate matched the input rate, and a new steady state would be reached. If the input then returned to the initial rate the amount stored would also return to the initial

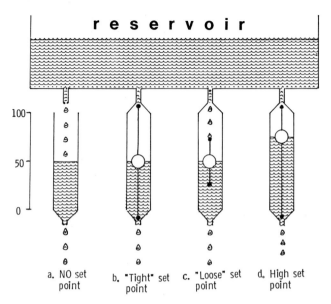

Fig. 6.8 Hydraulic analogy of various possible set-point control systems (see text for further explanation)

state. Thus, although the system has no set point, it will find and maintain a constant level of storage when offered a constant rate of input, but the level of storage will differ with different rates of input.

Cylinder 'b' illustrates a tight set-point regulation. In the equilibrium situation it behaves exactly like 'a', with 1 l/day dripping in and out, and 50 l stored, but if the input filling pressure is increased, and inflow and the amount stored starts to increase, the float moves upwards and cuts down the inflow so the initial rates of inflow and storage are maintained. Cylinder 'c' represents a loose set-point arrangement: over a range of storage from about 20–80 litres it behaves like 'a', but outside that range it behaves like 'b'. Cylinder 'd' is also regulated at a tight set-point like 'b', but the float is so placed that the volume stored is fixed at 75 litres rather than 50 litres.

Which of these systems most closely resembles the control of energy balance in man? This is a difficult question, since the performance of the different systems is similar at the set point, and differs only when there is pressure to depart from the set-point equilibrium. To test each model in man, therefore, it is necessary to know if the subject is at his or her set point. One possible protocol is to persuade a volunteer who is normally at constant body weight

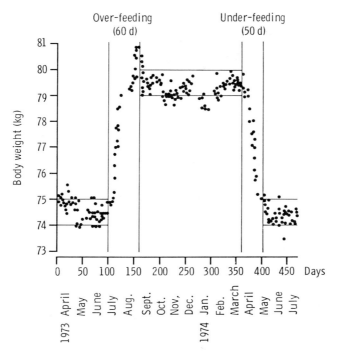

Fig. 6.9 Fluctuations in body weight in author induced by deliberate overfeeding and underfeeding (Data of Garrow & Stalley 1975)

to eat more, and see if body weight increases, and if it does to see if on stopping the deliberate overeating body weight reverts to baseline values. The results of such an experiment on the author are shown in Figure 6.9. During the overeating period body weight increased, but the excess energy stored was only about half the increased energy intake. After overeating stopped there was no tendency to revert spontaneously to baseline weight, which was regained only after a period of deliberate undereating (Garrow & Stalley 1975).

Unfortunately this study does not decide the existence or otherwise of a set point in body weight, since it has been argued that the period of overeating may have caused the set point to change, which makes it very difficult to disprove the existence of a set point. Recently Keesey (1987) has suggested that the natural set-point weight for an animal is determined by its RMR relative to body weight raised to the power of 0.75, as suggested by Kleiber (1961). In rats a normal value for RMR is 10 ml O_2.min/kg$^{0.75}$. If we compare the RMR of 111 women, ranging from very fat to very thin,

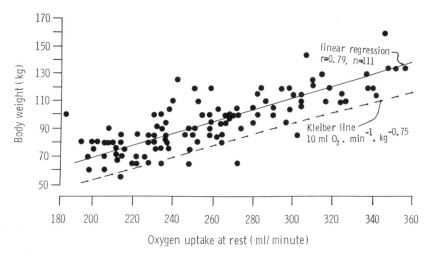

Fig. 6.10 Relation of resting metabolic rate to body weight in 111 women ranging from thin to very fat. Continuous straight line is regression line (r = 0.79). Broken curve shows weight at which subjects would have had relation of oxygen uptake to body weight suggested by Kleiber (1961)

with this 'set-point' line we obtain the relationship shown in Figure 6.10. All but six of the 111 subjects have a body weight above that predicted by the Kleiber line, but the best fit line through the points is virtually parallel to the Kleiber line, but displaced upwards by about 15 kg. This implies that 95% of the women are above the set point for body weight determined by their resting metabolic rate, that the average deviation is about 15 kg, and that those women who weighed least are (on average) just as much above their set point as those who weighed most. It is, of course, quite possible that the body weight of 95% of human subjects is above their set point as calculated from RMR, since depends on FFM, and the human species tends to have more fat (and hence a higher body weight) per kg FFM than most other species.

The relevance of the set-point theory to human obesity is that individuals are said to tend to revert easily towards their set point, but to oppose movement away from their set point by metabolic rate adaptations. We can predict, therefore, that since 95% of the women in Figure 6.10 were above their set point they would not experience any undue decrease in metabolic rate if their weight was decreased by (on average) 15 kg. This prediction is not supported by the experimental evidence. Figure 6.6 shows the RMR of these individuals at the beginning and end of a period of 21 days on a diet which supplied 800 kcal/day. The average decrease in body weight was about 6%, but the average decrease in metabolic rate was 14%. Contrary to the set point hypothesis they metabolically opposed a shift *towards* their set point. Furthermore there was a similar response (proportionately) among the heaviest and lightest women. If we examine the response of individual women this further weakens the evidence for set-point regulation of body weight.

Figure 6.11 shows the weight and metabolic rate of 27 women at the start and finish of the dieting period. These data are from a subsample of the series shown in Figure 6.10, but the axes for weight and metabolic rate are now reversed. These results were used by Keesey (1986) to support the set-point hypothesis, on the grounds that (at least in some women) weight loss is being opposed by a greater-than-expected decrease in metabolic rate, and thus the set-point weight was defended. However, this argument makes sense only if the subjects were initially at, or below, their set point: if they were above it this 'defence' is quite inappropriate. Furthermore we can see in Figure 6.11 that the women who do not 'defend' themselves against weight loss tend to be those with a lower body weight relative to metabolic rate. This is the group most likely to be at or below set point, in whom defence should be most vigorous.

For the reasons given above I find it very difficult to accept the set-point theory of body weight regulation in man. The observed changes in metabolic rate with changes in energy balance can be much more simply and consistently explained by a 'buffer' control system (Garrow 1974b), which tends to oppose and minimise any imposed weight change, as a chemical buffer opposes and minimises any imposed change in acidity or alkalinity.

During conditions of overfeeding energy expenditure increases, and thus limits weight gain. The biochemical basis for this increase is only partly understood: the increased energy intake increases the thermic effect of feeding, there are energy costs associated with the storage of nutrients, and the increased FFM associated with weight gain also increases RMR. However, these changes do not account for all the observed increase: there is an additional increase of about 10% in metabolic rate which is probably modulated by as-yet unclear endocrine changes involving thyroid and sympathetic tone. Whatever the mechamism these adaptations have been shown to occur to a similar degree in lean and obese subjects, whether they claim to be easy weight gainers or not (Daniels et al 1982, Webb & Annis 1983).

During underfeeding converse changes occur which cause a

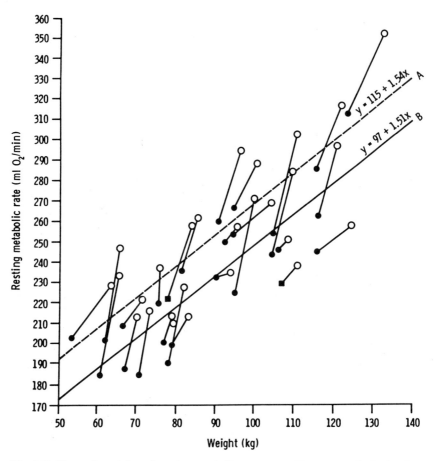

Fig. 6.11 Change in weight and resting metabolic rate among 27 women at beginning (open circles) and end (closed circles) of 3 weeks on diet supplying 3.4 MJ (800 kcal) per day. These are a subset (cited by Keesey 1987) of patients shown in Figure 6.6

decrease in metabolic rate and hence a limitation of weight loss. This was first documented by Benedict and his colleagues during studies on caloric restriction in normal volunteers more than 60 years ago (Benedict et al 1919), and has been found by every competent investigator since then who has looked for this effect. Some results from Benedict's classical study are shown in Figure 6.12. Normal young men were fed a restricted diet for a period of 126 days in order to achieve a 10% reduction in body weight. However, the experiment was interrupted at Thanksgiving and at Christmas, when they returned to their own homes. The effect of these brief periods of refeeding on RMR (or 'basal heat production' as Benedict calls it)

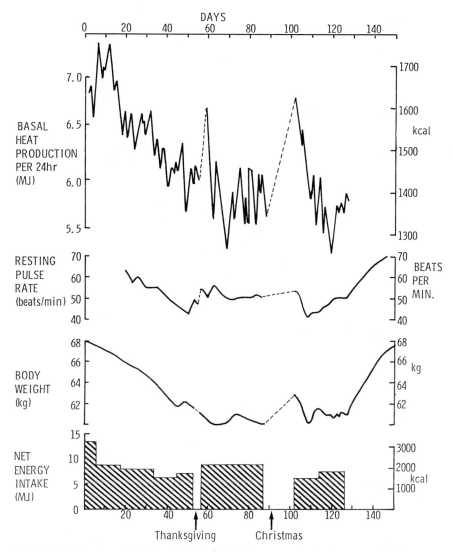

Fig. 6.12 Effect of restricted diet on basal metabolic rate, resting pulse rate and body weight in normal volunteers (Data of Benedict et al 1919). Experiment was interrupted at Thanksgiving and Christmas. After 126 days subjects ate ad libitum

is striking but short-lived: when the restricted diet was reimposed the RMR fell very rapidly to the level before the break.

The decrease in RMR during underfeeding is about 10%: similar to the percentage increase during a similar degree of overfeeding. As the results in Figure 6.11 show, the decrease in metabolic rate is similar for individuals of different body weight when subjected to the same degree of restricted energy intake. It is easier to explain these findings on the basis of 'buffer' regulation of body weight than by postulating a 'set point' regulation.

6.d GENETICS OF OBESITY IN MAN

In some strains of rodent, such as the Zucker rat, obesity is genetically determined: although it can be modified by feeding the tendency to obesity still emerges (Johnson et al 1973). In man genetic factors certainly influence the pattern of deposition of fat in children: monozygotic twins have more similar skinfold measurements than dizygotic twins (Brook et al 1975, Borjeson 1976) and the skinfolds of newborn babies of obese mothers are thicker than babies of thin mothers (Whitelaw 1976, Udall et al 1978). It may be that some families have a 'thrifty gene' (Neel 1962), but it is a mistake to assume that characteristics shared by families are necessarily genetically determined (Garn & Clark 1976): fat dog-owners tend to have fat dogs (Mason 1970), but in this case the explanation is obviously not genetic.

The findings from the Ten-State Nutrition Survey may be interpreted to support or refute the idea that genetic factors are important in determining obesity in children. Since more than 40 000 people were examined it is possible to trace obesity through family lines, with many parental and sibling fatness combinations (Garn & Clark 1976). If parents and children are classified as lean if they are below the 15th centile in skinfold thickness, obese if they are above the 85th centile, and medium if they are between these limits, it is possible to calculate the correlation between fatness in parents and fatness in their children. On average the children of two lean parents were leanest, and those of two obese parents were fattest, with intermediate parental combinations producing children of intermediate fatness. Children with one lean and one obese parent were of similar fatness to those of parents who were both of medium fatness. The distribution of triceps skinfold thickness according to the obesity of their children or parents is shown in Figure 6.13. It made little difference if it was the father or mother who was obese, nor were correlations of fatness significantly stronger for parents and children of the same sex than of the opposite sex.

This result is certainly compatible with the view that genetic influences are important, although it does not indicate any particular

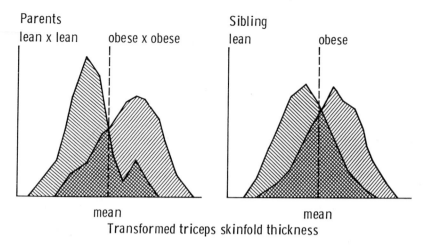

Fig. 6.13 Distribution of triceps skinfolds in children whose parents were both lean or both obese, or whose sibling was lean or obese (Data of Garn & Clark 1976, from the Ten State Nutrition Survey)

pattern of inheritance. However there are two findings from this large study which cast serious doubt on the importance of genetic influences. Analysis of similarities in fatness between spouses shows correlation as strong as that found between parents and children, which increased with time. This cannot be due to genetic influences, since spouses are not genetically similar, but presumably reflects the effect of family attitudes to food and weight. These attitudes would apply also to the children of the marriage, so it suggests that some, and perhaps most, of the parent-child similarity in fatness is due to environmental rather than genetic influences.

Another observation from the Ten-State Nutrition Survey which weakens the case for genetic determination of obesity concerns the relationship of social class to obesity. It has been well established that obesity is commoner among the lower socio-economic groups, which is not in itself an argument against genetic influences. It might be that genes associated with obesity occur unevenly across the social spectrum. However, in prepubertal girls, those of the lower socio-economic classes are leaner than those of more affluent parents, but at puberty the situation is reversed. Furthermore the influence of social class on obesity is stronger with women than with men. These findings are easier to explain on the basis of environmental influences than on the basis of heredity.

To distinguish between genetic and environmental effects on obesity it is necessary to compare the similarity of fatness among people who share genes or who share environments. The study of Stunkard et al (1986a) was based on 540 Danish adult adoptees, for whom information was available about the build of both biological and adoptive parents. Some of the results are summarised in Table 6.4. When the adoptees were grouped into three classes — thin, median and overweight/obese — there was a significant relationship between the weight class of the biological mother and the adoptee, but not between the adoptive mother and the adoptee. With the fathers the relationship was less strong, but there was still a significant trend, as the adoptee became more obese, for biological fathers to be more obese, but for adoptive father to be less obese. This study certainly suggests a genetic influence on body build, but the effect seems strongest in determining thinness rather than fatness — it is striking that of the thin adoptees only 18% had overweight or obese biological mothers, compared with a general rate of about 37% in the other classes. It is also intriguing that thin adoptees had significantly more overweight adoptive fathers as well as significantly fewer overweight biological fathers.

If genetic influences predispose to obesity they must do so either by reducing energy expenditure or by increasing energy output (the logic of this statement has been extensively discussed in 6.a. above.) Griffiths & Payne (1976) measured resting metabolic rate and total energy expenditure (by a heart rate method) of the young children of obese and non-obese parents. They found that the children of obese parents had a lower energy expenditure than children of non-obese parents, suggesting that the not-yet-obese children had inherited a 'thrifty gene' from their obese parents. This very interesting observation needs replication. Avons & James (1986) investigated in a respiration chamber the energy expenditure of men aged 17-27 years, who had normal-weight parents or one obese parent. There was no significant difference between the groups in RMR, thermic effect of food or response to standard exercises.

Table 6.4. Proportion of overweight or obese biological or (in parentheses, adoptive) parents, according to weight class of the adoptee. (Data of Stunkard et al 1986a)

Weight class of adoptee	Thin	Median	Overweight/obese
Mean QI of adoptees	17.8	23.0	31.4
Percentage overweight parents:			
Mother— biological	18	35	41
(adoptive)	(34)	(37)	(35)
Father— biological	35	38	49
(adoptive)	(57)	(53)	(45)

One investigation which helps to explain the familial aggregation of obesity is reported by Bogardus et al (1986). They demonstrated that when the resting metabolic rate of Pima Indians was regressed against FFM, age and sex 83% of the variance was explained, and this observation fits well with other workers. However they went on to show that a further 11% of the variance of RMR could be explained by the familial relationship of the subjects. This is the first time that evidence has been offered for a familial (but necessarily genetic) resemblance in energy expenditure.

When data on body build are available for many types of relationship — biological and adoptive sibships, cousin sibships, monozygotic and dizygotic twins — possible to undertake mathematical analyses comprehensible only to the expert (Longini et al 1984, Bouchard et al 1985). A most helpful review of this difficult area was given by Bouchard (1987). The problem is that inheritance may be genetic or cultural, and it is difficult to distinguish these possibilities. For example the total inheritance of percentage body fat, and of distribution of fat, may be 0.55 and 0.61 respectively, but some of this inheritance is due to a genetic–environmental interaction, and the true genetic inheritance is probably about 0.22 and 0.28 respectively.

From the therapeutic viewpoint is is useful to know that there is a genetic (and hence untreatable) component to obesity, but reassuring also that this component is not so large that, with suitable modification of the environment, normal weight cannot be achieved.

6.e INACTIVITY AS A CAUSE OF OBESITY

It is obvious that, other things being equal, an inactive person expends less energy than an active person, so inactivity could be a cause of obesity. However, it is very difficult to obtain data to show that inactivity really causes obesity, largely because habitual physical activity is so difficult to measure accurately, for the reasons given in the previous chapter. Certainly very obese people tend to be inactive, because they have a very low exercise tolerance, and cannot manage much exertion. On the other hand the exercise which obese people do undertake costs them more energy than the same activity undertaken by a thin person. Furthermore many non-obese people are also very inactive. Figures 6.14 and 6.15 show the estimated energy expenditure in leisure activity (Mcal/month) among men and

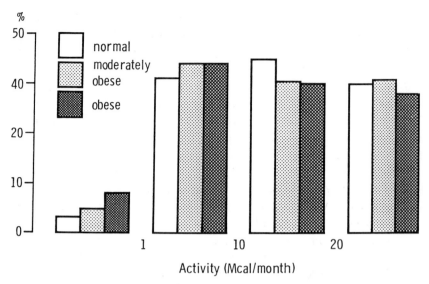

Fig. 6.14 Energy expenditure (Mcal/month) in leisuretime activities among men aged 39 years, related to tertiles of W/H² (Data of Braddon 1985)

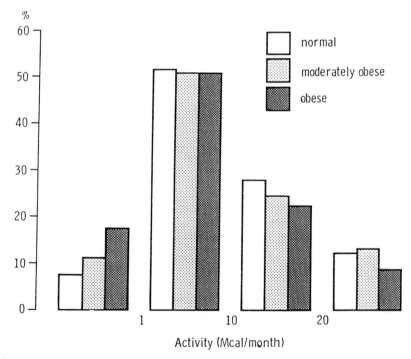

Fig. 6.15 Data similar to that in Figure 6.13, relating to women aged 39 years (Data of Braddon 1985)

woman aged 39 years who were surveyed by Braddon (1985). Among those individuals who took virtually no exercise (<1 Mcal/month) obese and moderately obese were overrepresented, but otherwise the pattern of leisuretime physical activity was quite similar for normal, moderately obese and obese subjects. The mean level of activity was 10 Mcal/month, or about 300 kcal/day. It is clear that the majority of obese people have a pattern of physical activity which is indistinguishable from that of the majority of non-obese people: namely a sedentary lifestyle.

Another argument has been advanced to suggest that inactivity is an important cause of obesity (Thompson et al 1982). It is well known that inactivity causes muscle wasting, and resting metabolic rate is closely related to the FFM, of which muscle contributes about half. Inactivity will therefore cause a low metabolic rate. There are at least two flaws in this argument. First, it is remarkably difficult to cause measurable muscle wasting simply by rest — for example by encasing a healthy limb in plaster of Paris for 6 weeks. Thigh muscles of trained athletes waste rapidly after knee injuries, but this involves effects other than simple inactivity. Second, patients who have spinal injuries and are therefore paralysed have no increase in body fat (Greenway et al 1969, Cardus et al 1985), and have a normal metabolic rate (Agarwal ct al 1985). It is therefore quite unlikely that inactivity causes any effect on energy expenditure by virtue of a change in FFM.

A publication by Mayer et al (1956) is often cited as evidence that inactivity causes obesity. These workers recorded body weight and estimated energy intake among various grades of workers in a jute mill in West Bengal. They assigned levels of energy expenditure to each job, so stallholders, supervisors and clerks who lived on the premises were 'sedentary', clerks who travelled to work various distances and mechanics were classified as 'light work', and so on through to workers heaving bales of jute whose work was 'very heavy'. The results were presented in the form shown in Figure 6.16. It is evident that sedentary workers have a paradoxically high energy intake and high body weight. This conclusion was particularly acceptable, since it confirmed previous work by Mayer et al (1954) on rats, who ate more if they were sedentary than if they were moderately active. However the conclusion is really not valid: if sedentary clerks are compared with clerks whose activity was described as 'light' it appears that the sedentary clerks ate more, but weighed less, than the more active clerks. This is difficult to believe.

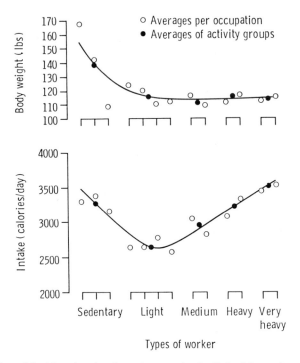

Fig. 6.16 Body weight (above) and estimated energy intake (below) in workers in jute mill in West Bengal (Data of Mayer et al 1956)

Probably a fairer conclusion is that errors in estimating habitual energy intake probably account for this paradoxical result.

The question remains: do people eat more if they are sedentary than if they are moderately active? To answer the question it is necessary to study subjects where they have access to palatable food ad libitum and where their energy intake can be covertly observed. The subjects must then be persuaded to alter their level of energy output by exercising without being aware that the investigators intend to study the effect on spontaneous energy intake. This very difficult protocol was achieved by Woo et al (1982a,1982b) on obese women, and by Woo and Pi-Sunyer (1985) on lean women. With increasing exercise the obese women showed a non-significant increase in energy intake, while the lean women showed a significant increase in energy intake. Neither study supported the hypothesis of Mayer et al (1956) that moderate exercise decreased energy intake when compared with the sedentary state.

On the available sketchy evidence it appears that inactivity may be a rather minor contributing factor in the aetiology of human obesity, but it is uncertain if people are obese because they are inactive, or inactive because they are obese. There is no evidence in man that moderate exercise decreases food intake, or that a sedentary lifestyle causes an increase in food intake. The role of exercise in treating or preventing obesity is discussed in Chapter 8.d.

6.f SOCIAL, CULTURAL, PSYCHOLOGICAL AND COGNITIVE FACTORS

Social and cultural factors affecting food intake

Food has an important social function, as well as a nutritive one. Food can have significance in many ways in different societies: to establish social status, to placate enemies, as religious symbols or to bind together families or communities (De Garine 1972). Strong flavours which are the mainstay of certain national cuisines are often unpalatable to people unaccustomed to them: for example Rozin (1976) points out that chili pepper is used in some Mexican villages applied to the mother's breast to promote weaning. Flavours may convey warnings that a particular food is dangerous to eat: rats which have eaten poisoned food will starve rather than eat food of a similar flavour even if it is not poisoned, and this phenomenon of bait-shyness must have had protective value in primitive conditions. It is obviously important that young animals should copy the eating habits of their parents to avoid poisonous food. This effect was dramatically illustrated by Wyrwicka (1976) who used implanted brain electrodes to change the eating pattern of a cat so that, when given the choice, the cat would prefer banana to meat. When kittens, who had a normal preference for meat, were put with this cat the kittens also chose banana. We probably underestimate the extent to which eating patterns in human children are learned from their parents, and this effect probably explains some of the familial aggregation of obesity.

Reports from New York (Goldblatt et al 1965), London (Silverstone et al 1969, Ashwell & Etchell 1974), Canada (Millar & Wigle 1986) and other places agree that there is an inverse correlation between social class and the prevalence of obesity. The only exceptions seem to be less affluent countries like India (Gour & Gupta 1968) and Germany (Pflanz 1962) where there is the usual negative relation between obesity and social class among women, but not among men. This implies that overweight is more socially acceptable among successful German men than among their wives.

The association of fatness with low income does not hold at all ages. Figure 6.17 shows that the triceps skinfold of girls from higher-income families is greater than that of less affluent children, but in adult life the curves cross over, and the poorer women are fatter than the richer ones. There is no obvious explanation for the increased prevalence of obesity in the poorer sections of many communities, not is it clear if the poverty causes the obesity, or the obesity causes the poverty. There is some social discrimination against obese people, but this could hardly account for increased obesity in lower social classes. There is some evidence from Denmark that obese military recruits perform less well in intelligence tests than normal-weight men of the same social class (Sorensen et al 1983). These results are shown in Figure 6.18. Again, it is difficult to explain this association. It might be that a genetic endowment which predisposed to obesity also was associated with lower intelligence, or that the person who is obese does not try to do as well as possible in an intelligence test.

Orbach (1978), in a popular book entitled 'Fat is a feminist issue' suggests that compulsive eating in women is a response to their social position. It is said to be the social duty of women to be attractive to men, to bear and care for children, to be the one who feeds and comforts her family and, when sacrifice is necessary, sacrifices

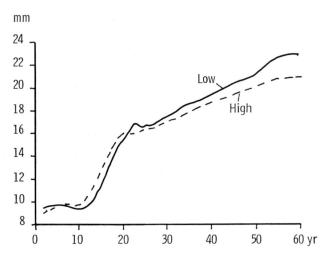

Fig. 6.17 Triceps skinfolds of girls and women of high or low income (Data of Garn & Clark 1976)

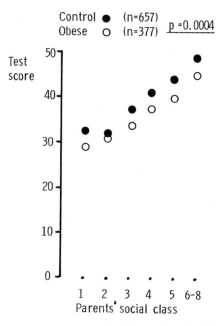

Control ● (n=657)
Obese ○ (n=377) p =0.0004

Fig. 6.18 Intelligence test score among normal-weight or obese Danish men (Data of Sorensen et al 1983)

herself. According to this ethic, fatness in a woman is evidence of greed, selfishness and a failure to fulfil her responsibilities. Brought up in this tradition, the adolescent girl may view with alarm and disgust the deposition of fat on breast, hips and thighs which is a normal part of the process of female sexual maturation. Adolescent girls who are seized by this anxiety are candidates for anorexia nervosa: they may starve themselves in order to reverse the processes of adolescent maturation (Crisp 1973). Anorexia nervosa occurs in about 1% of all schoolgirls aged 16–18 years, but is uncommon in males (Crisp 1973).

According to Orbach (1978) the woman who survives adolescence without developing anorexia nervosa is now subjected to remorseless pressure from the advertising media that she must look appealing, earthy, sensual, sexual, virginal, innocent, reliable, daring, myste-rious, coquettish and thin. So unreasonable a demand naturally provokes revolt among those who do not concur with the role of women as stated above, and one way of demonstrating the rejection of these standards is to be fat.

There is probably some truth in this analysis, but obesity also occurs in men, presumably for unfeminist reasons, so some obesity in women must occur for unfeminist reasons also.

Psychological factors in obesity

Interest in psychological factors which might predispose to obesity received a great impetus with the publications of Stuart (1967) and Schachter (1968). Stuart reported extremely good results in obese patients treated by behaviour modification, and Schachter showed that obese people eat for all sorts of reasons other than requiring food. Together these seemed to provide a theoretical basis for a new and effective treatment of obesity: obese people did not control their food intake accurately because they responded inappropriately by eating after many irrelevant stimuli, so if they could be taught to interpret food-related cues correctly their obesity should disappear. The next two decades showed that this was too optimistic a forecast. It was (and is) true that obese people eat in response to social and emotional pressures, and if they can be taught to eat only when they actually need food they lose weight. (The use of behaviour modification techniques in treatment is discussed in Chapter 8.) However, it is also true that normal-weight people eat in response to social and emotional pressures not connected with a need for food.

Many studies have been made on the 'eating disorder' which causes obesity. Frequently obese people report binge-eating, in which they eat huge quantities of food, far beyond the amount required to satisfy hunger, and only stop when further eating is virtually impossible. However, it is not clear if this is a characteristic of obese persons, or an effect induced by dietary restriction. Keys et al (1950) report many cases of non-obese subjects (prisoners, castaways, lost explorers) who have overeaten, sometimes to the point of causing death, when food is made available after a period of enforced semi-starvation. The volunteers for the experiments of Benedict et al (1919) and Keys et al (1950) overate when the experiment was over, and became fatter than they had been at the start of the underfeeding experiment. We therefore do not know if the eating patterns described by some obese patients differ from those which would be observed in non-obese subjects if the non-obese subjects were subjected to the same dietary restrictions as the obese patients.

Obese patients may be convinced that they have some mental

disease, and they seek referral to a psychiatrist. Not all obese people are sane, but neither are they all insane: psychometric testing has failed to identify any psychological disorder which is characteristic of obesity (Rodin et al 1977). In fact obese people show less abnormality on the personality inventory (MMPI) than patients with anorexia or bulimia (Scott & Baroffio 1986).

Cognitive factors in the regulation of body weight

Some variables, such as the serum calcium concentration, cannot be cognitively regulated because we do not normally know our serum calcium concentration, and if we did know it was too high or too low there is no action we can take to rectify the situation. Other variables, like the balance in our current account at the bank, are entirely cognitively regulated. If the balance moves out of an acceptable range we are made aware of the situation, and have to take some action to restore the appropriate balance. So far in this chapter various physiological factors which might affect energy balance have been considered, and none of them adequately explains the very precise long-term regulation of body weight which is achieved by some people. To explain this stability it is probably necessary to invoke cognitive control, i.e. people who maintain normal body weight over long periods do so by taking conscious corrective action when body weight strays out of the range which they regard as acceptable.

Let us consider a specific example. Dr R Passmore, a distinguished nutritionist, has a tail-coat made for him 44 years ago, and it still fits him. He cites this as evidence that over that time period his energy balance has not accumulated an error of more that 25,000 kcal (10 MJ), which over 16,000 days is an average error of less than 2 kcal (8 kJ) per day (Davidson et al 1979). How is this possible? Clearly he has not balanced energy intake and output to better than 2 kcal every day for 44 years, but has gained and lost imbalances of several megacalories to achieve the final overall balance. If long-term energy balance is more accurate than short-term energy balance, there must be something which detects accumulated errors in balance and initiates corrective action. In the case of Dr Passmore one candidate for this detector of imbalances is his tail-coat: suppose one year he found it did not fit him, what would he do? Would he ruefully note that his energy balance was at fault, and obtain a tail-coat of a different size, or would he alter his level of food intake or physical activity so he came to fit the tail-coat once more? If (as I think likely) he took the latter course this would be an excellent example of cognitive regulation of body weight.

Most people do not regulate body weight in the normal range by reference to a particular garment, and many people do not regulate body weight in the normal range at all. However, probably most households possess a bathroom scales, and those who do not can use coin-operated weighing machines in public places. The presence of these instruments indicates that there is a general desire in the population to be able to monitor their body weight. It is therefore at least a tenable hypothesis that the people who maintain a normal weight do so because they take corrective action when their weighing machine, tail-coat, spouse, or other monitoring device tells them that all is not well.

To test the hypothesis it would be necessary to compare over a long period the stability of body weight in a population who did not know, or care, what they weighed with another population, otherwise similar, who did know and care what they weighed. It is virtually impossible to carry out such a trial. A more possible test is to observe the fluctuations in weight with time in survey populations who were not particularly interested in their body weight. Figure 6.19 shows the weight variation (maximum to minimum weight) during 10 examinations over a period of 18 years in the Framingham population (Gordon & Kannel 1973). The average variation among men and women is 10 kg (22 lb), so most would

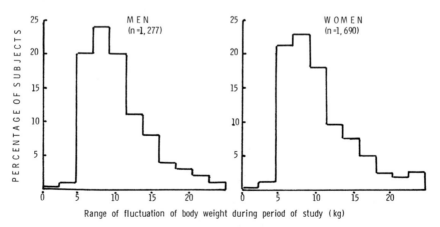

Fig. 6.19 Fluctuations in body weight during 18 years among men and women in Framingham study. Age at entry 30–59 years (Data of Gordon and Kannel 1973)

have failed Dr Passmore's tail-coat test. More women (4%) than men (3%) showed a variation of more than 20 kg during the study period, and it was quite rare to observe a variation of less than 5 kg (1% in both sexes). However this weight fluctuation was a short-term wobble on a fairly constant average, so the average final weight differed by only about 3 kg from the average weight at entry.

Evidence of large short-term fluctuation can be obtained from any longitudinal study of body weight in normal populations. Another example is shown in Figure 6.20. This is taken from a survey by Miall of 411 females living in the Rhondda Fach region of Wales. The survey was done to investigate the epidemiology of hypertension, and measurements were made on the same people of (among other things) weight in 1960 and 1964. The weights lie around the line of identity, showing that there was no very large change in average weight over the 4-year interval, but some people who weighed 90 kg in 1960 weighed 60 kg in 1964, and vice versa. The standard deviation for the entire group is 6.6 kg, so about one third of the women had changed in weight by more than that amount between the times of the two surveys.

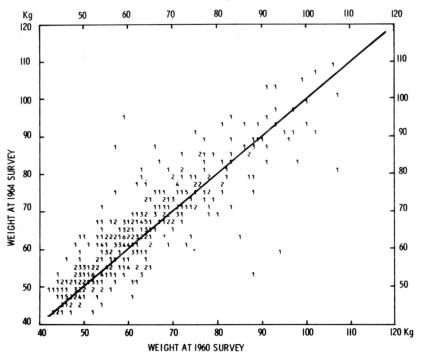

Fig. 6.20 Weight of 411 women surveyed by Miall in 1960 and 1964

A change of 6 kg in body weight is certainly too much to pass unnoticed by the average person, so we must conclude that most people, at some time, realise that they have gained or lost weight, and it seems likely that they will then take steps to do something about it. There is a large demand for popular literature on how to lose weight, so it is also reasonable to guess that many people take the appropriate action to restore their weight to the desired range. If this is so then cognitive factors explain why many people maintain energy balance rather accurately over long periods, although they fluctuate in weight by many kilograms in the short term. This is of great importance in understanding the aetiology of obesity, and gives a useful clue to treatment. If obese people are obese because they do not know, or care, that they are overweight then it is the task of the therapist, or health educator, to guide them to a more accurate assessment of their situation.

6.g SUMMARY: CONTROL OF ENERGY BALANCE IN MAN

A normal adult man has about 12 kg body fat, which represents an energy store equivalent to about 50 days energy requirements, so he has no need to match daily energy input and output as accurately as a rat, which has smaller stores relative to daily energy flux.

About one third of the adult population in affluent countries is overweight to an extent which causes a measurable decrease in health and longevity. The excess weight is 75% fat and 25% fat-free tissue. The RMR of obese people is, on average, greater than that of lean people of the same sex, age and height. Even when the RMR of obese and normal people is compared per kilogram fat-free mass the obese do not have a lower-than-normal RMR. It is debatable if there is a reduction in thermogenic response to some stimuli in obese people, but it is agreed that their total energy expenditure is greater than normal, because their resting metabolic rate is so high. They must therefore have a higher energy intake than normal to maintain body weight. This conclusion is passionately disputed by some people, but the evidence for it is compelling.

During periods of overfeeding or underfeeding energy output changes to limit weight change, i.e. metabolic rate increases during overfeeding and decreases during underfeeding. The biochemical basis for this adaptation is partly understood. This defence of body weight occurs with equal vigour in lean and obese people, and there is no good evidence that there is a 'set-point' body weight to which an individual tends to return because that weight is metabolically more strongly defended than any other weight. With weight loss metabolic rate decreases, but (in the long term) no more than would be expected as a result of the change in body weight and composition, unless excessive amounts of fat-free tissue have been lost. Genetic factors and inactivity probably play some part in the aetiology of obesity, but their influence is usually masked by other more powerful influences.

Physiological controls which regulate energy balance in the short term operate rather poorly in subjects who have ad libitum access to palatable food. In such circumstances long-term regulation of energy balance to achieve normal body weight is (or in some people is not) achieved mainly by cognitive control (Garrow 1974b).

7

Possibilities for the treatment of obesity

Treatment of obesity must be based on the principles set out above concerning the aetiology of obesity. Any successful treatment must create a negative energy balance, so the excess fat stores are burned off. If treatment was simply a matter of creating an energy deficit then total starvation would be the ideal solution, since during starvation the maximum possible energy deficit is created. However, starvation is not the ideal treatment for obesity, since it causes the loss of an excessive amount of lean tissue. The objective of treatment is to arrange things so that the tissue which is lost is of the same composition as the excess tissue which is stored, namely about 25% lean and 75% fat by weight. Theoretically there are seven ways in which this might be achieved, which are illustrated in Figure 7.1.

The energy intake of a typical person might be 10.5 MJ (2500 kcal) per day, of which about 95% is absorbed from the gut and 5% is lost in faeces. If the person is in energy balance this energy input is balanced by an equal output of 10 MJ, of which roughly 7.5 MJ will be resting metabolism, 1.0 MJ the thermic effect of food, and the remaining 1.5 MJ all other thermogenesis, including the energy cost of exercise. Obviously these values will vary between people, but they are reasonably typical values for the average sedentary adult.

The possible methods of treatment indicated in Figure 7.1 are:

a. Excise excess adipose tissue.
b. Decrease energy intake (ie reducing diet).
c. Increase energy loss in faeces.
d. Increase resting metabolic rate.
e. Increase dietary-induced thermogenesis.
f. Increase thermogenesis due to physical activity.
g. Increase other thermogenic stimuli.

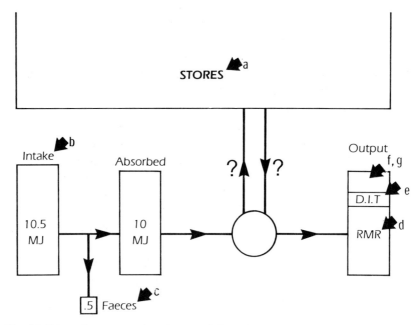

Fig. 7.1 Schematic representation of energy balance in man, showing the seven points at which it might theoretically be possible to intervene in order to treat obesity

This list of possibilities does not include some strategies which have been advocated for the treatment of obesity, namely drugs which have a direct action on lipolysis or lipogenesis, behaviour modification, and contingency conditioning. Reasons are given below for not considering these as primary treatments of obesity. Every possible effective treatment must act through one of the mechanisms listed in methods a–g above.

7.a EXCISION OF EXCESS FAT

One certain way to lose fat is to employ a surgeon to cut it off. However removal of 1 kg fat is quite a major operation, and a similar effect could be achieved quite easily, quickly and less painfully by dieting. It was at one time suggested that excision of fat prevented recurrence of obesity, since the fat cells were removed and therefore could not regenerate. It is now known that fat cells can be recruited from subcutaneous stromal tissue whenever there is a need to store excess fat, so this argument is invalid.

Fat which is accessible for excision is in a layer under the skin which varies from a few millimetres to several centimetres in thickness. Nerves and blood vessels supplying the overlying skin pass through this layer of subcutaneous fat, so it is difficult to remove significant quantities of fat without damage to the blood and nerve supply to the overlying skin. If skin flaps are raised to expose the underlying fat the final cosmetic result will almost certainly be worse that that before the operation.

To minimise damage to overlying skin various types of liposuction are practised in cosmetic surgery (Fournier & Otteni 1983). A hypotonic solution containing some hyaluronidase is injected into the area to be treated, and a cannula attached to a powerful suction machine is then inserted through a small stab wound to extract the injected solution together with some fat. Each surgeon has his own favourite design of cannula for this purpose (Kesselring 1983). The procedure is not without hazard: free fat is passed in the urine after the operation, and cases of pulmonary embolism have been reported (Grazer 1983). In my opinion the trauma involved does not justify the trivial amount of fat removed. I do not think this line of treatment holds any promise of value in the management of obesity in general, but there will no doubt be a continuing demand from fee-paying patients for this method of 'spot reduction'.

7.b LOW ENERGY DIET

This is the mainstay of conventional treatments for obesity, and in many cases excellent results are obtained. The primary disadvantage is that it requires considerable dedication for the obese person to refrain from eating normal quantities of food, and compliance is made even worse if the patient is subjected to advertising which suggests that weight loss can be achieved without the tedium of dieting. Another disadvantage is that the low-energy diet inevitably reduces dietary thermogenesis, thus reducing total energy expenditure somewhat. However dieting is certainly a strategy which will be included in future methods of treatment of obesity, since it is potentially the most powerful method for generating the required energy deficit. Practical aspects of this approach are considered in detail in Chapter 8.

7.c DECREASE INTESTINAL ABSORPTION OF ENERGY

Some clinicians are impressed by the apparently small energy intake of obese patients compared with normal-weight people, and conclude that obese individuals must be unusually efficient at extracting energy from the diet (Macnair 1979). If this were so it might be logical to try to decrease the ability of these patients to absorb energy from food, but the premise is false. Many studies have shown that in both obese and normal subjects about 92–97% of the energy of ordinary food is absorbed, so there is no possibility for obese subjects to have super-efficient absorption, and indeed they do not (Garrow & Wright 1980).

It is possible to cause significant malabsorption either by drug treatment or by surgical bypass of a large proportion of the small bowel. This certainly causes weight loss, but not, as was at first thought, without affecting food intake. Pilkington et al (1976) showed that patients after jejuno- ileal bypass learned to eat in a manner which controlled the diarrhoea. Careful balance studies demonstrated that weight loss was more due to decreased energy intake than decreased absorption. Bypass operations therefore work by forcing the patient to diet, but the diet which controls diarrhoea is not necessarily nutritionally desirable. Even if the diet supplies adequate nutrients malabsorption of fat, for example, necessarily leads to malabsorption of fat-soluble vitamins, and often to various forms of electrolyte imbalance. Finally, the energy which is not absorbed in the small bowel enters the large bowel and provides an unusually rich substrate for the growth of colonic bacteria, with resulting increased fermentation and flatulence.

Similar objections apply to drugs which are intended to inhibit the digestion or absorption of nutrients from the gut. There was recently a vogue for 'starch blockers', which were said to inhibit the action of pancreatic amylase, and thus prevent the digestion and absorption of starchy food (Hanssen 1982). There are several natural substances which inhibit alpha amylase in vitro but these are totally ineffective when taken by mouth before eating a starchy meal (Bo-Linn et al 1982, Garrow et al 1983). This result could have been predicted on theoretical grounds for several reasons. First, the enzyme inhibitor was itself a protein, and therefore would be digested in the stomach and would never reach the duodenum in active form. Second, it is virtually impossible to distribute the inhibitor throughout the starch in food in such a way that the amylase encounters the inhibitor before it has digested the starch. Third, the pancreas secretes a large excess of amylase, so even if 90% of the amylase had been inhibited there would still be enough left to digest the starch quite efficiently. New drugs are being developed which inhibit the digestion of sucrose (Cauderay et al 1985) or starch (Tappy et al 1986) but for the reasons given above I do not believe that treatments aimed at causing malabsorption hold promise for management of obesity, and they will not be discussed further.

7.d INCREASE RESTING METABOLIC RATE

The idea that obese subjects have a low metabolic rate is common in lay circles, and is even promoted in the fringes of the scientific literature (Cataldo 1985). In fact, every well-controlled study which has compared the measured metabolic rate of a group of obese and lean subjects has shown that on average the obese group had the higher metabolic rate.

Neverthelesss, the idea of increasing RMR as a treatment for obesity is quite attractive, and undoubtedly there are drugs which can achieve this. The foreseeable problems are that a large increase in metabolic rate would be hazardous for severely obese patients whose cardiovascular system was already under strain to cope with a normal metabolic rate. The poor exercise tolerance of these patients indicates how little increase in metabolic rate they can cope with, and a drug which increased resting metabolism would reduce their exercise tolerance still more. Furthermore it would be necessary to find a drug which increased resting metabolism without also increasing appetite, otherwise the patient would have done better simply to adopt the strategy of a low-energy diet. This possibility is therefore of doubtful promise for future methods of treatment, but possible applications of thermogenic drugs are discussed further in Chapter 8.

7.e INCREASE DIETARY-INDUCED THERMOGENESIS

A decrease in dietary thermogenesis (the increase in metabolic rate which normally follows a meal) has been reported to be a characteristic of obese subjects (Pittet et al 1976, Shetty et al 1981, Ravussin et al 1985, Segal et al 1985a). However, other investigators do not find this difference between lean and obese subjects (Nair et al 1983, Welle & Campbell 1983). Probably these conflicting results can be explained by differences in experimental protocol, or in the way that the lean and obese subjects were selected. It would probably be a fair to say that if there is a difference in dietary thermogenesis between obese and lean subjects the difference is quite small and hence difficult to measure.

It may be that a drug will be found which would increase dietary thermogenesis, but even if this were done it would probably not be very helpful in the treatment of obesity. Dietary thermogenesis accounts for roughly 10% of total energy expenditure, so even if were doubled this would only increase energy expenditure by 10%. Also a strategy based on increased dietary-induced thermogenesis would not work well in combination with a low-energy diet which, as stated above, is likely to be a component of future treatments of obesity. This approach is therefore not discussed further.

7.f INCREASE EXERCISE

Physical exercise is a powerful thermogenic stimulus, and it is enjoyable to many people. Unfortunately severely obese patients have a very poor exercise tolerance, so they are unable to take enough exercise to make much difference to their total energy expenditure. The idea that exercise causes a prolonged increase in metabolic rate after the exercise period has ceased, or that it enhances dietary-induced thermogenesis, is not supported by the experimental evidence (Pacy et al 1985). However, exercise confers other benefits to health apart from weight reduction (Fentem 1985), so overweight people who can and will take exercise should certainly be encouraged to do so. The use of physical training in preventing and treating mild obesity is discussed in Chapter 8.

7.g INCREASE OTHER THERMOGENIC STIMULI

Apart from food and exercise, the only stimuli which cause a significant increase in metabolic rate, and which are likely to be encountered in real life, are anxiety (Blaza & Garrow 1980) and exposure to cold (Wyndham et al 1968). To achieve an increase of more than 10% or so in metabolic rate a most unpleasant degree of anxiety or cold exposure must be used, so this is not an acceptable form of treatment.

7.h DRUGS ACTING DIRECTLY ON LIPOLYSIS OR LIPOGENESIS

In Figure 7.1 there are question marks against the arrows leading to and from the fat stores, to indicate that drugs which inhibited lipogenesis, or enhanced lipolysis, would not in themselves be helpful. Suppose a drug was produced which inhibited lipogenesis, but had no effect on energy intake or output, what overall effect would this have? The energy which would previously have been stored as fat would have to go somewhere, and it is by no means certain that the metabolic disposal of this energy would be by as benign a pathway as the synthesis of subcutaneous triglyceride. Similarly if lipolysis was enhanced without any change in energy intake or output, what would happen to the fatty acids which were released? It is hard to imagine any fate other than being deposited again somewhere as fat. If they were oxidised they would displace some other fuel, and in the end the same amount of fat would be synthesised, although not necessarily in as safe a place as subcutaneous adipose tissue. These approaches are therefore not at all promising. Ultimately all effective treaments of obesity must affect energy intake and/or output (see Chapter 6.a).

7.i BEHAVIOUR MODIFICATION

Behaviour modification has rightly been hailed as one of the most significant recent advances in the treatment of obesity. The features of this approach are that the therapist concentrates on the attitude of the patient to food and eating, the social circumstances which promote or inhibit eating, the effect of various non-nutritive stimuli, and so on. Since the emphasis of this type of therapy is explicitly not to insist that the patient should adhere to a diet, but rather that he should study exactly what and why he eats, the patient regards behaviour modification as an alternative to dieting. In fact, in so far as behaviour modification causes weight loss, it does so by altering energy intake (or output), and it is thus a special case of strategy b above (or f). For this reason behaviour therapy is not represented in Figure 7.1, or listed as a primary treatment strategy, but the value of behaviour modification techniques when using low-energy diets is considered in Chapter 8.

7.j CONTINGENCY CONDITIONING

This term is used to describe a somewhat heavy-handed type of behaviour therapy, which might less charitably be termed benign blackmail. A striking example was provided by Scrignar (1980) who describes a situation in which overweight policemen were required to lose at least 2 kg per month, or be penalised by loss of leave privileges or pay. This was very effective in causing weight loss until someone obtained a ruling that the arrangement infringed constitutional rights, and the sanctions were withdrawn and the excess weight was soon regained. Clearly the penalties, or threats of penalties, did not in themselves cause weight loss, but they motivated the policemen to adopt stategies affecting energy intake and/or output which caused weight loss. Monetary rewards or penalties are associated with weight loss (Jeffery et al 1978) and with success in stopping smoking (Stitzer & Bigelow 1984). The larger the sum of money involved the greater the effectiveness of these contracts.

Ethical problems arise with these forms of treatment: surely the patient must be free to keep to the diet or not, as he or she chooses? However obese patients often say that they wish to be bullied into dieting, since otherwise their will-power is inadequate to achieve the end result they require. In part it is legitimate for patients to seek help of this sort which may enable them to keep to the diet for a longer time, but the danger is that the patient will then expect the therapist to guarantee the success of the treatment. This is too much to ask, because ultimately it will always be the patient who decides whether or not a particular item of food will be eaten. The practical applications of these theoretical considerations are discussed further in the next chapter.

7.k HYPNOSIS

Hypnosis might plausibly help patients to keep to a prescribed diet, but there are no published trials comparing hypnosis with any other treatment for obesity (Mott & Roberts 1979). In most reports the weight loss achieved is similar to that achieved by conventional methods. In a recent study Cochrane & Friesen (1986) measured various aspects of the personality of 60 obese women who were undergoing treatment by hypnosis, but none of the variables (suggestibility, self-concept, quality of family origin, age of obesity onset, education level, socio-economic status or multi-modal imagery) related significantly to weight loss. This was about 3 kg at 1 month, and 8 kg at 6 months, and the weight loss was not affected by the provision of audiotapes to reinforce the hypnotic suggestion to one group of patients. We therefore do not know what part hypnosis played in the weight loss. We still need a good trial of hypnosis versus some other form of treatment, with random allocation of patients to the two treatment groups.

8

Practical treatment strategies

The theoretical possibilities mentioned in the last chapter can be reduced to a rather small number of practical strategies — to reduce energy intake by some form of energy-restricted diet, with or without the assistance of anorectic drugs, or to increase energy expenditure by physical activity or thermogenic drugs. Dietary treatments according to various formulae will be discussed first.

8.a STARVATION

There is no doubt that of all dietary measures the largest energy deficit, and consequently the greatest rate of weight loss, is achieved by total starvation (mean rates of weight loss about 2.7 kg/week are reported). These are attractive features, so intermittent starvation was advocated as a treatment for obesity (Bloom 1959), and later some were emboldened to use prolonged starvation (Drenick et al 1964, Runcie & Thomson 1970), extending up to a period of 315 days in one case. However enthusiasm waned with reports of unexpected sudden death in patients who were treated by prolonged starvation (Norbury 1964, Spencer 1968, Garnett et al 1969). There are still occasional case reports of patients who present with severe vitamin deficiency states after prolonged self-imposed fasting for weight reduction (Waterston & Gilligan 1986).

In the light of more recent knowledge we have come to realise that there is a fundamental theoretical flaw in starvation treatment. The excess weight in obese people is 75% fat and 25% FFM (see Chapter 3.f.), but the weight lost during starvation is roughly 50% fat and 50% FFM. Thus the starved obese person may eventually reach normal weight, but can never achieve normal body composition, since at normal weight he or she will have a deficit of FFM. Nitrogen

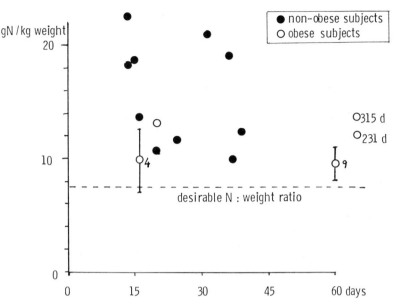

Fig. 8.1 Ratio of nitrogen loss to weight loss in subjects totally fasted for longer than 14 days (Data reviewed by Forbes & Drenick 1979)

balance data on all recorded cases of starvation for more than 14 days have been reviewed by Forbes & Drenick (1979). The ratio of N loss to weight loss according to the duration of the fast is shown in Figure 8.1. The range is from 10 g N/kg to about 20 g N/kg, with a mean value about 15 g N/kg, which indicates 50% FFM in the weight lost, since FFM has a nitrogen content of about 30 g N/kg. It should be noted in Figure 8.1 that the more obese subjects generally showed a lower nitrogen:weight loss ratio than non-obese subjects, but even with the most obese subjects the ratio was still above the desirable ratio of 7.5 g N/kg weight loss. For this reason, as well as the danger of sudden unexpected death, total starvation is not an acceptable treatment for obesity.

It is perhaps informative to interpret the weight loss data in terms of energy balance. Table 8.1 shows that the energy value of tissue with 75% fat : 25% FFM is 7000 kcal/kg, while tissue that is 50% fat : 50% FFM has a value of 5000 kcal/kg. If a person during starvation loses 2.7 kg/week of the former mixture, then total energy expenditure has been 18 900 kcal/week, or 2700 kcal/day. This is an improbably high energy expenditure for a starving person. If the weight lost is 50 : 50 fat : FFM then 2.7 kg represents an energy deficit of 13 500 kcal, or about 1930 kcal/day, which is altogether a

Table 8.1. Energy value of 1 kg tissue mixture which is 75% fat : 25% FFM (A) or 50% fat : 50% FFM (B)

| | (A) | | (B) | |
	Weight kg	Energy kcal	Weight kg	Energy kcal
Fat	0.75	6750	0.50	4500
FFM	0.25	250	0.50	500
Total	1.00	7000	1.00	5000

more plausible estimate of energy output. In practice the rate of weight loss provides a useful guide to the composition of weight lost. A rule-of-thumb is that (after the initial rapid loss when glycogen is being burned) a rate of weight loss between 0.5 kg and 1 kg/week is appropriate for most people, nearer the lower limit for patients who are old and short and not very overweight, and nearer the upper limit for patients who are young and tall and very overweight. These guidelines will be discussed further on the section dealing with conventional reducing diets.

8.b VERY-LOW CALORIE DIETS

Of course attempts have been made to preserve the attractive rapid weight loss seen in starvation, but to prevent the loss of FFM. This is the objective, and the claim, of proponents of very-low-calorie diets (VLCD), which is either attacked or defended with more passion than is usual in scientific debate (Wadden et al 1983, 1984, Howard 1984). Criticism relates as much to the way in which such diets are promoted and distributed, as to the properties inherent in the diets. There are considerable commercial interests involved, so each company will strongly defend the reputation of its own product, while equally vigorous criticism will always be forthcoming from an alliance of commercial rivals and those who think anything produced by the food industry must be bad. Furthermore a decade ago a 'liquid protein' diet was promoted (Linn & Stuart 1976) which used collagen as a protein source of a hydrolysate of very low biological value, which caused several deaths. Thus the public and physicians have learned to be wary of such preparations. It is undoubtedly true that there have been deaths among obese people losing large amounts of weight rapidly, and it may be that rapid massive weight loss always carries a danger of cardiac dysfunction, however it is achieved (Van Itallie & Yang 1984).

There is no generally accepted definition of what is meant by a VLCD; clearly it implies a regimen with less energy than a 'conventional' reducing diet (say 800–1200 kcal/day), but more than starvation. In practice most commercial diets provide about 400 kcal. The compositions of three VLCD commercially available in the UK are shown in Table 8.2. They all use protein sources of high biological value such as milk or egg protein. The similarity of their vitamin and mineral content is not a coincidence: each has been formulated to supply the recommended dietary allowance of these nutrients. Are such preparations safe?

The question cannot be answered either way, since the safety depends on the duration of use and the health of the user. Any reasonable person, including the manufacturers of VLCD, would be

Table 8.2. Composition of four very-low-calorie diets. Nutrients provided by the recommended daily amount of diet

Nutrient	Modifast	Cambridge diet	Uni-Vite microdiet	Nutroclin
Protein (g)	70	33	42	60
Carbohydrate (g)	30	42	35	54
Fat (g)	2	3	3	5
Energy				
kcal	410	330	330	500
kJ	1744	1380	1380	2090
Vitamins				
A (μg)	1500	1000	1000	2070
D (μg)	10	10	11	—
E (mg)	30	10	10	0.7
C (mg)	90	60	70	70
Folic acid (μg)	400	400	400	420
Thiamin (μg)	2250	1500	2000	920
Riboflavin (mg)	2600	1700	2000	1100
Niacin (mg)	20	18	19	19
B_6 (mg)	3	0.1	3	1.1
B_{12} (μg)	6	3	5	5
Biotin (μg)	360	200	200	250
Pantothenic acid (mg)	10	5	7	9
Minerals				
Calcium (mg)	915	800	900	980
Phosphorus (mg)	977	800	800	1000
Iodine (μg)	50	150	150	150
Iron (mg)	18	18	20	18
Magnesium (mg)	200	350	350	500
Copper (mg)	2	2	2	2
Zinc (mg)	15	15	20	15
Potassium (mg)	1500	2010	2010	2000
Sodium (mg)	920	1500	1500	1014
Manganese (mg)	4	4	3	—
Selenium (μg)	150	60	60	—
Chromium (μg)	150	60	60	60
Molybdenum (μg)	300	150	160	200

concerned if such a preparation was used for any length of time by a growing child or a pregnant woman, since any form of severe dietary restriction is inappropriate for such people. A diabetic or person on anti-hypertensive drugs would need to have expert advice to maintain good control while switching to VLCD. A patient with porphyria or gout might well precipitate an acute attack by taking VLCD. For reasons such as these a person planning to take VLCD would be well advised to seek competent, independent medical advice that they had no contraindication before starting.

Suppose there is no contraindication, are there still grounds for concern? I think so, as there would be about the use of total starvation to achieve rapid weight loss. It may be argued that total starvation is perfectly safe, since millions of people regularly undergo periods of starvation for religious reasons and come to no physical harm, and probably gain spiritual benefit. On the other hand prolonged starvation will inevitably cause death if continued long enough, so it is clearly not safe. The paradox arises because the human species is adapted to cope with a certain degree of dietary deprivation, and only shows harmful effects when the deprivation goes beyond the range of adaptation. The question is not, therefore, if VLCD represent an immediate threat to life or health (which they do not) but if the deprivation associated with VLCD is within the scope of the range of adaptation of normal people. More specifically, is the composition of the weight lost on VLCD the correct composition which will eventually return the overweight person to normality in terms of body composition and metabolic rate?

If the weight loss takes place in a metabolic ward where the intake and output of energy and nitrogen are very carefully monitored it is also possible to use the energy balance or nitrogen balance data to calculate the ratio of fat to fat-free tissue in the weight lost. The loss of FFM can also be calculated from the change in body density, or body water, or body potassium (see Chapter 3). All five of these methods of calculation have been applied to a group of 19 obese women, and the calculated loss of fat and FFM on average agrees well between the methods, but estimations of the composition of weight loss by change in density, water or potassium are subject to errors of 2 kg or more (Garrow et al 1979). Nitrogen balance gives reproducible results, but it requires meticulous technique, and does not reveal changes in glycogen stores, which cause relatively large changes in weight due to the water associated with the glycogen. Furthermore the composition of weight lost differs considerably from one individual to another (Durrant et al 1980, Finer et al 1986). Therefore to obtain a reliable picture of the composition of weight lost on a given diet it is desirable to have data obtained by several methods on a large group of subjects over a long period, but such ideal data are usually not available.

One of the earliest investigations into the composition of weight lost on a 'strict reducing regimen' was that of Passmore et al (1958). The diet provided 390 kcal/day (25 g protein, 41 g carbohydrate and 14 g fat) which is not very different from modern VLCD, but it was derived from natural foods. The seven patients were in Grade III (mean QI 45.8). The weight lost was about 16 kg in 6 weeks, and the composition was calculated to be 73–83% fat. This seems a very satisfactory result, but unfortunately the method for calculating the change in body composition involved the assumption that body carbohydrate stores were negligible, so any energy loss not accounted for by protein loss must have been fat loss. If we recalculate the results on the reasonable assumption that 1 kg protein loss was associated with 5 kg loss of FFM, then the composition of weight lost would have been, on average, 73% fat and 27% FFM, which is still a very acceptable result.

There are conflicting reports about the protein losses in patients on VLCD. Wechsler et al (1984) claim that the nitrogen loss incurred in the first 3 weeks is made good by nitrogen gain thereafter, while Baird (1981) reports a mean negative nitrogen balance up to the sixth week.

The nitrogen balance study of Wilson & Lamberts (1979) was conducted on 11 obese patients (average QI 37.5) who took a diet similar to the Cambridge diet for 4 weeks. Their calculations are based on the assumption that 1 kg FFM contains 40 g N, which is an improbably high figure: the evidence points to 30 gN/kg, or possibly 33 g N/kg, being about correct. The patients lost on average 10.0 kg in 4 weeks. The negative nitrogen balance was initially about 7 g/day, and decreased by the fourth week to 1.3 g/day. Therefore during the last week the weight loss was about 356 g/day, and nitrogen loss about 1.3 g/day, which is equivalent to about 43 g/day FFM, indicating that 12% of the weight loss was FFM. The cumulative nitrogen loss over the whole 4 week period was on average 73 g N, implying a loss of 2.4 kg FFM, or 24% of weight loss as FFM. Wilson and Lamberts note that these nitrogen losses are larger than those reported by Baird et al (1974), but the latter study had not measured faecal and integumental nitrogen loss, and also patients had been studied after a period of starvation, which would have caused nitrogen retention to be more favourable.

Several investigators comment that within a group of subjects who are fed under identical conditions there are often wide variations in nitrogen balance. The report of Yang & Van Itallie (1984) is particularly helpful, since they measured nitrogen balance on 6 subjects (average QI 48.7) over 64 days on a diet supplying 600–800 kcal/day and either 68 g or 121 g of protein. The different protein levels made no significant difference to the nitrogen balance. At the end of the study the cumulative weight loss was about 22 kg, but in one subject the cumulative nitrogen loss was only 90 g N, giving a very satisfactory figure of 4.1 g N/kg, while another subject lost 279 g N, giving a ratio of 12.7 g N/kg, or about 42% fat-free tissue. The cumulative deficit over the first 16 days of the study predicted only 40% of the variance in total nitrogen loss, so the initial response does not predict the ability of the individual to adapt to a low-energy diet with efficient conservation of body protein.

These studies indicate that very obese patients on VLCD lose about 7 kg in the first 2 weeks, and about 2.5 kg/week thereafter, and the composition of the weight loss is, on average, about 75% fat and 25% FFM. There are no data about the composition of weight lost by moderately overweight, or even normal-weight, subjects who take VLCD. By analogy with the results obtained with starvation, or with conventional reducing diets, we would expect that loss of FFM would be greatest in the first week or two of the diet, and that the less obese the subject the higher the proportion of weight loss which would be FFM. On theoretical grounds the type of person most at risk to lose an excessive amount of lean tissue is the slightly-overweight subject who takes VLCD for short periods repeated many times. However there are no publications describing nitrogen balance on such a protocol.

If excessive protein loss occurs, is it permanent, and does it matter? Again the data are inadequate to answer the question definitively: it would be unethical to induce excessive loss of lean tissue to study the long-term consequences, but the available scaps of evidence are not reassuring. The loss of lean tissue by the volunteers studied by Keys et al (1950) was not made good by refeeding. Some survivors of prison camps never regain a normal lean body mass, and patients who recover from anorexia frequently have a struggle to avoid obesity because they have a low lean body mass and hence a low metabolic rate. The patients treated by Finer et al (1986) with a 400 kcal diet showed a depression of metabolic rate which was significantly related to the rate of weight loss, whereas the patients of Dore et al (1982) who lost a similar amount of weight more gradually on an 800 kcal diet did not. Presumably these differences in response relate to the proportion of lean tissue lost, since RMR is very closely related to the lean body mass.

In view of this circumstantial evidence the onus should be upon those who advocate VLCD to show that the weight loss does not contain an excessive amount of lean tissue and hence lead to depressed metabolic rate, or alternatively that the lost lean tissue is readily restored without increase in adipose tissue. I do not know any publication which provides this evidence to date.

Many obese patients, and some doctors, believe that energy requirements in certain 'refractory' obese patients are as low as 800 kcal/day, so of course only a diet supplying less that 800 kcal can be expected to cause weight loss. The premise is false: in a recent study reporting 'unexpectedly low levels of energy expenditure in healthy women' (Prentice et al 1985) the lowest daily energy expenditure was 1466 kcal in a woman who was only 95% of ideal body weight. Among obese subjects energy expenditure is greater than normal (see Ch. 6), and among 400 obese patients admitted to a metabolic ward for investigation we have never found one who did not have an energy expenditure over 1200 kcal/day, and usually much more (Garrow et al 1978). Therefore the argument that VLCD are necessary because obese patients cannot otherwise lose weight is true only if obese people can keep to the VLCD but could not keep to a conventional reducing diet.

There are many publications which report patient compliance; for example Isaacs & Parry (1984) report that 217 out of 335 patients in general practice completed a 4-week course of Modifast, with an average weight loss of 6.6 kg. Under metabolic ward conditions the expected weight loss in 4 weeks would have been about 10 kg, so evidently many of these patients did not restrict their intake to Modifast alone. Wadden et al (1985) compared the acceptability over 4 weeks of a VLCD in liquid formula form, or a similar diet derived from lean meat, fish or fowl. Weight losses were about 8 kg, indicating quite good compliance, and were not significantly different between the two types of VLCD, although the liquid formula was rated less acceptable. Wadden & Stunkard (1986) in an outpatient trial compared the effect of VLCD with and without behaviour therapy. The effect of the behaviour therapy component will be discussed later, but the weight loss on VLCD for 2 months averaged about 11 kg, whereas about 20 kg weight loss would have been expected with perfect compliance. Van Gaal et al (1985) report an average weight loss of 14 kg in 6 weeks among 15 outpatients on a trial of Nutroclin, which can be compared with an expected loss of about 16 kg: this indicates good (but not perfect) compliance. Apfelbaum (1987) reports an average weight loss of 7 kg in 3 weeks.

The largest weight losses obtained with VLCD regimens are reported by Andersen et al (1984) in a comparison between VLCD and gastroplasty. The diet provided 341 kcal (1.4 MJ) and 34 g protein daily, and after 8 weeks on this diet the patients switched for 2 weeks to a diet supplying 900 kcal (3.8 MJ) of high-protein, low-fat, low-carbohydrate foods. The patients were also allowed to take diethylpropion (up to 25 mg 3 times per day) if they found that they were too hungry to keep to the diet. The maximum weight loss was attained after 3–21 months (mean 9 months) when the mean weight loss was 22.0 kg, which was not significantly different from the mean loss of 26.1 kg in the group treated by gastroplasty. However regain of weight was greater in the VLCD group: after 18 months the mean weight regain was close to the mean maximum weight loss, whereas the gastroplasty patients regained about 10 kg in the year after maximum weight loss and then stabilised.

These reports of outpatient compliance with VLCD are no doubt influenced by the patients' selection procedure, the level of monitoring of the patient, and the enthusiasm of both patients and therapists. Bistrian (1978) suggests that compliance with ketogenic diets is good because they are particularly anorectic and mood-elevating. However, Rosen et al (1985) failed to find any difference in the effect on mood or appetite of isoenergetic diets which were, or were not, ketogenic. Unfortunately there seems to be no published controlled trial of compliance to VLCD versus a conventional reducing diet.

Quite a strong argument can be made for VLCD on the grounds that a very obese patient is more likely to succeed in losing a lot of weight if removed entirely from normal eating and transferred onto a bland diet of known composition. However this advantage can be more safely and inexpensively obtained by using a diet consisting of 1200 ml milk, with suitable iron and vitamin supplements, which is discussed in a later section of this book.

8.c CONVENTIONAL REDUCING DIETS

Conventional reducing diets supply about 800–1200 kcal

(3.4–5.0 MJ)/day, based on a selection of normal foods. There are three guiding principles in designing such diets:

1. The diet must supply less energy than the patient's maintenance requirements, otherwise there will be no weight loss.
2. The diet must supply all nutrients requirements apart from energy, and conform with good nutritional principles, otherwise it will eventually lead to malnutrition.
3. The diet must be (as far as possible) acceptable to the patient, otherwise the patient will not comply with dietary advice.

The practical implication of these principles will be considered in turn.

In the UK the average national diet is continuously kept under review by the National Food Survey, operated by the Ministry of Agriculture, Fisheries and Food. Each year the food purchases for 1 week of about 7000 randomly chosen households are analysed. This does not give a complete picture of food intake, because alcohol and food purchased outside the home is not included, but from these data it is possible to construct a fairly reliable account of total intake of energy and other nutrients, and of the food groups which contribute to this total. The average British diet in 1984, the most recent year for which analyses have been published, is shown in Table 8.3. The average daily intake is about 2192 kcal and 65 g protein. The contribution of different food groups to this total is shown in Figure 8.2.

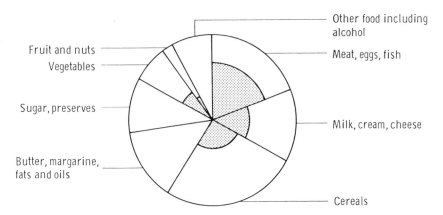

Fig. 8.2 Contribution of food groups to energy and protein intake in average household in UK (Data of National Food Survey 1984). Area of each segment indicates contribution of that food group to total energy intake, and shaded area indicates contribution of food group to protein intake. Numerical data on which diagram is based are shown in Table 8.3

Table 8.3 Energy (kcal), protein (g), fat (g) and saturated fat (g) content of (A) the average British diet, (B) a conventional reducing diet, and (C) 1800 ml whole cow's milk (Data on average British diet from National Food Survey 1984)

Food group	(A) Average				(B) Conventional				(C) Milk			
	Energy kcal	Protein g	Fat g	S. fat g	Energy kcal	Protein g	Fat g	S. fat g	Energy kcal	Protein g	Fat g	S. fat g
Meat	321	21	24	10	250	16	19	8	—	—	—	—
Egg	37	3	3	1	45	4	4	1	—	—	—	—
Fish	28	3	1	—	32	3	1	—	—	—	—	—
Milk, cream, cheese	297	15	19	12	255	15	16	8	1170	59	69	43
Bread and cereals	610	17	10	4	230	8	6	3	—	—	—	—
Butter	86	—	10	6	—	—	—	—	—	—	—	—
Margarine	121	—	14	4	74	—	8	2	—	—	—	—
Fat and pils	108	—	12	4	—	—	—	—	—	—	—	—
Sugar and preserves	167	—	—	—	—	—	—	—	—	—	—	—
Potatoes	102	2	—	—	160	4	—	—	—	—	—	—
Other vegetables	82	3	—	—	45	3	—	—	—	—	—	—
Fruits and nuts	61	1	1	—	100	1	1	—	—	—	—	—
Other (and alcohol)	172	—	—	—	—	—	—	—	—	—	—	—
Total	2192	65	94	41	1191	64	55	22	1170	59	69	43

Principle 1 above could be satisfied by halving the intake of each item in the diet to create a reducing diet with half the normal energy value. The energy sources of a person taking such a diet are indicated in Figure 8.3. The intake of all nutrients, including protein, is halved, so this diet is unlikely to satisfy principle 2. For a well-designed reducing diet is necessary to restrict particularly those foods which provide energy and relatively little in the way of other nutrients, such as sugar, fats and oils. In the past general carbohydrate restriction was advocated, but we now realise that complex carbohydrates have a valuable role in human nutrition. The energy sources for a person on a conventional reducing diet are indicated in Figure 8.4.

In Figures 8.2–8.4 the contribution of food groups to protein intake is indicated, because, next to the energy content, the protein content of the diet is of most importance in achieving weight loss of the appropriate composition. Also, better nitrogen retention is achieved when the diet is taken in several small meals, rather than in one larger meal. The interaction of these two factors on weight loss and nitrogen balance is illustrated in Figures 8.5 and 8.6. A total of 38 obese women were studied on a metabolic ward for 3 weeks. During the first week all patients were given a diet supplying 800 kcal (3.4 MJ) daily with 13% of the energy as protein (i.e. 26 g protein) served as three equal meals per day. In the second and third weeks, in balanced crossover design, either the protein concentration was altered to 10% and 15% served as 3 meals per day, or the meal

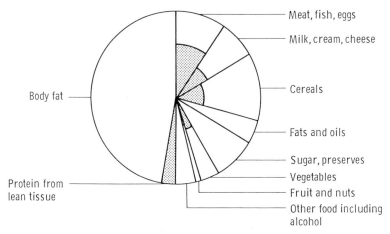

Fig. 8.3 Energy sources for individual consuming half-quantities of diet shown in Figure 8.2. Note that remaining half of energy requirements are supplied by body fat and lean tissue

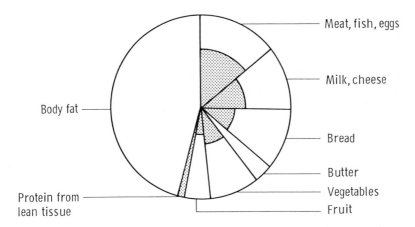

Fig. 8.4 Energy sources for individual consuming a conventional reducing diet as shown in Table 8.3. Energy intake is reduced by about 50%, but protein intake is maintained by selecting relatively high-protein foods

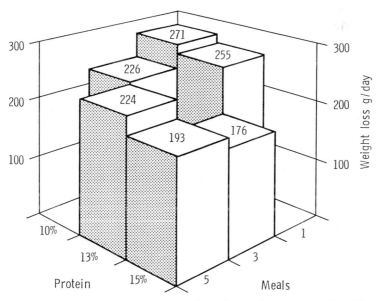

Fig. 8.5 Weight loss among 38 obese women given diet supplying 800 kcal (3.4 MJ) per day with either 10%, 13% or 15% of energy as protein, and served as 1, 3 or 5 meals per day (Data of Garrow et al 1981). Infrequent meals of lower protein concentration were associated with more rapid weight loss

frequency was altered to 1 or 5 meals per day of 13% protein, or both these changes were made so the second and third weeks were on either one meal of 10% protein energy, or five meals of 15% protein energy. It is evident from Figure 8.5 that the most rapid weight loss

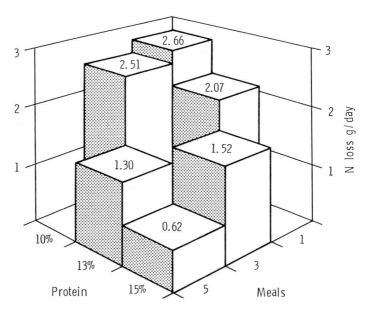

Fig. 8.6 Nitrogen loss among subjects whose weight loss was shown in Figure 8.5. More rapid weight loss on infrequent meals of low-protein concentration is entirely accounted for by more rapid loss of fat-free mass, not of fat

(271 g/day) was achieved on the one-meal 10% protein regimen. However Figure 8.6 shows that this situation arose because on this regimen much more nitrogen (and hence FFM) was lost.

We can calculate the contribution of FFM to weight loss in the patients taking 5 meals with 15% protein: 0.62 g N is equivalent to 20.5 g FFM, which is 10.6% of the weight loss of 193 g/day, while in the patients having 1 meal of 10% protein a loss of 2.66 g N indicates 87.8 g FFM, which is 32.4% of the weight loss of 271 g/day. Other things being equal, therefore, it is desirable to maintain a high protein : energy ratio in reducing diets. However one of the things which is not equal is the cost of high-protein foods: this is illustrated in Figure 8.7. If the average cost of energy and of protein is designated 1.0, then energy from high-protein foods such as meat, fish and eggs is more than twice as expensive. Fruit and vegetables, although nutritionally desirable, are expensive energy sources when compared with sugar and fats which have less desirable nutritional characteristics.

One final point about conventional reducing diets concerns the satiating effect of dietary fibre. Since all reducing diets are (by definition) deficient in energy, it is desirable to make them as

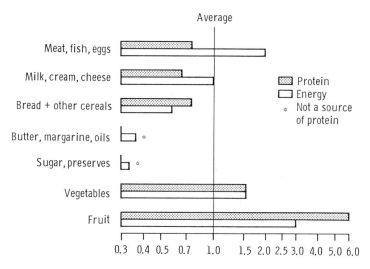

Fig. 8.7 Relative cost of energy or protein when derived from different food groups, related to average cost of energy and protein in diet as a whole. Energy from meat, fish, eggs, vegetables and fruit is much more expensive than energy from sugar or fats.

satiating as possible. The evidence about the effect of fibre on hunger has been mentioned already in section 4.c., and the therapeutic effects of fibre will be mentioned again in later chapters dealing with conditions such as diabetes. If it is true that fibre increases satiety this should increase the acceptability to the patient in line with principle 3 above. However, it is difficult to find hard evidence that high-fibre reducing diets are really more satiating than isoenergetic diets of lower fibre content.

The results of a study by Bryson et al (1979) are shown in Figure 8.8. Ten normal subjects were offered a free lunch of bread, butter and jam at weekly intervals for 4 weeks. On two of the occasions the bread was white (70% extraction) with a low fibre content, and on the other two occasions the bread was wholemeal. The average lunchtime energy intake on these two types of bread did not significantly differ, but individual subjects maintained a characteristic energy intake at that meal which ranged from 500 kcal to over 1500 kcal. Recorded energy intake for the subsequent 24 hours was also unaffected by the fibre content of the bread taken at lunchtime.

It appears that the only controlled trial comparing high-fibre and low carbohydrate diets which has been reported so far is that of Baron et al (1986). They found that among 135 overweight outpatients the weight loss at 3 months was rather greater among those

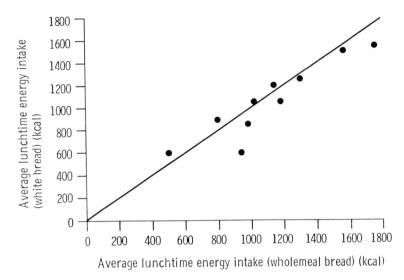

Fig. 8.8 Average lunchtime energy intake of bread, butter and jam by normal volunteers (Data of Bryson et al 1979). Energy intake at that meal, or during following 24 h, not significantly different whether bread was white or wholemeal

on the low-carbohydrate diet (5.0 kg vs 3.7 kg). It is therefore not established that a high fibre content in the diet contributes significantly to satiety, although fibre has other valuable characteristics which are discussed elsewhere.

In the sections dealing with starvation (8.a.) and with VLCD (8.b.) stress was laid on the composition of weight lost, specifically on the g N/kg weight loss. We therefore need to check that this is satisfactory with conventional reducing diets. Figure 8.9 shows the nitrogen : weight loss ratio among 21 women who were on a diet supplying 800 kcal (3.4 MJ) for 3 weeks (Durrant et al 1980). There is a significant ($p < 0.05$) decrease in this ratio with increasing body fat, as there was among subject who were totally starved (see Fig. 8.1). However the average ratio is about 7.5g N/kg weight lost, which is the ratio appropriate for 75% fat:25% FFM, whereas among patients starved for a similar time the ratio was about 15 g N/kg weight lost.

8.d MILK DIET, JAW WIRING AND WAIST CORD

In 1973 severely obese patients were exhorted to keep to a reducing diet, and perhaps given anorectic drugs which were amphetamine

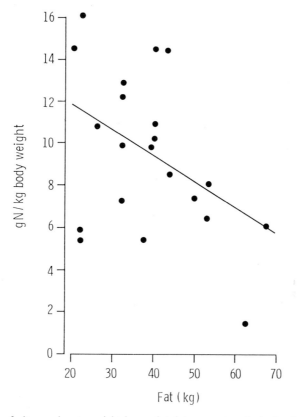

Fig. 8.9 Ratio of nitrogen loss to weight loss, related to percentage body fat, in 21 women on a diet supplying 800 kcal (3.4 MJ) for 3 weeks. As in the case of starvation, fatter subjects conserve nitrogen more efficiently (Data of Durrant et al 1980)

derivatives. If that did not work the alternative treatment on offer was the jejuno-ileal bypass operation, which was even then becoming notorious for the long-term metabolic disturbances which it caused. It was in this climate of opinion that I tried jaw wiring as an alternative treatment for patients who described themselves as compulsive eaters (Garrow 1974a).

The technique of jaw wiring is illustrated in Figure 8.10. After careful examination of the teeth, and treatment of any caries or gum infection, eyelets of thin stainless steel wire are prepared as shown at (a), and passed between adjacent molar teeth (b). The ends of the wires encircle the bases of two teeth and are secured by being twisted together (c). Eyelets are fixed close to the gum margin, usually two pairs on each side of the mouth. Stainless steel wire of a heavier gauge (d) is laced through pairs of eyelets fixed to the upper and

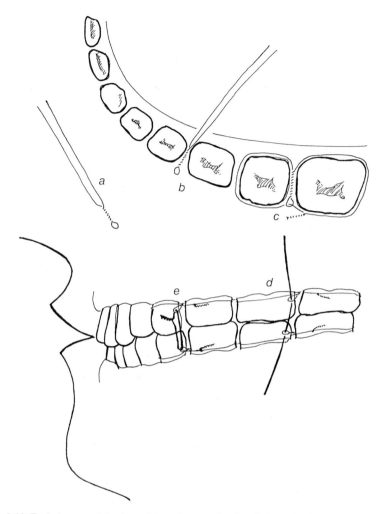

Fig. 8.10 Technique used for jaw wiring. See text for description of technique.

lower jaws and twisted to hold the jaws together (e). Recently stainless steel brackets cemented to the teeth have been used, instead of the circumferential eyelet wires, to anchor the tie wires.

The short-term complication from this procedure is pain which may originate in four ways. First, the gums may be bruised, or one of the circumferential wires may be pressing on the edge of the gum, rendering it ischaemic. Second, the teeth may ache as a result of the sideways force on them. Third, there may be a spasm of the masseter muscle which occurs reflexly when the jaw cannot be opened normally. These three sources of discomfort can all be avoided if the patient is given a sedative dose of diazepam (usually 20 mg, repeated twice if necessary) orally immediately after the wires have been applied. This prevents muscle spasm, and enables the patient to sleep until the pain from teeth and gums has subsided, which usually takes about 12–24 hours. A fourth source of discomfort may occur 2–4 days after wiring: this is ulceration of the buccal surface of the lip by a protruding loop of wire. However carefully the wires are applied there may be slight movement in the first 2 days which causes an end of wire to protrude. The patient should be warned to report immediately local tenderness from this cause, which can be treated by pushing the wire out of the way, and perhaps smoothing the surface with dental wax while the mucosa recovers.

Later the fixation technique was changed to use stainless steel brackets cemented to the teeth between which the wire loops are attached. This is preferable, since it avoids trauma to the gums and is less likely to give rise to gingival problems. This procedure caused very gratifying weight loss with zero mortality, and jaw wiring with various modifications was taken up in other centres (Kopp 1975, Rodgers et al 1977, Harding 1980). Drenick & Hargis (1978) reported a case of a woman who nearly choked after this procedure, but otherwise there were no reports of dangerous ill-effects. The procedure of jaw fixation for various orthodontic procedures is well established and not hazardous, although normal-weight patients having this procedure also lose a significant amount of weight (Harju & Pernu 1984). However by 1979 it was evident that most of the patients who lost weight with the jaw wiring procedure regained it when the wires were removed, so a policy of gastroplasty to maintain weight loss was tried (Fordyce et al 1979). This is not without hazard, and it is very difficult to design the gastroplasty so that a satisfactory weight is maintained, so by 1980 the treatment policy had changed again to jaw-wiring plus waist cord (Garrow & Gardiner 1981). The results to date are summarised in Table 8.4.

Thirty-five obese patients (36 female, 2 male) were offered the jaw wiring-waist cord package between September 1979 and December 1984. Of these 9 patients dropped out during the jaw wiring phase, 12 did not continue with the waist cord either because they became pregnant, or required an abdominal operation, or dropped out of the clinic, and the remaining 14 still wear their waist cord. The initial characteristics (age and excess weight) of these three groups are not significantly different, but there is a trend for those who stayed with the treatment to be younger, initially more overweight, and to have

Table 8.4 Characteristics of 38 obese patients (36 female, 2 male) treated by jaw wiring and waist cord (Data of Garrow & Webster 1986b)

Jaw wiring: Waist cord: n:	Dropped out Not applied 9		Completed Dropped out 12		Completed Continuing 14		Not done Continuing 3	
	Mean	SD	Mean	SD	Mean	SD	Mean	SD
Age (y)	30.6	6.3	31.8	8.7	27.2	7.3	35.7	4.9
Weight (kg)	101.9	17.8	111.8	15.5	118.0	11.7	118.3	11.7
Wt/height^2 (kg/m^2)	40.0	4.1	43.4	5.6	46.4	5.2	43.5	4.1
Excess wt (kg)	38.4	12.9	47.3	13.8	54.1	11.2	50.3	11.2
Duration of wiring (months)	—	—	9.0	3.1	11.1	3.6	—	—
Weight lost (kg)	—	—	36.8	11.1	42.4	7.4	41.7	16.5
Follow-up (months)	—	—	—	—	35.6	22.3	20.7	3.1
Overall wt loss (kg)	—	—	—	—	32.8	12.7	33.0	12.1
Overall wt loss (as % excess)	—	—	—	—	61.9	23.4	64.3	11.0

had their jaws wired for longer than those who dropped out. We have a follow-up after unwiring of at least 1 year (mean 35.6 months) of those who continue to wear the waist cord. Of the average loss of 42.4 ± 7.4 kg achieved during the jaw wiring phase an average of 32.8 ± 12.7 kg remains at follow-up. We also have 3 patients who lost a similar amount of weight without jaw wiring, and who have maintained a similar proportion of their weight loss with a waist cord 20 months later.

Geleibster et al (1986) have shown that an abdominal belt, 20 cm × 152 cm, alters food intake, abdominal pressure and gastric emptying rate in normal volunteers, but this is probably a different effect from that caused by a waist cord 2 mm in diameter. Patients who use the waist cord successfully report that they use the discomfort of a tight waist cord as a cue to restrict food intake for the next few days. They have usually had experience of unnoticed weight gain, especially when on holiday, and are reassured that they will not gain weight without due warning from the cord.

An adjustable waist cord was used by Simpson et al (1986) to prevent weight regain during periods between intermittent protein-sparing fasting. They reported that 14 subjects with the waist cord lost an additional 4.8 kg during 11.4 months follow-up, while 17 subjects without a waist cord regained 6.6 kg of the weight they had lost. They conclude that an adjustable waist cord is a valuable aid to successful and permanent weight loss in some subjects.

These results obtained by jaw wiring and waist cords are encouraging, but still leave room for improvement. Compared with other series the duration of jaw fixation in our series (11 months) is longer than that of Rodgers et al (1977) and Bjorvell & Rossner (1985) who both had a mean fixation time of about 7 months, and consequently the weight loss is also greater (42 kg compared with 26 kg). The average rate of weight loss in all three series is around 1 kg/week. which is within the desirable range in Figure 9.1. All the authors cited above agree that the technique is simple, safe and cheap.

The problems concern drop-outs and weight regain after the wires are removed. It is difficult to compare drop-out rates between series, since the selection procedure will greatly affect drop-out rate. The patients shown in Table 8.4 were given a very full explanation of the jaw wiring and waist cord procedure, and had opportunities to talk with other patients on the same programme, but still about half dropped out. However, the results with those who continued to wear the waist cord are strikingly better than those recorded elsewhere in the literature.

During the 13 years in which the jaw wiring regimen was developed the milk diet was a by-product: it was fortunate that there was a readily available fluid of high nutritional value which jaw-wired patients could take. However it soon became evident that many patients — even those without wired jaws — found it a very easy diet to keep to. The obvious deficiencies are iron and vitamins, but this problem is easily rectified with 1 multivitamin capsule BPC and 200 mg ferrous sulphate daily, or the equivalent in liquid form for patients whose bite is so closed that there is no room to insert these small tablets.

It also seemed undesirable that the diet should provide 53% of energy in the form of fat, and 33% as saturated fat, since this is the type of diet which causes hypercholesterolaemia. However there were no marked changes in the blood lipid of patients on the milk diet, and review of the literature revealed two studies which actually claimed that milk had a hypocholesterolaemic effect (Howard & Marks 1977, Hepner et al 1979). It will be seen from Table 8.3 that 3 pints (1800 ml) of milk has an energy and protein content similar to that of a conventional reducing diet of 1200 kcal (5 MJ), and 2 pints (1200 ml) provides about 800 kcal (3.4 MJ). The difference with milk is that it is very cheap, convenient, and does nothing to stimulate appetite. In section 4.c it was shown that appetite is very responsive to variety in the diet, so a diet consisting of milk as a sole energy source is about as monotonous, and hence unappetising, a diet as is possible to devise. Patients on milk comment that they get bored with it, but they are not hungry, and some find this a situation they can more easily control.

In the case of patients who have lost a massive amount of weight with jaw wiring and milk diet it is particularly important to check that they have not lost excessive amount of lean tissue, and thus suffered an undue decrease in metabolic rate, since this would make it very difficult for them to maintain their weight at a level at which the waist cord would be comfortable.

A study of 19 women who had lost on average 30.8 kg (from 104.5 kg to 73.7 kg) was undertaken by Dore et al (1982). Before weight loss these women had an RMR of 290 ± 33 ml O_2/min, which was in good agreement with the metabolic rate predicted by the formula described in section 6.a. (Dore et al 1982). After weight loss the average metabolic rate was 234 ± 26 ml O_2/min, which again agreed well with the predicted metabolic rate for their new weight

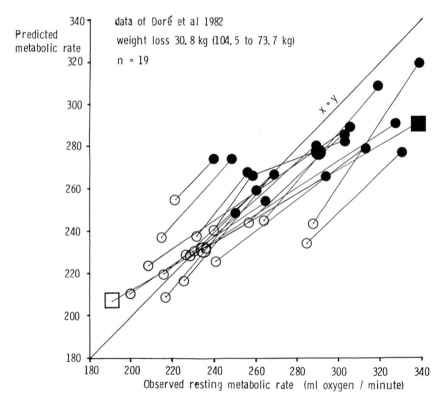

Fig. 8.11 Relation of observed resting metabolic rate to that predicted from formula of Dore et al (1982) among 21 obese women before (open symbols) and after (closed symbols) they lost weight. Average weight loss was 30.8 kg (Data of Dore et al 1982)

and body composition. The values before and after weight loss are shown in Figure 8.11. In most cases the decrease in metabolic rate is as predicted, but one individual, shown by square symbols, lost weight most rapidly (from 112.1 kg to 63.7 kg in 10 months) and her metabolic rate which was initially 5% higher than predicted subsequently was 7% lower than predicted. Unfortunately she became involved in a national slimming competition, and achieved greater weight loss by periods of starvation, but at a high price in terms of reduced metabolic rate. Her loss of FFM was excessive, but the other patients in this series lost on average 75% fat and 25% FFM.

Therefore the available evidence suggests that weight loss achieved at the rate indicated in Figure 9.1 (i.e. with 800–1200 kcal milk) is not associated with an excessive loss of lean tissue, or an excessive decrease in metabolic rate. After weight loss the metabolic rate of all but one of these patients agreed with that which would be expected in women of similar age, weight and FFM who had not previously lost weight.

8.e SURGERY TO CAUSE INTESTINAL EXCLUSION

The original surgical procedures for the treatment of severe obesity had the humane intention of allowing the obese patient the satisfaction of eating normally, yet achieving weight loss because the food was only partly absorbed from the gut. To this end most of the absorptive area of the bowel — namely the ileum — was short-circuited, and weight loss was indeed achieved. For example a series of 30 patients achieved a weight loss of 28 kg which was maintained over a follow-up period of 10 years (Werner et al 1985). However the mechanism was not what had been intended: if the absorptive capacity of the bowel is seriously impaired then normal eating leads to catastrophic diarrhoea, so the weight loss was achieved mainly because it forced the patient to eat less. The loss of energy in faeces explained only a very small proportion of the weight loss (Pilkington et al 1976).

There were (and still are) many versions of the intestinal bypass operation, but the more complex the pattern of anastomosis the more suture lines are at risk of breaking down and the longer and more difficult the operation. Also malabsorption brings with it problems of deficiency of fat-soluble vitamins, calcium and magnesium, and

inappropriate absorption of oxalate. Such patients require careful
and prolonged supervision, and this aspect of the procedure is
already straining the resources of one department with 180 patients
who have had the operation, now with an average age of 42 years
(McFarland et al 1985). To perform more operations would merely
add to this inexorable burden.

For all these reasons recent authoritative reviews from Sweden
(Olsson et al 1985), the USA (Halverson & Printen 1986) and the
UK (Shearman & Baddeley 1986) agree that the operation of choice
is some form of gastroplasty, which limits the rate of food intake,
rather than the small-bowel bypass operations which caused malabsorption. The rival versions of this operation are shown in Figure
8.12. In both procedures a pouch (p) with a capacity of about 50 ml
is separated from the main body of the stomach by a double line of
staples (s), the only exit from the pouch being via a small reinforced
stoma about 12 mm in diameter. In the 'horizontal banded gastroplasty' (Fig. 8.12a) the line of staples is horizontal and the stoma is
at the greater curvature of the stomach, while in the 'vertical banded
gastroplasty' (Figure 8.12b) the line of staples is vertical and the
stoma is at the lesser curvature. In both cases the stoma is reinforced
by a loop of silastic tubing threaded over a non-absorbable suture,
so the stoma cannot distend with time. The weight loss produced
by these two operations is similar, but more difficulties with
constructing a stoma of the right size are reported with the horizontal

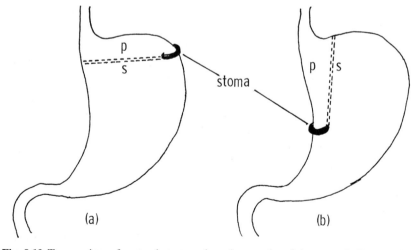

Fig. 8.12 Two versions of gastroplasty to reduce the capacity of the stomach (See text for
description of the techniques)

version than the vertical version (Shearman & Baddeley 1986). However the size of the pouch or stoma do not necessarily relate to the clinical outcome (Andersen & Pedersen 1984).

The rationale of gastroplasty is exactly the same as that for jaw wiring: it limits the patient's ability to eat large meals. However, while jaw wiring stops incoming food at the lips, gastroplasty eventually limits food intake by causing vomiting. This is altogether a less benign procedure, and all the reviews on gastroplasty cited above report some problems with vitamin and electrolyte depletion. Of course these can be overcome with good medical management, but we must remember that the sort of patient who qualifies for operations of this sort cannot be relied upon to report promptly and responsibly when things go wrong. Some patients lose weight extremely quickly, and this places a strain on the ability of the liver to cope with the flux of fatty acids from adipose tissue. Cases of sudden and unexpected death have been reported in patients after gastroplasty, with severe fatty infiltration of the liver (Cairns et al 1986).

With skilled surgeons and anaesthetists gastroplasty can be performed on severely obese patients with low operative mortality and good weight loss. The psychosocial consequences of the massive weight loss associated with these operations is, in general, favourable (Stunkard et al 1986b). However there must always be greater risks with this procedure than with jaw wiring, which seems to be a better option if it is technically possible. Apart from any other consideration, it appears that any gastric operation increases the risk of gastric cancer some 40 years later (Viste et al 1986).

A recent development is the insertion of an artificial bezoar to limit the capacity of the stomach. First reports using a cylindrical plastic bubble about 200 ml in volume are encouraging (Schreiber & Guyton 1986, Garren et al 1987), the main complication being ulceration of the stomach in 1.6% of patients so treated. Follow-up results are disappointing: McFarland et al (1987) report that patients who lost 11 kg in 3 months with an intragastric balloon regained this weight in one year, even with the inflated balloon in situ.

8.f ANORECTIC DRUGS

Amphetamine, and the chemically related compounds phentermine and diethylpropion, will reduce or abolish hunger for some hours if given in adequate dosage. The mechanism of action is on the

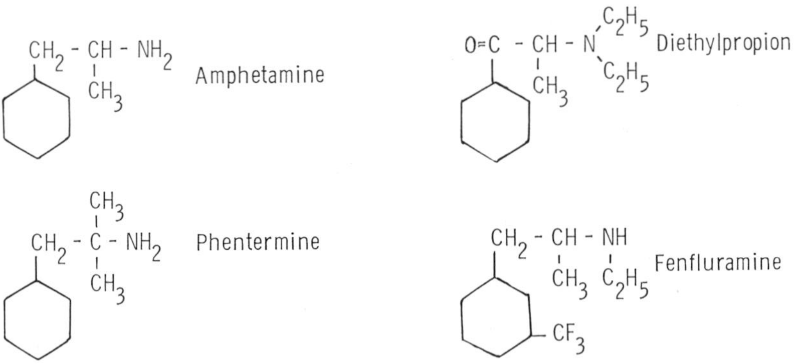

Fig. 8.13 Four anorectic drugs. Amphetamine, phentermine and diethylpropion are central stimulants and act on adrenergic pathways. Fenfluramine is non-stimulant and acts through serotinergic pathways.

adrenergic neuroreceptors in the brain, and the anorectic effect is associated with central stimulation and euphoria. For this reason these drugs have some danger of abuse, and their prescription is subject to governmental regulations, although addiction or dependence rarely occurs among patients who receive these drugs on medical prescription.

Fenfluramine, although it appears structurally similar to amphetamine (see Fig. 8.13) has very different pharmacological action. It acts by promoting the release of serotonin (5-hydroxytryptamine), and enhances satiety, rather than reducing hunger, and it has no stimulant action. The most important undesirable side effects of fenfluramine are depression if the drug is stopped suddenly and, in some cases, pulmonary hypertension. It has recently been discovered that the anorectic activity of fenfluramine resides in the dextro-isomer, so it may be that dextro-fenfluramine will have fewer side effects.

A new drug, fluoxetine, acts by blocking re-uptake of serotonin, and thus enhancing serotonergic neurotransmission. The pharmacology and clinical trials of these drugs were reviewed at a meeting on 'Drugs regulating food intake and energy balance' in Rome in September 1986 which will be published by John Libbey: the interested reader is referred to these proceedings.

The problem about anorectic drug treatment of obesity (apart from any side effects of the drugs used) is that although weight is lost when the drug is given (typically 4 kg in 10 weeks), it is very rapidly regained on stopping the drug. There is also a very high drop-out rate in many trials. The question is whether possible to achieve and maintain a clinically significant weight loss by the use of anorectic drugs given over a period of many months. The trial of Steel et al (1973) compared several drugs over a period of 36 weeks with only 23% drop-out rate. The greatest weight loss (12 kg) was achieved with either fenfluramine of phentermine. Stunkard et al (1980) compared various treatment schedules. When fenfluramine was given to simulate 'doctor's office medication' the weight loss was 6 kg in 6 months, but when another group of patients were given fenfluramine, and also met weekly for 1.5 h in groups of 8–10 persons led by a clinical psychologist, the average loss was 14.4 kg. Thus the manner of giving the drug doubled the weight loss.

A valuable feature of the study of Stunkard et al (1980) is that the patients were followed up 1 year after the end of the active treatment phase: the patients who had lost 14.4 kg in 6 months with fenfluramine regained 8.6 kg in the next 12 months. These results compare unfavourably with those obtained by behaviour therapy, which are discussed later. However, an attempt to combine behaviour therapy with anorectic drug treatment was very unsuccessful.

Patients often ask for an anorectic drug to 'get them started' on a reducing diet, but this is not a good plan. The early phase of dieting is associated with relatively rapid weight loss, which is itself reinforcing to the effort to diet. If the drug is given at this stage the rapid weight loss will be wrongly attributed to the effect of the drug. If anorectic drugs are to be used they would be most valuable in helping patients to maintain weight loss which had been started by a reducing diet, but it is not clear that they can be relied upon to have this effect either.

It seems reasonable to suppose that some patients, if given access to effective anorectic drugs, will lose weight better than those without this help. To seek evidence for this hypothesis Gilbert & Garrow (1983) allocated obese patients randomly to one of three therapies: conventional dietary advice, or dietary advice plus behaviour therapy, or dietary advice plus an anorectic drug (which was 75 mg slow-release diethylpropion). The drug group each 4 weeks received active drug or placebo, according to a double-blind protocol. Initially there were 95 women and 20 men in the series, but by the end of 12 months only about 20% were still attending the clinic, and the attrition rate was not significantly different between the treatment groups. However, at 12 months after enrolment in the trial 80 of the 95 women, and 18 of the 20 men, were traced and weighed: the

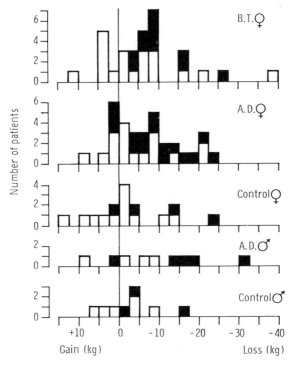

Fig. 8.14 Weight change after 1 year of treatment by conventional dietary advice alone (control), or with additional behaviour therapy (BT), or additional anorectic drug treatment (AD) among 80 obese females and 18 obese males. Those patients who were attending clinic 6 months after enrolment are shown by solid squares, and those who had dropped out at 6 months by open squares (Data of Gilbert & Garrow 1983)

change in weight of each patient between enrolment and follow-up 12 months later is shown in Figure 8.14. The striking feature of the results is the variation in response to each treatment: within each group there was at least one individual who gained more than 5 kg, and one who lost more than 15 kg. The patients who were still attending the clinic at 6 months tended to lose more weight than those who dropped out in the first 6 months, but the largest individual loss was in a woman who was allocated to the behaviour therapy group, dropped out, but had lost 37.8 kg a year later.

The weight loss at 1 year among the patients offered anorectic drugs was greater than that for the control group offered dietary advice alone: 6.3 ± 8.3 kg vs 1.6 ± 7.6 kg for the women, and 12.0 ± 7.8 kg vs 2.8 ± 6.7 kg for the men. However although each of the patients in the drug group could have collected 12 prescriptions for drugs the average was only 3.3 prescriptions for women, and 3.2

prescriptions for men. Tablet counts on returned bottles indicated that on average the women took 23 tablets/28 days of diethylpropion, and 20 tablets/28 days of placebo, whereas men took 20 diethypropion or 22 placebo/28 days. In no case was the difference statistically significant. When mean weight losses on active drug or placebo were compared there were 20 patients who lost more on active than placebo, and 11 who lost more on placebo than active drug: again the difference is not significant (P = 0.11).

It appears, therefore, that patients given anorectic drugs achieve modest, but significantly greater weight losses than control groups, but it is not clear why this is so. When the drug or placebo is supplied in double-blind fashion the patients do not seem to use the two preparations differently. This suggests that at least some of the efficacy of the anorectic drug is a placebo effect — it encourages previously failed dieters to try again with renewed hope. This explanation also helps to explain the great difference in effectiveness between the 'doctor's office medication' and group treatment medication in the trial of Stunkard et al (1980).

An effective anti-obesity drug would be commercially very valuable to the pharmaceutical company which produced it, so there are many drugs which are tried and found wanting. One disappointment was the failure of opiate antagonists to cause useful weight loss. It has been shown in animals that an effect of eating is to release endorphins which interact with opiate receptors to cause a pleasant sensation. However, naloxone or the longer acting naltrexone have not been found to be useful in treating human obesity (O'Brien et al 1982, Silverstone 1987). Likewise evening primrose oil was found to be no more effective than placebo in causing weight loss (Haslett et al 1983).

8.g THERMOGENIC DRUGS

Two of the objections to reducing diets, or any surgical or drug treatment aimed at reducing energy intake, are first, that it is unpleasant to be deprived of maintenance requirements of food, and second, that the resulting diet may be deficient in nutrients. If the necessary negative energy balance could be achieved by increasing energy expenditure, while leaving intake constant, it would be possible to find a treatment for obesity which avoided both the problems mentioned above.

There are many drugs which increase energy expenditure, of which one of the first to be used was dinitrophenol, a drug which uncouples oxidative phosphorylation. It fell from favour because in large doses it is very toxic, but at least one group is now reconsidering its use (Bachynsky 1987). The active thyroid hormone, tri-iodothyronine (T_3) has also been used to increase metabolic rate, but unfortunately it causes severe loss of FFM when used in this way. Figure 8.15 shows the cumulative nitrogen balance in 3 obese patients on a diet supplying 800 kcal (3.4 MJ) per day. The study concerned the effect of rest or exercise on weight loss and nitrogen balance (there was no discernible effect on either variable), but when T_3 was given to one patient to increase daily energy output to the same extent as the exercise programme had done there was a dramatic loss of nitrogen (Warwick & Garrow 1981). It has been

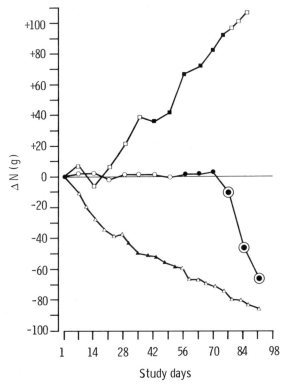

Fig. 8.15 Cumulative nitrogen balance in 3 obese patients in metabolic ward on diet supplying 800 kcal/day for 3 months. During periods shown by open symbols they undertook an exercise programme designed to increase energy expenditure by 20%, which did not affect nitrogen balance. However, during period marked by double circles 1 subject took 120 μg tri-iodothyronine daily, which increased energy expenditure to a similar extent, but also caused a severely negative nitrogen balance (Data of Warwick & Garrow 1981)

suggested that small doses of T_3, just enough to prevent the fall in metabolic rate with dieting, may be helpful in maintaining the rate of weight loss without excessive loss of FFM (Welle & Campbell 1986, Rozen et al 1986). This treatment, when added to a VLCD caused a loss of 8.1 kg in 18 days, compared with 6.94 kg in a placebo control group, and nitrogen balance is reported to be unaffected. However, on thermodynamic grounds it is difficult to accept that the tissue lost was 75% fat, because this implies that the patients had an energy expenditure around 3000 kcal/day, which is improbably high.

Sympathomimetic thermogenic drugs have been re-examined in view of the interest in brown adipose tissue and the 'thermogenic defect' which is alleged to contribute to obesity. In animals intravenous infusions of catecholamines stimulate the thermogenic action of brown adipose tissue, but in man a more convenient way to increase sympathetic tone is to use the drug ephedrine, which was for many years a treatment for asthma. A trial of ephedrine for 3 months in unselected obese outpatients did not significantly affect weight loss, but patients on the higher dose (50 mg t.i.d) showed significantly more side effects than the placebo control group (Pasquali et al 1985). However, Astrup et al (1985) used 20 mg t.i.d. for 3 months in 5 obese women and showed an increasing thermogenic responsiveness during chronic treatment with the drug. Body weight reduction was 5.5 ± 0.3 kg after 12 weeks. Other beta-adrenoreceptor agonist drugs are under trial, but it is not yet clear if they will be clinically useful.

It is evident from the above brief review that no clinically satisfactory thermogenic drug has been produced so far. The drugs available are either dangerous if used at dosages which cause clinically significant weight loss, or else are of such low potency that their contribution is negligible. Probably the ideal specification for a thermogenic drug would be that it increased metabolic rate by a maximum of 15–20% (to reduce the danger of toxic overdosage), that it did not increase appetite (or else energy balance would be re-established at a higher rate of energy flux), that it did not cause loss of lean tissue, and that it had no undesirable side effects. Suppose such a drug was invented, and it caused clinically significant weight loss in obese people. Inevitably, as weight was lost energy expenditure would decrease, so a new equilibrium must be reached even while the patient continued to take the drug. If the drug was stopped the regain of weight seems at least as certain as it is following the cessation of an anorectic drug. Furthermore the ideal specification set out above will be difficult to meet: so far there has been no method found for increasing energy expenditure which does not increase appetite also. My assessment is that it is unlikely that a thermogenic drug will be found which is both effective and safe in the treatment of human obesity.

8.h. PHYSICAL TRAINING

The case for physical activity to treat or prevent obesity has been strongly put by Allen & Quigley (1977) and by Thompson et al (1982). Five arguments are advanced to show that exercise should be a better form of treatment than dietary restriction. These arguments can be summarised thus:

1. Dietary treatment of obesity is usually ineffective, because a decrease in food intake leads to a decrease in metabolic rate, which results in a plateauing of weight loss, even if the restricted diet is maintained.
2. Most dietary surveys show that obese people do not eat more than normal, but they are less active. Thus an exercise programme is directed at the causal abnormality of obesity.
3. Extreme inactivity is associated with a paradoxical increase in food intake, so changing from a sedentary lifestyle to a moderately active one will actually decrease food intake.
4. Inactivity leads to muscle wasting, but exercise will increase lean tissue mass and hence increase metabolic rate.
5. The true energy cost of exercise is much more than the energy expended during the exercise, because exercise causes a prolonged elevation of RMR.

These argument seem to present a strong case, but we have already seen that some of them are not founded on true observations. The counter-arguments can be summarised thus:

1. Dietary treatment of obesity is invariably effective if the diet is well designed and accurately followed. Of course metabolic rate decreases with weight loss: the subjects shown in Figure 8.11 decreased in weight from 104 kg to 74 kg, and their metabolic rate decreased from 290 ml O_2/min to 234 ml O_2/min. However in the unlikely event that a group of subjects who weighed 104 kg

were reduced to 74 kg by an exercise programme they too would show a similar decrease in metabolic rate.

2. The fallibility of dietary surveys has been discussed in Chapter 4.b. The evidence that obese people have (on average) a higher energy intake than lean people, and therefore must have a higher energy intake to maintain body weight, is summarised in Tables 6.1 and 6.2, and discussed in Chapter 6.a. There is no good evidence that obese people spend less energy in physical activity than lean people (see Chapter 6.e).

3. The paradoxical effect of inactivity on food intake, proposed by Mayer et al (1956), has never been demonstrated in man, and the studies of Woo et al (1982a, 1982b) and Woo and Pi-Sunyer (1985) have failed to provide any support for this hypothesis.

4. If an activity causes loss of lean tissue and hence decrease in RMR these changes should be marked in patients paralysed by spinal cord injuries, but in fact they are not found (Greenway et al 1969, Agarwal et al 1985).

5. The effect of exercise on subsequent RMR depends critically on the intensity of the exercise. Hermansen et al (1984) report elevation of metabolic rate by 19.4% for 12 h after prolonged severe exercise in 1 subject. In a later report the same group report the effect on subsequent resting metabolic rate of 80 min exercise at 70% maximum oxygen uptake in 8 healthy young subjects (Maehlum et al 1986). This work load is equivalent to an oxygen uptake of 2.4 l/min, (152 watts) since the maximum oxygen uptake in these subjects averaged 3.3 l/min, which is not in the class of Olympic champion runners or cyclists who may achieve oxygen uptakes over 5 l/min, but considerably above average fitness. The total oxygen consumption in the following 12 hours was 26 litres (i.e. 14%) higher than on a control day without exercise.

Bielinski et al (1985) used a protocol similar to that in counter-argument 5 with young athletes with a maximum oxygen uptake of 4.5 l/min. They exercised for 3 hours at 50% of maximum (ie about 2.3 l/min, or 12 kcal/min), and their energy expenditure was increased by 40 kcal over the 4 hours after exercise, compared with non-exercising condition. One of the 11 subjects showed an elevation of RMR 4.7% the following morning. However this study has been criticised by Pi-Sunyer & Segal (1986) on the grounds that the subjects were given more to eat on the exercise days than the control days, in order to cover the energy cost of the exercise. The increased intake will itself have an influence on increasing RMR (Woo et al 1985).

Freedman-Akabas et al (1985) exercised fit and unfit men and women for 20 min at the aerobic threshold, which was about 2.4–2.9 l/min for unfit to fit men, and 1.6–2.2 l/min for unfit to fit women. They subsequently found no sustained increase in RMR in either trained or untrained subjects.

The 24-hour energy expenditure of lean and obese subjects exercising in a direct calorimeter for 30 min at a work load of 50 W increased over the resting control measurement by the amount of energy expended while riding the bicycle ergometer, suggesting that there was no sustained increase in metabolic rate after the exercise ceased (Blaza & Garrow 1983). A study designed to see how quickly metabolic rate returned to baseline after stopping exercise on a bicycle ergometer was undertaken by Pacy et al (1985). The results are shown in Figure 8.16. Each of the 4 subjects did 2 exercise runs

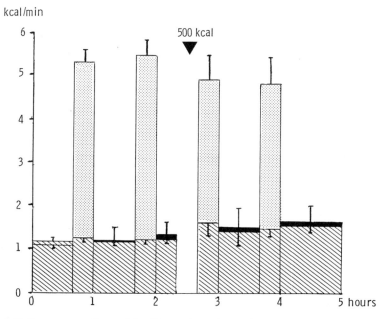

Fig. 8.16 Energy expenditure of 4 subjects who each exercised for 20 min in the hour for 4 h (stippled columns), and took a meal supplying 500 kcal in the middle of the third hour of experiment. Resting metabolic rate after exercise was not significantly different from that on control rest days (shaded area) except during first 10 min after stopping exercise. There is no interaction between exercise and food in causing extra thermogenesis (Data of Pacy et al 1985)

and 2 control runs. During the exercise experiments they rode a bicycle ergometer for 20 min in each hour, with an energy expenditure of about 5 kcal/min (oxygen uptake about 1.1 l/min), and they took a meal providing 500 kcal in the middle of the third hour. The energy expenditure after exercise fell to a level not significantly different from the control days within 10 min of stopping. It seems, therefore, that a measurable increase in RMR some hours after exercise is not seen unless the exercise is of an intensity and duration beyond that which the average person can achieve.

Lennon et al (1985) report that a 12-week programme of 30 min self-selected exercise daily, or prescribed exercise training on alternate days, decreased the decline in metabolic rate among obese subjects on a reducing diet. However their data show that this is so only if metabolic rate is related to body weight, which also goes down. The absolute change in metabolic rate was a decrease of 6%, 4% and 2% in control, daily exercise and prescribed exercise groups, and the change in FFM was a decrease of 2%, 1% and 2% respectively. Therefore, if metabolic rate was expressed either in absolute terms, or in relation to FFM, there was no evident effect of the exercise in maintaining metabolic rate. A similar conclusion can be drawn from the study of Warwick & Garrow (1981) of the 3 subjects whose nitrogen balance was shown in Figure 8.15. The effect of exercise and of tri-iodothyronine on RMR is shown in Figure 8.17. The relative effect on nitrogen balance of a negative energy balance caused by increased exercise or reduced intake has been investigated by Goranzon & Forsum (1985). They found no difference in the rate of nitrogen loss with the method used to generate the negative energy balance.

It is claimed that one of the benefits of regular exercise is the feeling of well-being it induces. Of course people who habitually go jogging enjoy jogging, just as those who go fishing enjoy fishing, and birdwatchers like watching birds. The question is: will habitually sedentary people who are persuaded to take regular exercise come to enjoy it for its mood-enhancing effect? The answer seems to be: Probably not. Six sedentary females who took part in a 10-week jogging programme for research purposes did not enjoy it, and did not intend to continue with it, although they were pleased by their increased physical fitness (Lawson et al 1986). Hughes et al (1986) tested the effect of exercise on mood in 14 men, using a crossover design, and failed to find any significant benefit attributable to the exercise. We must conclude, therefore, that although exercise is

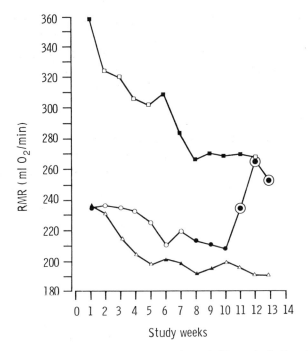

Fig. 8.17 Resting metabolic rate in the 3 subjects shown in Figure 8.15. Exercise does not affect decrease in metabolic rate

mood-enhancing to some people, this is not an effect which is reliably obtained.

This review of the effect of exercise in the treatment of obesity is largely negative, but this is not to say that exercise has no benefits to health. The valuable aspects of exercise will be discussed in connection with diabetes and heart disease in later chapters. However, it is not enough to advise 'exercise': the various health benefits which may be derived depend on the intensity, duration and frequency of the exercise performed (Haskell 1985).

8.i BEHAVIOUR MODIFICATION

Until the mid-1960s the approach of psychologists to the problem of obesity had been to investigate the tensions, hostility, insecurity etc. which might be expressed in overeating. However Stuart (1967) put the case for behaviour therapy, which is based on the assumption that behaviour is acquired and maintained by environmental events, and can be relearned in a more appropriate form if the environment is manipulated in an appropriate way; specifically that obese people eat in response to many inappropriate cues, and if eating can be limited to specified times, a particular room in the house, using a specific place setting etc. then obese people will gain control of their eating pattern. He reported excellent results in 8 patients (mean weight loss 17.1 kg in 12 months) but at enormous cost to therapist and patient. They were seen 3 times a week for 5 weeks, then every 2 weeks, the individual patient recorded her weight 4 times a day, and the therapist was available at all times to guard against failure. This level of attention is impractical for any but a small minority of patients with enough time and money to invest in the enterprise.

Attempts to make the treatment by behaviour therapy more widely available have been reviewed by Stunkard (1985). The important behavioural principles can be set out in a manual, and groups of patients can be supervised by suitably trained lay leaders. This strategy has been well established in commercial weight-loss groups. The important principles are:

1. Record food intake, and the circumstances associated with eating.
2. Make eating a pure experience, not something done while watching television, or waiting for a bus. Limit stimuli which are associated with eating.
3. Eat slowly.
4. Take more exercise.
5. Learn more about nutritional requirements, and the energy and nutrient content of foods.
6. Learn to cope with self-defeating thoughts about dieting by learning counter-arguments which will reinforce success.
7. The goals of treatment are set by negotiation between patient and therapist, and the treatment programme may vary from patient to patient according to circumstances.

It is notable that dietary prescription ('eat this, do not eat that') is studiously avoided. The emphasis is on learning more about the factors which make a particular person eat a particular diet, and how that situation can be changed if change is desired. The reasoning is that if patients go on a diet, they will sooner or later go off the diet, and the benefit will have been lost. However, if patients learn to control eating, this skill should be available (perhaps after some rehearsal) whenever it is needed.

As might be expected from the above discussion, behaviour tharapy on its own causes rather gradual but sustained weight loss.

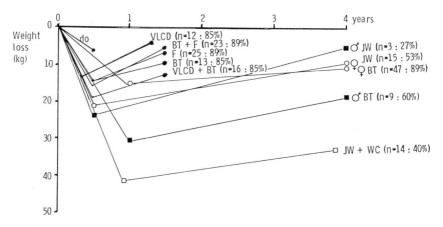

Fig. 8.18 Summary of weight loss achieved during treatment, and on later follow-up, by behaviour therapy (BT), very-low-calorie diet (VLCD), fenfluramine (F), jaw wiring (JW) and waist cord (WC). Number of patients and percentage followed up are shown (data of Stunkard et al 1980, Bjorvell & Rossner 1985, Wadden & Stunkard 1986 and Garrow & Webster 1986b)

Therefore it is a good system for moderately obese people who do not have much weight to lose. However, the objective of recent studies has been to see if a combination of behaviour therapy with some other treatment would be effective: the treatment to achieve more substantial weight loss and the behaviour therapy to assist the patient to maintain this weight loss. Figure 8.18 summarises the results in the most successful studies so far in which behaviour therapy has been used alone or in combination with other treatments. Unfortunately many papers on behaviour therapy are projects by students of psychology who treat a group of patients for a few weeks until there is a statistically significant result, but such publications throw no light on the effectiveness of the treatment in substantially overweight (grade II or III) patients.

By far the most successful series treated with behaviour therapy (apart from the 8 patients of Stuart 1967) have been those of Stunkard et al (1980), Wadden & Stunkard (1986) and Bjorvell & Rossner (1985). None of these series used pure behaviour therapy: Stunkard et al (1980) used a registered dietitian who 'provided extensive nutritional counselling, based on a 1000–12 000 kcal (4.2–5.0 MJ) diet with a food exchange plan'. The subjects in the 'behaviour therapy only' group of Wadden & Stunkard (1986) 'consumed a 1000–1200 kcal diet of their own choosing'. The patients of Bjorvell & Rossner were trained in low energy cooking by a dietitian, they had a 600 kcal diet in hospital for some time and were given 'shopping exercises', and patients who relapsed were readmitted to hospital. The weight loss achieved after 6 months by Stunkard et al (1980) was 10.9 ± 1.0 kg, by Wadden & Stunkard (1986) was 14.3 ± 6.7 kg, and by Bjorvell & Rossner (1985) in 1 year was 15.0 ± 10.9 kg among women and 30.9 ± 18.6 kg among men. These rates of weight loss are very satisfactory, and similar to the best results obtained by anorectic drugs or jaw wiring, but not as rapid as those reported with exclusive use of VLCD.

The superiority of the behaviour therapy approach become evident with the long-term results. The patients treated by Stunkard et al (1980) with behaviour therapy maintained weight loss well, so after 1 year follow-up they were 9.0 kg below starting weight, while patients treated with fenfluramine, who had initially lost more weight than the behaviour therapy group (14.5 kg vs 10.9 kg), were at 1 year after treatment only 6.3 kg below baseline. The combination of fenfluramine and behaviour therapy also failed to produce lasting weight loss (4.6 kg 1 year after treatment).

In the study of Wadden & Stunkard (1986) the behaviour therapy group maintained 9.5 kg of their initial 14.3 kg loss after 1 year. A comparison group who had VLCD for 2 months lost initially 14.1 kg at 4 months, but regained to 4.7 kg below baseline after 1 year, but when behaviour therapy and VLCD were combined the loss at 4 months was 19.3 kg, and 1 year later was 12.9 kg. Clearly the behaviour therapy had both increased the effectiveness of the VLCD and greatly helped to maintain the weight loss.

The patients studied by Bjorvell & Rossner (1985) included a group treated by jaw wiring, which was maintained for about 7 months. Their weight loss was initially 21.5 kg for women and 23.7 kg for men, but at 4-year follow-up the 15 women (53% of initial group) were only 9.4 kg below baseline, and the 3 men (27% of initial group) were 5.1 kg below baseline. By contrast the groups treated with behaviour therapy had maintained most of their weight loss: women who had lost 15.0 kg at 1 year were 11.5 kg below baseline at 4 years, and the corresponding results for men were 30.9 kg and 18.4 kg. We can therefore conclude that behaviour therapy which is used in conjunction with dietary advice can produce significant and prolonged weight loss.

However, Figure 8.18 also shows that the best results for weight loss and maintenance so far among patients treated non-surgically have been in the jaw wiring-waist cord group of Garrow & Webster (1986b): the 14 patients (40% of initial group) lost 42.4 kg in 11 months with jaw wiring, and were 32.8 kg below baseline 47 months after the start of treatment.

9

Investigation and treatment of grade III obesity

The principles of treatment apply to all grades of obesity, but in practice treatments which carry greater risks, and require greater use of resources (such as surgery) are justified only in the more severe grades of obesity, while other treatments (such as physical training) are applicable only to the less severe grades of obesity. Table 9.1 provides an overview of the applicability of the various treatments discussed in the previous chapter according to the grade of obesity of the patient. Obviously, the boundaries between grades are arbitrarily chosen, and a treatment strategy which would be appropriate for a patient at the upper limit of one grade would also be appropriate for a patient at the lower limit of the next grade above. However it is hoped that the classification used in this book will provide a useful guide to the best treatment choices. In this and the next three chapters a policy for investigation and treatment is suggested in greater detail.

Table 9.1 Selection of treatment strategy appropriate to grade of obesity.

Treatment strategy	Grade III	Grade II	Grade I	Grade 0
Diet				
starvation	NO	NO	NO	NO
very-low-calorie	Poss	NO	NO	NO
conventional	YES (1)	YES (1)	YES (1)	NO
milk	YES (2)	YES (2)	Poss	NO
jaw wiring/cord	YES (3)	Poss	NO	NO
exclusion surgery	Poss	NO	NO	NO
Drugs				
anorectic	Poss	Poss	NO	NO
thermogenic	NO	NO	NO	NO
Physical training	NO	Poss	YES	YES
Reassurance	NO	NO	Poss	YES

(1), (2) and (3) indicate first, second and third choices of treatment within grade of obesity.

PREVALENCE OF GRADE III OBESITY

In a representative sample of adults in the UK about 0.1% of men and 0.3% of women were over $W/H^2 = 40$. In the Harrow Slimming Club (Seddon et al 1981) about 5% of members were in grade III, and in the hospital obesity clinic 34% of patients attending are in grade III. These are severely obese patients who are almost always to some degree disabled by their obesity. They have almost all had various forms of treatment in the past, and frequently describe the hospital referral as a 'last hope' of successful treatment.

INVESTIGATION OF GRADE III OBESE PATIENTS

a. Weight history and expectations.

First, measure the patient's weight and height, so the W/H^2 index can be calculated. Next ask the set of ten questions listed below, from which the patient's motivation and expectations can be assessed. It is best to ask the questions and record the answers without comment, but if a question is evaded persist in asking it again.

1. 'Why do you want to lose weight?' This may be rephrased 'What benefits do you think you would gain from losing weight?' or 'What things do you want to do, but are unable to do on account of your present weight?' Try to obtain specific examples, rather than generalisations like 'I hate being fat' or 'I just feel generally uncomfortable'. Do not accept second-hand reasons: you want to know what reasons the patient has, not his or her doctor, friends or relatives.
2. 'What weight do you think you should be?' Usually patients will give an estimate near the upper part of the desirable range of weight-for-height. Those who have been to slimming clubs will promptly quote the mid-point of this range for their height, since this is a target weight they have been given by a club leader. If the weight given is unusually high or low ask why they have this target: low estimates of ideal weight are usually related to weights at some halcyon period of youth, and high estimates to the weight they were immediately prior to the onset of their present disabilities.
3. 'Are you on a diet at present?' The immediate answer to this

question is worth recording: often it will be modified later. If the answer is 'yes', find out the nature of the diet, and for how long it has been observed. Is it simply 'being careful what I eat', or is there a defined calorie limit, or does it involve the conscientious ingestion of diet pills without any actual restriction on food intake?

4. 'Is your present weight the maximum you have ever been?' If not what was the maximum, how long ago, and how was it reduced?

5. 'Tell me about the longest time you have ever kept strictly to a reducing diet?' Record the nature of the diet, the duration, the weight loss achieved — from what weight to what weight, how long ago this effort was made, and why it was abandoned. This information may have been obtained already in answer to question 4.

6. 'If you keep strictly to a diet, how quickly do you think you should lose weight?' If the answer is 'I don't know', or 'Quite quickly at first, I should think, from my weight', try to get a quantitative answer by asking: 'After the first week or two, when you may lose weight quicker, do you think it is reasonable to expect on average to lose one, two, four pounds per week, or what?' Sometimes it is impossible to obtain any quantitative reply.

7. 'Tell me about your family'. This deliberately vague question will elicit whatever aspect of the family the patient thinks is most relevant to the present problem, namely 'Both my parents are overweight' if genetic factors are considered important, 'I have two girls and a boy' if obesity is attributed to childbearing, or 'My eldest boy works night shifts and my husband is a milk-roundsman' if the social pattern of the family is such that meals are being prepared every hour of the night and day. If necessary elicit information on all these aspects, find out who does the shopping and cooking, and if other members of the family are inclined to be helpful in keeping the patient on a diet.

8. 'Are you on any medication at present?' Note particularly anorectic drugs, diuretics, antidepressants, thyroid preparations, analgesics for arthritis, oral hypoglycaemic agents, steroids, contraceptives and anti- hypertensive drugs.

9. Do you expect to lose weight without dieting?' Usually the reply is 'Of course not', but the question will sometimes reveal that the patient has pinned hopes on some magic cure. If this is so the fact must be unearthed or the entire interview will be a failure,

since (from the patient's viewpoint) the only topic of real interest
was never mentioned.

10. 'What work do you do?' The answer gives an indication of social
circumstances and intellectual ability, and may reveal special
circumstances (extensive travelling, shift work, business enter-
taining, employment in catering) which will affect the patients
ability to adhere to a diet.

It takes about 10 minutes to obtain answers to these 10 questions
from the averagely articulate patient. This process does not represent
a complete examination in itself, but I have found that there is a
higher yield of useful information about obese patients from these
10 questions than from all the subsequent examination and laboratory investigations. It may be useful to draw attention to questions
which are excluded from this list, although they occur in other
screening questionnaires, such as that of Levitz & Jordan (1973).
The patient is not asked about her body image, or what she thinks
other people think about her, although this information may be
volunteered. She is not asked about the age of onset of her obesity
or if at any period she was underweight. She is not asked about the
ill-effects of previous dieting attempts, but again these may be
volunteered. She is not asked about the psychological antecedents
of her obesity, temptation foods, bingeing and feelings of guilt.
There are three reasons for excluding questions of this sort. First,
they take much longer than the 10 rather factual questions listed
above, because they are matters of opinion which provoke many
supplementary questions from the patient about exactly what the
question means and to what period it refers. Second, I do not think
the answers, when they are obtained, are of any practical help in
planning the appropriate line of treatment. Third, if the initial questions are directed to matters of social acceptability, age of onset of
obesity, and psychological aspects of eating behaviour, the patient
may reasonably infer that these are the factors which determine prognosis or which are likely to be changed by treatment. I believe that
this inference is untrue and should not be fostered by questions
which have no compensating advantage.

b. Routine medical history and examination.

The questions directed towards previous attempts and failure to lose
weight should be followed by the normal systematic enquiry about

general health at present, previous health and investigations, smoking and drinking habits, and (where relevant) menstrual function. Physical examination of very obese patients is unsatisfactory, particularly when listening to the chest or palpating the abdomen, since the fat layer may obscure all but the grossest abnormality. However, there is no excuse for not taking the blood pressure, observing the skin for evidence of thyroid or adrenal disease, noting operation scars, examining the hips and knees for evidence of osteoarthritis, and the ankles for oedema. The ocular fundi should be examined, and the urine tested for protein and sugar.

With this information it is possible to judge if the obese patient is simply an obese patient, or if there is significant pathology in addition to, and separate from, the obesity. Only a minority of obese patients, will have a second pathology, but it is important to detect it. A thin patient with a bulging stomach due to an ovarian cyst will soon be diagnosed, but in an obese patient the diagnosis may not be considered. Obese patients may be weak from anaemia, leukaemia or renal failure and never be investigated because their symptoms were plausibly explained by obesity. Breathlessness and pain in weight-bearing joints are common features of severe obesity, but they may indicate other disease if the disability is disproportionate to the degree of obesity.

c. Special investigations.

Severely obese patients are often pathetically willing to be investigated: they are desperate, they regard hospital referral as their last chance of successful treatment, and often they have low self-esteem and consider that they must go along with whatever is suggested. This excessively docile attitude is a temptation to research workers to carry out tests far beyond the needs of diagnosis or management.

From the patients' viewpoint the facts which need to be established are as follows:

1. What is the body composition of the patient? It is known that body weight exceeds the normal range by some 45 kg (100 lb) at least, but is this excess mainly fat, or is there a large amount of excess water also?
2. What is the patient's metabolic rate? This is of importance for several reasons. First, the metabolic rate is the main determinant

of total energy expenditure, especially in very obese patients who are relatively inactive (see Chapter 5.c.). Second, the metabolic rate should check with predictions based on body composition: if it does not it raises the possibility of some disorder of energy metabolism. Finally, it is necessary to try to calculate the energy expenditure which the patient will have after weight reduction, because this is the factor which will be most important in determining how easy it is to maintain the reduced weight.

3. Does the patient have any other major disability other than obesity? If the ability of the patient to live an active independent life is anyway limited by old age, irreversible damage to weight-bearing joints, chronic bronchitis, mental subnormality, or any such disability which will still exist after weight loss, then the benefit to the patient of weight loss is correspondingly reduced. In this connection the significance of depression in severely obese patients is difficult to assess: are they obese because they are depressed, or vice versa? In my experience, if there is good evidence that the patient was not very obese at the time when treatment for depression was started, it is very likely that the patient will still be depressed after weight loss. However a measure of unhappiness is a natural feature of any person disabled by obesity, and is not a contraindication to treatment. I have often been wrong in guessing to what extent depression would be improved by weight loss.

The tests which should be applied to answer questions 1 and 2 above have been described in Chapters 3 and 5. The minimum and most convenient measurements are total body potassium to assess lean body mass, and measurement of RMR on at least three occasions as an inpatient on a reducing diet. It is useless to make random measurements of metabolic rate on outpatients on an unknown diet.

The practical application of these tests can be illustrated by two examples. Let us suppose the patient is a woman of 32 years, weight 115 kg, height 1.6 m, total body potassium 3000 mmol, and resting metabolic rate 300 ml O_2 /min. Her predicted metabolic rate is 285 ml O_2/min which checks well with the observed value. Her W/H^2 is 44.9, and to achieve W/H^2 of 25 she would need to weigh 64 kg, a loss of 51 kg. Her total body potassium indicates a lean body mass of 50 kg, which is quite high for a woman of her age and height, and it also implies that she has a body fat of 65 kg. At rest she will use about 2100 kcal (8.8 MJ) per day. The rule-of-thumb estimate of the energy value of her excess weight (51 kg x 7000 kcal) is that somehow she needs to expend 357,000 kcal (1500 MJ) more than she eats. This is roughly equivalent to suggesting that she should take a diet supplying 1000 kcal (4.2 MJ) per day for 1 year, making an allowance for the fact that her metabolic rate will decrease with weight loss.

In this example the arithmetic is favourable: there is at least a chance that by the age of 33 this woman could achieve a normal weight, with a greatly improved quality of life ahead of her. If we had chosen a woman of the same weight and height, but aged 55, with a total body potassium of 2200 mmol, and with an oxygen uptake of 210 ml/min the outlook would be much less favourable. Her lean body mass is about 37 kg, so she is much more obese: her body fat is about 78 kg. Her daily resting energy expenditure is only about 1500 kcal (6.1 MJ) per day, so to generate an energy deficit of 357,000 kcal (1500 MJ) on a diet supplying 1000 kcal/day would take more than twice as long as for the former example. Here the arithmetic is unfavourable: she is being asked to make a much greater effort in the hope of attaining normal weight at age 57, and even at that weight she would still be more obese, and have a much lower energy requirement than the younger woman.

It is the function of a doctor to try to make life more tolerable for the patient. The jeremiads about the impossibility of treating obesity do not distinguish between those situations in which there is a good chance of obtaining worthwhile benefit (as in the first example above), and those in which quite modest objectives are appropriate (as in the second example). The actual disability suffered by the patient is relevant to the assessment of the case. If, in the second example, the woman was disabled by osteoarthritic knees, weight loss of about 15 kg would be a very sensible objective, which would be attainable, and which would bring considerable relief to the patient. In the first example (unless there was some other pathology complicating the prognosis) it would be wise to aim for a weight loss of 40–50 kg whether or not she had disability attributable to her obesity. Her chance of losing weight will never be greater than it is now, and if she does not lose weight the chances of developing complications will steadily increase, so there is every reason to tackle the problem vigorously as soon as possible.

Those readers who are accustomed to the American idea of a 'work-up' of the obese patient may be surprised that this section does not list tests of insulin, cortisol and catecholamine secretion, X-rays of the pituitary fossa, and so on. It is rather rarely that these tests yield abnormal results which actually help with management. Of course grossly obese people have raised plasma insulin level, and impaired glucose tolerance: if these changes are found (or even if they are not found) I cannot see how that helps in the management of an individual patient. The more often these tests are advised in textbooks the more difficult it is for the doctor to defend himself in court against a charge of negligence if he has not done them. It is ironical that, despite batteries of tests in the 'work-up', the two that really matter — a measure of metabolic rate and of body composition — are the ones most frequently omitted.

TREATMENT OF GRADE III OBESITY

Table 9.1 indicates some lines of treatment which are inappropriate for grade III obese patients. Starvation is never appropriate, although severely obese subjects fare better than thinner people. Thermogenic drugs are particularly inappropriate for severely obese patients, since they already have a reduced exercise tolerance. Any further increase in their already high metabolic rate will diminish exercise tolerance still further, and may lead to death. Physical training is inappropriate for the same reasons as thermogenic drugs: it is impractical and possibly dangerous in severe obesity. The time for physical training will come as the grade III obese patient reduces into the grade II or grade I range. Reassurance is certainly inappropriate: everything should be done to encourage the Grade III obese person to tackle the problem sooner rather than later, since with time the health risks will become greater and weight loss will become more difficult to achieve.

All the other treatment strategies are worth considering, since everything possible must be done to help the patient.

Conventional reducing diet

The first choice, as with other grades of obesity, is the conventional 3.4-5 MJ (800-1200 kcal) diet. The nutrient composition of a 1200 kcal version of this type of diet is shown in Table 8.3(B). The distribution of energy is about 21 : 41 : 38 between protein : fat : carbohydrate — this is a higher proportion of fat energy than is recommended for healthy weight-maintenance diets, but inevitably a person on a reducing diet will use a large proportion of fat as a fuel, most of which is their own body fat. This diet translated into items of food is shown in Appendix 1: to adjust the total energy value between 1200 kcal and 800 kcal the number of slices of bread (or exchanges) is adjusted appropriately.

Although the conventional reducing diet is the first option for treatment of grade III obesity, it is foolish to expect that such advice will be sufficient to achieve satisfactory weight loss in the great majority of cases. Virtually all grade III patients have had such advice before, and if it had worked then they would not now be grade III. However it is essential to establish why it did not work in the past, since on this information future strategy is planned. Previous failures on conventional diets fall into three categories:

1. The patient could not keep to the diet, and therefore did not lose weight.
2. The patient kept to the diet for a few weeks, but was dissatisfied with the rate of weight loss achieved.
3. The patient kept to the diet, but lost no weight.

Intermediate and mixed forms occur, but for purpose of discussion these three types of failure will be discussed in turn.

Patient could not keep to diet

First check that the previous diet was well designed — if it was a crank diet with no scientific basis then failure with such a diet should not prevent the patient giving a conventional diet a serious trial for at least 4 weeks. If the previous failure was on a conventional diet, why was it not possible to keep to it? Sometimes the reason transposes to a matter of unsatisfactory weight loss, which is discussed below.

Often patients offer as an explanation that they 'have no willpower'. If they were imprisoned without access to any food which was not allowed on the diet all would be well, but if the food is available they fall to temptation. A patient may feel very guilty about this weakness. Feelings of guilt are not helpful in this situation, because somehow the patient has to regain control of eating and recover self-esteem in order to be convinced that the effort to regain normal weight is possible and worth while. In a hospital obesity clinic it is easy to point out that none of the patients coming to the clinic is good at dieting, if they were they would not need to come to the clinic. Restricting energy intake below maintenance requirements is a difficult feat to achieve and maintain for many months, but there are tricks which increase the chance of success.

First the grade III patient must be certain that there is no way to lose their excess weight without reducing energy intake. It is easy to show that the patient with, say, 50 kg to lose is not going to achieve much energy deficit by exercise. Often patients have heard of surgical procedures for weight loss, and regard these as preferable alternatives to dieting. It is necessary to point out that surgical procedures which cause weight loss, such as jaw wiring or gastric exclusion, do so because they force the patient to eat less — the principle is still the reducing diet, but forced upon the patient by some surgically induced disability. That may in the end be the treatment with the best chance of success, but the conventional reducing diet should be given a trial first.

The procedures of behaviour therapy and contingency conditioning are often helpful to the patient who is convinced of the need to diet, but whose will-power is deficient. It is obviously useful to recruit the help of other members of the family and of colleagues at work to reduce the exposure of forbidden foods to the patient. Keeping an accurate diet diary with the circumstances in which food was eaten indicates the situations in which the diet is likely to be broken, so steps can be taken to provide extra support to the patient at these danger times. The process is one of continual guidance and encouragement which makes considerable demands on the therapist.

At the back of the mind of the patient there is always the option of just giving up and accepting their obesity and whatever penalties that may bring. In grade I obesity this may be a sensible plan in some situations which are discussed later, but it is always a poor choice for Grade III obese patients. They are almost always already suffering from some physical disability, and the situation will get worse unless weight loss is achieved. As the patient gets older weight loss is more difficult to achieve, and it confers smaller benefits, so the grade III patient should be given every encouragement to work hard at losing weight on a properly designed diet, since this effort will be well repaid by benefits in the future.

Weight loss was unsatisfactory

The rate of weight loss which is acceptable is the key to the successful treatment of severely obese patients. Very often patients come to the clinic who have lost, or have been promised that they will lose, about 3 kg/week or more with some diet or drug treatment, and they are unwilling to settle for anything less. Of course it is possible to achieve such rates of weight loss temporarily, but the obese person who has 50 kg to lose must burn their excess energy stores of about 350,000 kcal. In order to lose 3 kg/week of this material it would be necessary to maintain a negative energy balance of 3000 kcal/day, which is clearly impossible, since few people have a total energy expenditure as much as 3000 kcal/day.

Figure 9.1 indicates a range of desirable rates of weight loss in obese patients: the upper line shows 2 kg/week for the first 4 weeks and 1 kg/week thereafter, and the lower line is half that rate. In general younger, taller and more overweight patients can expect to achieve rates of weight loss near the upper line, and older, shorter and less obese patients may have to settle for something near the lower line. Patients who complain they cannot achieve a satisfactory

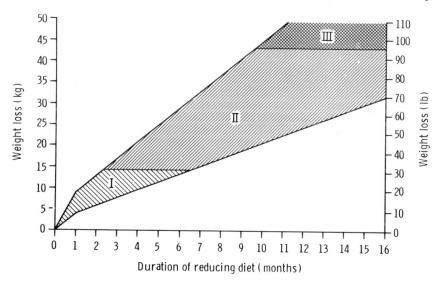

Fig. 9.1 Range of desirable rate of weight loss in obese patients in order to achieve loss of the appropriate 75% fat : 25% fat-free tissue. Younger and taller patients may achieve rates at upper limit of range: older and shorter patients will probably be near lower limit of range. Shaded areas show the length of treatment required for patients in grade I, II or III to reach $W/H^2 = 25$. For explanation of grades see Figure 1.1

rate of weight loss usually have in mind rates faster than the upper line of Figure 9.1. It is necessary to point out that (for the reasons given above) rates above that zone do not indicate loss of fat, which is what the severely obese person needs to do. There are, of course, patients who will not accept this explanation. They should be told to come back when they have satisfied themselves that it is true, because unless patients accept the rates shown in Figure 9.1 as a reasonable target it will not be possible to find a satisfactory line of treatment.

The patient who diets but does not lose weight

Patients coming to a tertiary referral centre include individuals who apparently defy the laws of thermodynamics: despite maintaining an energy intake of, say 800 kcal/day over a year they have gained weight. If such a patient is in grade III it is necessary to admit him or her to a metabolic ward to discover what is wrong. Either the patient must have an energy expenditure less than 800 kcal/day (which has never yet been recorded in a human adult) or else the diet was incorrectly calculated. Unless it is established which explanation is correct, it is not possible to plan the appropriate treatment. It is necessary to have a ward on which the diet supplied to patients is accurately known, and this means that there must be a good diet kitchen, and a system to ensure the patients do not go off the ward and obtain food elsewhere, nor do visitors bring extra food into the ward. A suitable arrangement is described by Garrow et al (1978). Three weeks is about the minimum time required to establish the rate of weight loss on a reducing diet, since over shorter periods other factors (such as water shifts relating to diuretic therapy of menstrual function) may obscure the true rate of weight loss.

When it is established that weight loss in the range shown in Figure 9.1 can be achieved on a conventional reducing diet a significant step forward has been made, but the patient may still find it almost impossible to keep to such a diet for the year or so which is required to achieve normal weight. In such situations other procedures may be required.

Milk diet

The energy, protein and fat supplied by 1800 ml (3 pints) of whole cow's milk are shown in column (C) of Table 8.3. The energy and protein content is not very different from the conventional diet, but there is more fat, and in particular saturated fat. Substituting semi-skimmed or skimmed milk would reduce the energy and fat content. The diet is inexpensive, does nothing to stimulate appetite, and is readily available almost anywhere. Both the patient and his or her family can easily check if the diet is being adhered to: if the patient is drinking milk or the acaloric fluids mentioned in Chapter 8.d. then all is well, but if the patient is having any other energy source then this is not permitted on the diet.

Many grade III obese patients find this milk diet much easier to keep to than a conventional reducing diet, presumably for the reasons given above. It is often possible for the patient to distance themselves from normal food, and thus reduce temptation to break the diet. Certainly any patient who says that he or she cannot keep to a conventional reducing diet because it is too expensive, or too much trouble to calculate and prepare, should be advised to try the milk diet. In the case of lactose intolerant patients the equivalent in yoghurt is often better tolerated.

Jaw wiring and waist cord

The idea of using a milk diet originally arose in connection with jaw wiring (Garrow 1974a), but subsequently it proved a valuable treatment in its own right. Jaw wiring is obviously one way to make it more likely that the patient will keep to the milk diet, but it is not a solution which should be tried without careful exploration of other options. Patients who have heard about the treatment through television or magazine articles often have too great faith that jaw wiring will enable them to become effortlessly thin, and have given too little thought to what will happen when the wires are removed. Some believe that having volunteered for such a drastic procedure they will earn a moral right to eternal thinness.

The outcome of jaw wiring is determined by thermodynamic considerations, rather than moral principles. If, having had the jaws wired, a grade III patient keeps to a milk diet, the subsequent weight loss will be identical to that which would have been achieved on the same milk diet without jaw wiring. The only function of the jaw wiring is to increase the chance that the diet will be kept: it certainly does not make it certain that the diet will be kept, since it is possible for virtually any food to be homogenised and drunk by a patient whose jaws are wired. It is also important to realise that patients have their jaws wired because they are otherwise particularly unsuccessful at dieting, and usually after weight loss they are still not good at dieting. There is no experimental basis for the idea that the 'stomach shrinks' after several months on a milk diet, so reduced intake will be permanent. It is therefore unethical to undertake jaw wiring in an obese patient unless a waist cord is part of the package deal, and suitable supervision can be provided both before and after the jaw wiring period (see Ch. 8.d).

Any candidate for jaw wiring, therefore, should try to keep to a milk diet for at least 2 months before being considered for the procedure. They should talk to other patients who have had the procedure, and who are at various stages in the programme. The patients who have been treated at the Clinical Research Centre, Harrow, have all been admitted to the metabolic ward for 3 weeks so that measurements of body composition and metabolic rate could be made, and they could be screened for other metabolic disease apart from obesity. If these tests are satisfactory, and the patient (and spouse if any) agree to the conditions set out below, and the dental condition of the patient is satisfactory, then jaw wiring is undertaken by a dental surgeon experienced in this technique. There are three conditions. First, that the patient should not remove the wires for any reason, and report immediately to the hospital if a wire accidentally breaks. Second, the patient undertakes to come at least monthly to the medical outpatient clinic for supervision. Third, the patient agrees to wear a waist cord indefinitely after the wires are removed, unless there is a good reason to remove it (e.g. pregnancy or an abdominal operation). This arrangement has been associated with very large and sustained weight losses in grade III patients.

Exclusion surgery

In patients who are unwilling to have their jaws wired, or who are dentally unsuitable, reduced energy intake may be achieved by one of the surgical procedures described in Chapter 8.e. However grade III patients are not good surgical or anaesthetic risks, so abdominal surgery as a first line of treatment should be avoided if possible.

Apart from the immediate operative mortality, the other problem associated with exlusion surgery concerns the nutritional state of the patient in the long term. An operation which reduces a grade III patient to near-normal weight must cause quite a severe limitation on food intake, so it is fortunate if the reduced patient is able to take an adequate diet. Surgical treatment of severe obesity requires at least as careful long-term follow-up and supervision as medical treatments.

Anorectic drugs

The efficacy of anorectic drugs is poor in achieving the weight loss required by grade III patients. However, it is possible that anorectic drugs may be helpful in association with some of the other treatments described above.

Very-low-calorie diets

The limitations of VLCD have been described in the previous chapter. However, if they are to be used at all they are safest when given to severely obese patients who have relatively great efficiency for nitrogen conservation. If, for any reason, the other lines of treatment described for grade III obesity are not available, then a VLCD would be better than leaving the patient untreated.

10

Treatment of grade II obesity

Grade II obesity affects about 6% of men and 8% of women among the population of the UK between the age of 16 years and 64 years. Thus its prevalence is some 30 times greater than grade III obesity. The mortality rate at the mid-point of grade II (i.e. at $W/H^2 = 35$) is about twice that among people in the desirable range of weight-for-height, so grade II obesity represents a very serious public health problem. In view of the relatively large number of patients involved, compared with grade III obesity, it is not logistically possible to refer all grade II patients to units with special interest and facilities for investigating obesity, so it is a problem which must usually be tackled with the resources in the health district. It is still necessary to take the weight history, medical history and examination described for grade III patients (see p 186–189). The special investigations described for grade III patients are relevant to grade II also, if the resources are available and the need arises (see 'Refractory' grade II obesity below).

TREATMENT OF GRADE II OBESITY

The treatment strategy for Grade II obesity is summarised in Table 9.1. The points on which the strategy differs from that for grade III are that VLCD and exclusion surgery are not considered as possible treatments, since the health dangers of grade II obesity are not so great that the risks in these treatments are justified. Jaw-wiring is possible as a last resort, and physical training may be useful.

The first choice treatment is the conventional reducing diet, for the reasons given in the previous chapter. Most grade II patients will have had experience of dieting unsuccessfully before, but they should be persuaded to try again. The target rates of weight loss shown in Figure 9.1 apply also to grade II patients. Since they may have 15–45 kg to lose the duration of dieting to achieve desirable weight is likely to be less than the year which it takes grade III patients to reach the desirable weight range.

Since grade II patients probably will not have had the intensive dietary education which grade III patients receive in the metabolic ward, it is all the more important to provide good outpatient supervision. Each patient needs to have an individual explanation of a suitable reducing diet, adapted if necessary to meet any special requirements (taste, cost, religious beliefs, etc.). Principles borrowed from the discipline of behaviour therapy should be used (see Chapter 8.i). The patient should be encouraged to keep a record of everything eaten or drunk at least for the first 4 weeks of treatment, and at any other time if weight loss is not being maintained at a satisfactory rate (see Fig. 9.1). The support of family and colleagues should be enlisted, and the reasons for failure to keep to the diet must be discussed in a courteous and constructive manner: it is quite unhelpful to scold or make fun of patients.

It is the job of the therapist to guide and encourage the patient, but with grade II or III obesity it is very rarely ethical to console the patient by saying that weight loss is not very important, so not to worry too much. Weight loss is important for the reasons given in Chapter 1, so reassurance is inappropriate.

Every patient should be seen at least every 4 weeks: shorter intervals may be better, but use more resources, and longer intervals are associated with much less satisfactory rates of weight loss. For patients in employment a visit every 4 weeks is a reasonable frequency to get time off work. The patient does not live in a dietetic vacuum, but will pick up tit-bits of dietary advice from friends, relatives and magazines: sometimes this advice is highly misleading, so it is necessary to check weight loss every 4 weeks, and to find out if the diet presents any problems.

The causes of dietary failure are the same as for grade III: not keeping to the diet, or being dissatisfied with the rate of weight loss, or not losing weight at all despite keeping to the diet. The same negotiations are necessary to agree the rates of weight loss shown in Figure 9.1 as a reasonable target. If the problem is that the patient cannot keep to the diet, the appropriate response depends on the age and medical condition of the patient. A young grade II patient with a family history of diabetes or hypertension should have a full explanation of the hazards of not losing weight, and as much support as possible from family and colleagues to assist with keeping to the diet. However, a grade II patient who is over 60 years old, and who says that he or she finds dieting too difficult, may opt for taking a chance on the consequences of this degree of obesity. It often happens that such a patient returns to the clinic after a few months, perhaps with chest pain, or pain in weight-bearing joints, having decided that perhaps dieting is a better option after all. If this happens all encouragement should be given to get the patient started on the diet with constructive support from the household and friends.

Milk diet

Some grade II patients find the milk diet very satisfactory. It requires very little effort or expense, and reliably causes weight loss. It is only very rarely that jaw wiring is indicated for grade II patients.

Physical training

Although physical training has very little effect on weight loss it confers health benefits which are discussed in later chapters of this book. Patients should therefore be encouraged to take regular aerobic exercise such as swimming, walking or jogging as their exercise tolerance, recreational facilities and lifestyle permit. This has the added benefit of providing some positive reinforcement with weight loss, since weight loss of 10 kg will have quite marked effects on exercise tolerance, so the level of exercise can be increased as weight decreases.

Anorectic drugs

These have low priority in the treatment of grade II obesity, but a few patients find them helpful, particularly in special situations, such as when they are dieting and also trying to give up smoking. It is certainly better for a grade II patient to take anorectic drugs than to give up the attempt to diet, or to decide to continue smoking. The problem is that weight gain almost always occurs when the drug treatment is stopped, and anorectic drugs added to behaviour therapy actually produce a worse long-term result than behaviour therapy alone (see Fig. 8.18).

'REFRACTORY' GRADE II OBESE PATIENTS

Clinicians working outside special centres, who do not have access to facilities for measuring metabolic rate, will encounter some grade II patients who absolutely insist that they have an intake of (say) 800 kcal/day for many weeks without weight loss. This is highly improbable (it has never happened yet in the experience of the author) but if the view is strongly held by the patient it is an effective bar to successful treatment. If every 'refractory' grade II patient was referred to a specialist centre for a measurement of metabolic rate a great deal of time and money would be wasted, since the vast majority have perfectly normal oxygen uptake (say 220 ml/min or more). However, if the clinician simply tells the patient that the diet history must be wrong this causes much ill-will, and does nothing to help patient. The latter will probably seek help from a charlatan who accepts the diagnosis of a very low metabolic rate, and prescribes an inappropriate treatment, such as a VLCD.

If any medical practitioner in this dilemma seeks my advice I suggest the following screening test. Suppose the patient insists that he or she has been keeping accurately to a diet of 800 kcal, or 1000 kcal, or 1200 kcal/day without weight loss, then the following arrangement is made. First check that the patient is not on medication (such as diuretics) which might cause large fluctuations in body water. Next, record an accurate weight at the start of a period of 3 weeks, during which the patient undertakes to keep to a milk diet equivalent in energy to the diet on which he or she has failed to lose weight (600 ml whole cow's milk = 400 kcal). Record the weight at the end of this period. If the weight loss is less than 2 kg (4.5 lb) then I will be happy to admit the patient for the investigations described for grade III patients. However, the vast majority of grade II patients do not require admission because they lose more than this amount. The test can be repeated as often as required.

MAINTENANCE OF WEIGHT LOSS IN GRADE II PATIENT

The price of maintaining weight loss is vigilance, but fortunately this does not have to be constant vigilance. A grade II patient who has reduced to grade I or 0 must be warned that weight regain is always a threat, and it is much easier to cope with a small amount of weight regained than a large amount. Sometimes patients suggest that they should reduce to below the target weight, so then they will not have to worry about gaining a few pounds. This is a risky policy: in the first place they will have unnecessary dificulty in reducing below target weight, and if they then do not worry about weight regain they will soon be back at target weight and rising fast.

It is a much better policy to set a threshold — say 5 kg above minimum weight — below which the patient plans to stay. This is the weight which can be gained on holidays and such times, but will have to be lost before the next such occasion. Some patients monitor progress by weight checks every few weeks, or more frequently by the fit of garments such as a particular pair of jeans which becomes unwearable when weight gain is excessive. A waist cord is essentially a built-in pair of jeans, for those who cannot trust themselves to check weight gain when it occurs. It is commonly observed that after a holiday there is a reluctance to consult a weighing machine, but the waist cord is ever present and will give warning of weight gain without any action on the part of the patient.

If and when weight gain to the threshold value occurs, the process of losing it and getting down to target weight again involves exactly the same techniques as were described above to achieve the initial weight loss.

11

Management of grade I obesity

Grade I presents two difficulties which have not been encountered in discussing the more severe grades of obesity. The more important one is that since the potential patients in this grade outnumber the potential therapist by several hundred to one, it is impractical to offer treatment on a one-to-one basis, nor would it be an efficient use of therapist time to do so. This problem can in part be overcome by the use of suitably structured groups, which are discussed later. The lesser problem is that since the amount of weight the grade I patient needs to lose is relatively small — less than 15 kg — it is more difficult to demonstrate that the conventional reducing diet is superior to treatments which are designed to strip glycogen stores rapidly. With glycogen-stripping techniques the grade I patient may lose 5 kg in 10 days, and be highly satisfied, since a loss of about 5 kg was the original target. That is all right, but the trouble starts when, at some later time, the patient complains that he or she is now unable to lose 10 kg in 20 days. Of course this is not possible, because the first 5 kg contained virtually the total body glycogen stores, and the next 5 kg needs to consist of adipose tissue with an energy density 7 times greater than the glycogen : water mixture.

The strategies appropriate for the treatment of grade I patients are the conventional reducing diet and exercise (see Table 9.1). Jaw wiring and anorectic drugs are not to be considered for obvious reasons.

In principle there is no reason why advice on a reducing diet and exercise, and on the principles of behaviour therapy, should not be given to grade I patients by the general practitioner. In practice, however, many general practitioners are opposed to this type of work. Bolden (1975), in an article entitled 'Against the active treatment of obesity in general practice' concludes: 'Because the present methods of treatment are so inefficient, I propose that weight reduction programmes for the average patient in general practice are worthless. We, as a profession, are hidebound by our traditions. It is time we took a long hard look at fruitless areas of therapeutic activity and asked ourselves if our efforts might not be better directed elsewhere.'

We do not know what proportion of general practitioners agree with this view. Where, for example, would their efforts be better directed? If it is beneath the dignity of general practitioners to treat obesity, whose job should it be? Some light on these questions is given by the survey of Ashwell (1973) who analysed the replies of 2333 people to a questionnaire from the Consumers' Association about methods of slimming. Most of those replying were grade I obese. Only 1362 of the respondents, 1117 women and 245 men, had received advice from a doctor about weight loss. About half the women, and a quarter of the men, had specifically sought advice about their weight: the remainder had gone about some other problem and been advised to lose weight. It appears, therefore, that in more than half the cases it was the doctor who suggested weight loss. Furthermore, since only 7% of the patients were advised to join a slimming group, 1% were referred to a hospital obesity clinic and 9% were advised not to worry about their weight, it follows that the general practitioner himself offered treatment to the remaining 83% of patients. Since we do not know the actual excess weight, and other medical problems of these patients, it is impossible to say if this was a reasonable arrangement.

It is certainly not reasonable that (if the replies are to be believed) only 28% of patients were asked to go back at regular intervals to be weighed. This is hard to understand. It takes very little time to weigh a patient. The measurement can easily be done by a trained assistant. The doctor who does not keep an accurate record of the patient's weight change every 2–4 weeks cannot claim to be treating obesity seriously, and has no right to complain if the results are poor.

The two advantages which a general practitioner has over the leader of a slimming club are the prestige which goes with a medical degree and the ability to prescribe slimming drugs. The former is more important, since the potency of drug treatment seems to be linked more with charisma than pharmacology (see section 9.f). It is significant that among the patients surveyed by Ashwell (1973) only one fifth of those who had been given slimming drugs thought they were the best way to achieve permanent weight loss, but over half said that dieting without drugs, but with the encouragement of a slimming group, was the most effective method. It is a pity, therefore, that doctors who do not want to weigh their obese patients regularly because, like Bolden (1975), they think their efforts would be better directed elsewhere, do not more readily refer their patients to slimming groups.

ROLE OF SLIMMING GROUPS IN THE TREATMENT OF GRADE I OBESITY

The great majority of slimming groups are sponsored by a commercial organisation, and at least one of their objectives is to make a profit from their members. It may be that the reluctance of doctors to refer patients to a slimming group comes from a desire to protect the patient from commercial exploitation. One solution is for the general practitioner to set up his own group. Craddock (1973) reports several such ventures, but does not give the results achieved. Coupar & Kennedy (1980), a clinical psychologist and general practitioner respectively, formed a non-fee-paying weight-control group of 16 members with a starting weight of 81.1 ± 13.2 kg for the 9 members who subsequently attended the group, and 75.9 ± 7.7 kg for 7 who dropped out. After 10 months the attenders had an average weight loss of 6.2 kg, and by 18 months this has decreased to an average loss of 5.2 kg, while the non-attenders had on average increased weight by 2.8 kg 18 months after the start of the group.

The results are less good than those reported by Garrow (1975) and by Ashwell (1978) for commercial slimming clubs. The average weight loss of members answering questionnaires was as follows; Weightwatchers (UK) 11.8 ± 7.9 kg, Slimming Magazine Club 8.6 ± 5.4 kg, Silhouette Club 7.3 ± 4.6 kg, TOPS (Take Off Pounds Sensibly) 6.6 ± 7.2 kg, and Weightwatchers (Australia) 8.2 ± 6.4 kg. However, these data must be interpreted with caution: only 56.8% of members who were sent questionnaires replied, and it may be that those who did not reply were less successful than those who did. Furthermore the replies will tend to report the 'best' weight loss achieved, which is not the same as the weight loss at some arbitrary time from starting, such as 10 months, or 18 months.

A truer picture would emerge if commercial slimming clubs kept a prospective record of a random sample of their membership from the time of enrollment, but, as Dwyer and Berman (1978) point out, there are several reasons why this is not likely to happen. They sent questionnaires to members of a slimming club 2 years after enrolment and obtained only 28% replies. These studies involve extra trouble and expense both for the organisers of the slimming club and for the members surveyed, and it is not in the commercial interests of the club that 'failures' should be documented. There is natural reluctance on the part of the members who constitute these 'failures' to fill in long questionnaires from which they can receive no benefit. If one club submitted to a thorough examination of its long-term results, and these were published, competing commercial concerns would claim better results without having to substantiate these claims.

In view of the great difficulties in getting complete unbiased data about the performance of commercial slimming clubs the report of Seddon et al (1981) is of particular interest. In the Harrow Health District, London, a non-profit-making slimming club was set up using local health authority premises, and with trained dietitians as group leaders. The club meets one evening per week for two hours, usually between 1930 and 2130 h. Members pay £15.00 (about $US 22.00 at 1986 rate of exchange) for a 10-week course, and recurrent costs are covered when there are at least 14 members in the group. The group size is limited to 30 maximum: the first 14 courses had 249 members. The initial payment ensures the financial viability of the course, and provides an incentive for members to attend regularly. For regular attenders the total cost is less than that of commercial clubs which typically charge an enrolment fee and a weekly charge of about £3.00.

The age and obesity index of the first 249 members to enrol in the Harrow Slimming Club is shown in Figure 11.1. Of the membership 43% (108/249) were grade I obese, 42% were grade II, 5% were grade III and 10% grade 0. The age distribution ranged from the teens to the seventies. The course began and ended with a meeting run entirely by the group leader, and meetings 2–9 included either a film show relevant to weight loss and nutrition, or a talk by some visiting expert: physician, physiotherapist or psychologist. The attendance and weight change among members is shown in Figure 11.2. Despite the advance payment, 6 of the members did not return after the first meeting, so no data about weight change are available for them. Eight members gained weight: none of these attended more than 4 sessions. The remainder showed some weight loss: the maximum loss was 25.7 kg in a man who attended every session. The average weight loss for the 243 members who attended more than 1 session

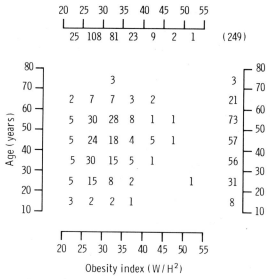

Fig. 11.1 Age (y) and QI (W/H²) among 249 people enrolling in first 14 courses of Harrow Slimming Club (Data of Seddon et al 1981)

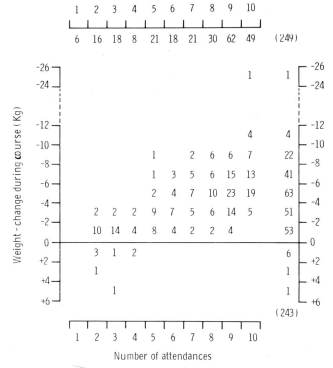

Fig. 11.2 Number of attendances (out of 10 possible) and weight change achieved by 249 people attending first 14 courses at Harrow Slimming Club (Data of Seddon et al 1981)

was 4.4 kg, and it is evident from Figure 11.2 that those members who attended more sessions tended to lose more weight.

At the end of the course, members who had attended at least 5 sessions were entitled to enrol in a follow-up course for another 10 weeks at which they were weighed weekly and counselled, but no formal instruction was given. This option was taken up by 110 members, and on average they attended 9.2 follow-up sessions. The average weight loss during the follow-up course was 0.6 kg, ranging from a gain from the end of the main course of 6.6 kg to a further loss of 20.0 kg. There was no significant relationship between the weight loss achieved on the main course and on the follow-up course.

These data illustrate the great variability in response which is seen with almost any form of treatment for obesity. Some members did very well: 131 members (53%) lost more than 4 kg in 10 weeks which must be regarded as satisfactory progress. There is no reason to believe that they would have done better if they had come to a hospital clinic. At the slimming club they received 20 hours of teaching and advice in 10 weeks, and had the benefit of discussion within the group, while at hospital in 10 weeks it is unlikely that they would have spent as much as 2 h in total actually talking to the doctor or dietitian. The cost to the health service of providing this amount of treatment is very high, but at the slimming club it is virtually zero, since the subscription fee covers the hire of films and sessional payment to the dietitian. On economic grounds, therefore, the case for the slimming club system is very strong.

The main argument against the slimming club is that perhaps some of the 118 members who failed to lose 4 kg in 10 weeks would have benefited from more intensive investigation and treatment, particularly those who attended regularly but failed to lose much weight. In this situation the hospital can provide a back-up service to take over the management of those club members who really need to lose weight, who really try, but do not achieve weight loss.

There can be no doubt that a proper integration of non-profit-making slimming clubs with professional dietitians as group leaders, backed up by a hospital service for special cases, is a practical and economical way of providing care for the large numbers of moderately obese people in the community. The treatment of obesity inevitably involves prolonged supervision with many follow-up visits, and if these visits must be made to a hospital in normal working hours this requires a major sacrifice for people in employment or looking after small children. The locally based slimming club is more economical for the patient, as well as for the health service. It is notable that the weight loss and attrition rate in the series reported by Seddon et al (1981) compares favourably with that reported by Stunkard & Brownell (1980) for work-site treatment of obesity. It may be that the system of a cost-covering down payment by the members, the convenient siting and timing of club meetings, and a thrifty desire to get good value for money combine to reduce the drop-out rate from the slimming club.

Since virtually any sustained weight loss is acceptable in grade I patients it is not necessary to specify the energy value of the reducing diet with any accuracy. If it is a nutritious diet which is causing a weight loss of about 0.5 kg (1 lb) per week, that is all that need be asked. The principles described in section 8.c. involve weighing portions of food, and calculating the energy value, which is tedious. Many people prefer approximate methods which work on the principle that if certain types of food are excluded from the diet the total energy content of the diet must decrease. A survey by the Consumers' Association showed that men preferred a 'no counting' method, and women living with a family a 'low carbohydrate' method (Rudinger 1978).

'NO COUNTING' DIET

All items of food are grouped into three categories: 'free' foods, which can be taken in unlimited quantity; 'restricted' foods, which can be taken in limited quantity, and 'forbidden' foods, which must be cut out completely.

Free foods are:
    Meat, eggs, cheese, poultry (without thick sauce or stuffing);
    Fish, boiled or steamed, not fried;
    Salads, without mayonnaise;
    Vegetables, cooked any way;
    Potatoes, not roast, fried or chip;
    Fresh fruit, or fruit bottled without sugar;
    Tea, coffee, Oxo, Bovril, Marmite, water;
    Condiments, Worcestershire sauce, saccharine.
These foods are the important protein sources, and either have a low energy value (like fresh fruit, vegetables and salads) or else are sufficiently expensive (like meat) to prevent vast overconsumption.

Forbidden foods are:
   Sugar, syrup, chocolate, sweets, cocoa, jam, honey, peanuts;
   Cakes, buns, biscuits, pastry, pies, tinned fruit;
   Spaghetti, rice, macaroni, semolina, puddings, ice cream;
   Alcohol, sweetened fruit juice.
These foods are concentrated energy sources, with relatively small contributions to essential nutrients in the diet.

Restricted foods are:
   Bread, butter, margarine, breakfast cereals, milk, cream, fats and oils.
These are staple foods which are sources of dietary fibre and of fat-soluble vitamins. Typically the allowance of bread is 3 slices (about 4 oz, or 100 g). The allowance of butter, margarine or cream is 1 oz (30 g), and of milk 1/2 pint (300 ml) to include that taken in tea or coffee. The allowance of restricted food can be varied to achieve the desired rate of weight loss. A short alcoholic drink, or a half-pint of beer, is roughly equivalent to a slice of bread and can, if necessary, be substituted.

The advantage of this type of diet is that there are only three types of food — bread, butter and milk — which have to be taken in measured quantities: all other foods are either free or forbidden. It is therefore very easy to calculate. The disadvantage is that if the only choice of food available is 'forbidden' food, the dieter must either starve or break the diet.

'LOW CARBOHYDRATE' DIET

The objective of this diet is to permit the consumption of virtually any food but, by limiting carbohydrate intake, to reduce total energy intake (Yudkin 1974). To use the diet it is necessary to refer to tables published by Slimming Magazine, or in some do-it-yourself slimmers' books (Yudkin 1958, Allan 1974, Rudinger 1978). These give 'carbohydrate units' (CU) for items of food, each unit is equivalent to about 5 g carbohydrate. For example 1 oz (30 g) of bread is 70 kcal and 3 CU, of sugar is 110 kcal and 6 CU, of roast beef is 55 kcal and 0 CU, of butter is 225 kcal and 0 CU, and of cheddar cheese is 120 kcal and 0 CU. It is suggested that the allowance of carbohydrate should be about 50 g (10 CU) per day. For the purpose of this diet alcohol is accorded carbohydrate equivalence, so 1 pint

(580 ml) of pale ale is 180 kcal and 9 CU, a single whisky is 50 kcal and 2.5 CU, and a glass of white wine is 125 kcal and 6 CU.

The diet enables the skilful slimmer to eat a great variety of food, and whatever the fare provided by a generous host it is theoretically possible to eat something and still remain within the limits of the diet. The weakness of the diet (and to a lesser extent of the 'no counting' diet) is that the skilful slimmer can observe the restrictions but maintain a high energy intake, for example by eating large quantities of cheese, which is zero-rated for carbohydrate units. Also it promotes the idea that some foods, such as meat, cheese, butter and margarine, are 'not fattening' despite their high energy content.

EXERCISE PROGRAMME

It is doubtful if group calisthenics have any part to play in the management of grade I patients. If the level of exercise is graded to that tolerable to the oldest and least fit of the group it will have little value to the younger and fitter members, and if different levels of exercise are used for different members this will cause embarassment and disaffection among the less fit. One of the reasons for joining a slimming group is to achieve better health and physical fitness, so the group leader should encourage each member to establish a personal quantitative measure of fitness at the outset, such as the maximum distance walked in 10 minutes, the number of stairs climbed without breathlessness, etc. The choice of fitness standard depends on the training and lifestyle of the subject, but it should involve aerobic exercise such as walking, cycling, jogging, stair-climbing or swimming rather than violent anaerobic exercise such as weight training.

The training programme must be gentle and gradual, so as not to cause injury or discouragement to the subject. Increasing exercise in the course of normal life is often more acceptable than setting aside time solely for physical training: very considerable increases in fitness will be achieved by sedentary people who start to use the stairs rather than a lift, or who walk or cycle to work rather than using motorised transport. It must be emphasised that the objective of the exercise is to increase fitness, not to lose weight, otherwise exercise and dieting will be used as alternative strategies to achieve weight loss, which they are not. The combination of weight loss and physical training will produce very gratifying increases in physical fitness, as assessed by the subject's personal fitness standard.

REASSURANCE

If no one ever increased in obesity above grade I, then obesity would not be a major public health problem. It follows that it does not matter very much if many people in grade I never achieve grade O, so long as they do not increase to grade II or III. However complacency about grade I obesity is misplaced, especially among young people, since the health hazards of overweight are so much greater in young people than in people over 50 years old. It is a matter for the clinical judgement of the group leader how hard individual members should be pushed to lose weight, and to what extent they should be reassured that it is all right to settle for their present weight. The judgement depends on many factors: mainly age and the presence of diseases associated with obesity, such as diabetes, heart disease or hypertension, or a family history of these diseases. It probably does not matter much if a fit grade I subject aged over 50 years does not lose weight: such people may wish to attend a slimming group for social support, and that seems a perfectly reasonable arrangement.

12

Management of grade 0 obesity

Bruch (1974) has an excellent chapter on what she calls 'thin fat people', i.e. formerly obese people who need the help of a psychiatrist because they find that the Promised Land of slimness does not come up to expectations. She cites the example of Beryl, a young woman who had reduced her weight from 114 kg to 61 kg and thereby gained the approval of her father. Although she now looked beautiful she was not satisfied: 'I want to be underweight so I can stop worrying about what I eat. I still cannot eat sweets like ordinary people. The minute I eat sweets my system craves a lot. I have to do one or the other, either diet — or go hog wild on sweets and all that stuff'. Her ambition to be so slim that she can eat sweets in unlimited quantity can never be fulfilled. She is already as slim as she can reasonably be, and however much she starved it would merely serve to reduce her metabolic requirements still further. Whatever benefits weight loss may bring, the ability to eat ad libitum without weight gain cannot be one of them.

This being so, was the effort to lose weight worth while? Usually the answer is 'yes'. People forget the disadvantages of obesity when they become thin. It is not as if the person who has reduced in weight has exchanged a carefree existence as a fat person for the tyranny of perpetual dieting. Even as a fat person it was not possible to eat unlimited sweets with impunity, and there were other disadvantages as well. Probably a psychiatrist such as Bruch sees a higher proportion of formerly obese patients who had totally unrealistic ideas about the benefits of weight loss, and who consequently suffered greater-than-average psychological trauma when these expectations were not fulfilled.

'Fat people are apt to blame all their difficulties on being fat and they hope for a new lease on life after they get thin.' (Bruch 1974). It is the responsibility of the therapist not only to guide the patient honestly about the means to achieve weight loss, but also about the realistic consequences of weight loss for that particular patient. The items which can reasonably be included in the prospectus are discussed in Chapter 1.e. Weight loss is usually a good bargain, but it should not be over-sold, or the therapist will lay up trouble for both himself and the patient in the future.

The way to make it as easy as possible for formerly obese patients to stay thin is to ensure that in the process of losing weight they do not lose an excessive amount of lean tissue. Of course their energy requirements after weight loss will be less than before weight loss, but they should not be less than that of a group of people of similar age, weight and FFM who have not lost weight (see Chapter 6.a).

Not all grade 0 patients are formerly obese: there is an important group of young women who demand specialist attention about their obesity although they are not, and never have been, obese. They are not thin enough to justify the diagnosis of anorexia nervosa, but they have the same morbid fear of weight gain. Some of these patients conform to the description of 'bulimia nervosa' (Russell 1979).

Compulsive eating is not clearly defined: it is not simply eating in response to hunger, it may far exceed the amount needed to satisfy hunger, and it is always associated with feelings of protest and self-criticism. The eating binge does not bring relief from the stress which precipitated it, and the compulsive eater reports heightened anxiety during the binge, because the situation is out of control, and it is not clear what can bring it to an end. About one-third of the patients coming to a hospital obesity clinic describe episodes of compulsive eating which have terminated previous attempts to diet, especially when 'crash diets' have produced a rapid weight loss which suddenly ceased. Compulsive eating is reported in these circumstances by both men and women, but among patients at a hospital obesity clinic women outnumber men by about 7 to 1.

Anyone who has personal experience of a restricted diet — not necessarily a low-energy diet, but any diet which has an abnormally high or low content of any major nutrient — realises that prolonged dietary restriction is very annoying, and whatever type of food is forbidden on the diet becomes unreasonably attractive. One does not have to invoke feminist concepts to explain the tensions which arise when a young woman of normal weight struggles unsuccessfully to force her weight to a still lower level in order to achieve a more acceptable figure. Non-existent obesity (or even genuine obesity) is often used as a whipping-boy for all sorts of dissatisfaction with social success: if only he or she were thin, then. . . . The supposed consequences of thinness are often highly improbable, especially in a grade 0 obese person who is only trying to lose a few pounds.

It is clearly inappropriate to give the normal-weight compulsive eater advice on a reducing diet, and still worse to prescribe anorectic drugs. It is important to try to find out why this person is trying to lose weight, what they would regard as an ideal weight, and what they expect to be able to do at this ideal weight which they cannot do now. Often patients have never formulated answers to these questions, and when they do so it provides some insight into their problem. When these questions are posed patients often keep returning to some alarming experience of weight gain which they fear will recur unless they are vigilant: having dieted for 2 weeks they put back all the weight they had lost in a single weekend. This experience is generalised to the conclusion that to maintain weight they can only eat 'normally' for 2 days in 14.

In this situation reassurance may help, backed by some scientific evidence. Yes, it is possible to gain one or two kilograms in one or two days by suddenly repleting empty glycogen stores. However, it is quite impossible to gain fat at the rate of a kilogram per day, since this would require an excess of intake over expenditure of more than 9000 kcal (28 MJ). In the long run weight can be maintained if, and only if, energy input matches energy output. The truth of this statement can be demonstrated in a metabolic ward, but it is impracticable to use such expensive facilities simply to allay the anxiety of normal-weight people about their metabolism.

Grade 0 compulsive eaters often benefit from a period of inpatient treatment in a metabolic ward in which the diet is strictly regulated. It demonstrates that they can maintain weight on a reasonable diet, and they do not have to worry about bingeing, since they are given no opportunity to binge. Some bulimic patients have asked to be fitted with a waist cord, and apparently find it helpful because they persuade themselves that they cannot binge because it would become too painful. This is not true, but if it serves as a psychological prop to the patient it does more good than harm.

The role of exercise in the management of grade 0 obesity is also largely psychological. Since the patient is convinced that her energy requirements are low, she is always at risk to gain weight, so she will adopt some strategy to avoid this calamity. Of the available options regular exercise is far healthier than a reducing diet or, worse, a policy of purging or vomiting. The bulimic patient is probably already quite active, and it is a good plan to encourage this. Thus her physical fitness will improve, and nothing disastrous will happen to body weight nor will her electrolyte balance be endangered, as it would be if she took purgatives or made herself vomit.

13

Management of obesity with non-insulin-dependent diabetes

The two diseases which make the biggest contribution to the excess mortality associated with obesity are coronary heart disease (CHD) and non-insulin-dependent diabetes mellitus (NIDDM). Since the former disease is such a common cause of death the excess deaths among obese people are mostly due to CHD, which will be discussed in the next chapter. However, the relative risk of death from NIDDM (compared with that of normal-weight people) is very greatly increased among obese people. For example in the American Cancer Society survey (Lew & Garfinkel 1979) the total mortality rate among men above 140% of average weight was 1.87 times that of average-weight men, but mortality from diabetes in these men was 5.19 times the mortality from diabetes in normal-weight men. The corresponding figures for women similarly overweight are 1.89 times greater total mortality, but 7.90 times greater diabetes mortality.

Diabetes mellitus occurs in two forms: insulin-dependent diabetes mellitus (IDDM) arises from a more of less total failure of the beta cells in the islets of Langerhans in the pancreas, so virtually no insulin is produced. This form usually starts in childhood, and without insulin the patient goes into diabetic coma and dies. Non-insulin-dependent diabetes mellitus (NIDDM) is much the most common form of diabetes; its onset is usually in adult life, and patients rarely go into diabetic coma. The islets of Langerhans appear normal microscopically, and indeed secrete more insulin than in a normal person, but this insulin does not have normal effectiveness in controlling carbohydrate metabolism, and other aspects of metabolism in the body.

NIDDM is a disease which affects susceptible people: its incidence increases with increasing age and increasing obesity. The work of Leslie & Pyke (1985) indicates that the susceptibility to the disease is genetically determined, since if one twin of a monozygotic pair becomes diabetic the other almost always does so too, but with dizygotic twins the linkage is less strong. This susceptibility is commoner in black people than white.

The three-dimensional histograms shown in Figure 13.1 are constructed using the analysis by Bonham & Brock (1985) of data from the 1976 National Health Interview Survey in the USA. One of the questions asked was: 'Does anyone in the family have diabetes or sugar diabetes?' Positive responses from people below the age of 17 years were excluded, which left about 70 000 people over the age of 20 years who reported that they had diabetes. In this analysis prevalence rates are reported by race, sex, age and obesity. Cut-off points were selected in order to obtain adequate numbers in each cell. Age groups were 20–44 years, 45–54 years, 55–64 years and

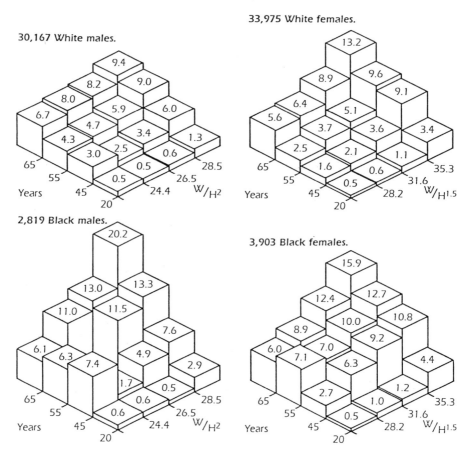

Fig. 13.1 Prevalence of reported diabetes acording to race, sex, age and obesity status (Analysis of Bonham & Brock 1985 of data from 1976 National Health Interview Survey)

65 years and over. The index of obesity for men was W/H^2 , and the 60th, 80th and 90th centiles were 24.38, 26.50, and 28.48 respectively. For women the index used was $W/H^{1.5}$, and the same centile points fell at values of 28.23, 31.57, and 35.28 respectively. For simplicity these values have been rounded to the nearest decimal place in Figure 13.1.

Both black and white men and women in the lowest age and obesity groups have a low prevalence of reported adult-onset diabetes, but in both sexes and races the prevalence increases both with increasing age and increasing obesity. This effect is seen more strongly in women than in man, and more in Blacks than in whites (Bonham & Brock 1985). In both sexes and races the prevalence increased from about 0.5% to about 6% with increasing age in the least-obese section of the population (roughly corresponding to grade 0 obesity), but with increasing obesity at each age the prevalence is higher. Among the black population the sample size was smaller, so the progression of increasing prevalence is less smooth. This study illustrates very clearly that young obese people have a prevalence of diabetes which would be expected at a much greater age among normal-weight people.

It is remarkable that the effect of obesity in predisposing to NIDDM emerges so clearly in the study cited above, since figures for prevalence, and even more so reported prevalence, tend to underestimate the contribution of obesity to the aetiology of NIDDM. This point can be shown by comparing the prevalence with the incidence of NIDDM in the Pima Indians. This group of pleasant people have lived for many centuries in the extremely hot and dry Sonoran desert in southern Arizona. Survival in that land is possible only because the Gila river provides water for irrigation, so the Pima Indians, unlike many other American Indian tribes, have for many generations been a separate, settled, trading and farming community on the banks of the river. These are conditions in which special genetic traits may emerge under evolutionary pressure, and the most well-studied trait of the Pima Indians is their susceptibility to NIDDM, which is among the highest in the world (Bennett et al 1976). Of all Pimas over the age of 35 years about 50% have diabetes. Diabetes is here defined by a plasma glucose concentration over 200 mg% (11.1 mmol/l) 2 hours after an oral load of 75 g glucose.

Figure 13.2 shows the relation of obesity to age- and sex-adjusted prevalence rates of NIDDM among the Pima Indians (Knowler et

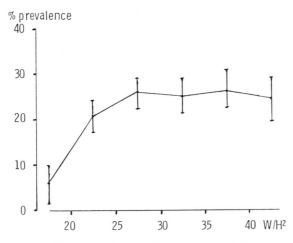

Fig. 13.2 Age- and sex-adjusted prevalence of diabetes in Pima Indians according to obesity status (Data of Knowler et al 1981)

al 1981). It appears that, while there is clearly a reduced prevalence among very thin Pimas, NIDDM is roughly equally prevalent in normal-weight and obese individuals, so these data give no indication that obesity has much to do with the aetiology of NIDDM.

However, Figure 13.3 shows that obesity is very highly correlated with the *incidence* of NIDDM. These results are based on data from 3137 subjects who were examined at least twice, normally at intervals of about 2 years. The W/H^2 value refers to the body build *before* the diabetes was diagnosed. The reason for the lack of association between obesity and the prevalence of NIDDM is that many patients lose weight rather rapidly at the time of onset of the disease, so cross-sectional studies do not detect their previous obesity.

The observation that fat people are more likely to develop NIDDM than thin people does not prove that the fatness causes the NIDDM. It might simply mean that the genetic make-up which predisposes to NIDDM also predisposes to fatness, or even that the NIDDM caused the fatness. This last explanation is not tenable, since we have already seen that obesity preceded the onset of NIDDM.

Sims et al (1973) attempted the definitive experiment to see if obesity could cause NIDDM in normal people with no family history of NIDDM. They overfed 19 male volunteers in the Vermont state prison so they increased body weight by 21% and body fat by 73%. After weight gain these men had significantly increased fasting blood

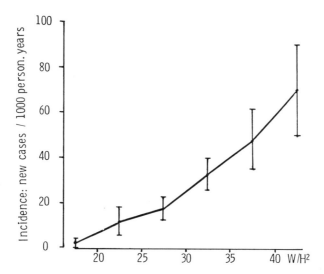

Fig. 13.3 Incidence of new cases of diabetes among Pima Indians according to obesity status. Compare this with Figure 13.2 which failed to indicate importance of obesity in precipitating the onset of diabetes (Data of Knowler et al 1981).

glucose, insulin and triglyceride concentrations, significantly decreased glucose tolerance to both oral and intravenous glucose loads, and a significantly increased insulin response to oral or intravenous glucose and to intravenous arginine. In short, although they had not become diabetic they showed the changes of insulin resistance which are characteristic of NIDDM, and which are also seen in spontaneous obesity.

Is the insulin resistance seen in obesity the same as the insulin resistance seen in NIDDM? The exact mechanism of insulin resistance is still a matter for continuing research, and this work is too complex to be described in any detail here. Briefly, insulin resistance in vivo is measured using clamp techniques. In a euglycaemic insulin clamp study, plasma insulin concentration is increased and maintained at about 100 u/ml above basal levels by an infusion of 40 U/min of insulin, and glucose is infused at a rate sufficient to maintain basal levels of glucose. Meanwhile the hepatic glucose production rate can be measured by infusing tritiated glucose, and onserving the dilution of the tritium label by unlabelled glucose coming from the liver. A similar technique can be used with a constant glucose infusion and variable insulin (a glucose clamp study). These can be done with the steady level of glucose or insulin at normal or at elevated levels.

DeFronzo et al (1985) have compared the insulin resistance of obese and diabetic subjects using these techniques and they conclude that 'The primary cause of the impairment of glucose metabolism in obesity is insulin resistance, whereas both insulin resistance and insulin deficiency contribute to the glucose intolerance in diabetes mellitus' and 'The metabolic abnormalities that characterise both the obese and diabetic state appear to be quite similar.' There are also striking similarities in the effect of insulin resistance in obese and diabetic patients on protein metabolism (Nair et al 1987).

It is probably fair to suggest that the scheme shown in Figure 13.4 indicates the sequence of events which decides if a person born with a liability to NIDDM develops the disease or retains normal glucose tolerance. If the individual becomes obese (step a) this will have the effect observed in the Vermont study, namely insulin resistance (b), which is initially compensated for by increased insulin secretion, but which still does not control glucose and lipid metabolism adequately (c). If this goes on long enough the capacity of the beta cells to secrete insulin at much higher than normal rates becomes exhausted (d) and thus the situation is reached that reduced insulin secretion is associated with insulin resistance, and this is characteristic of NIDDM (e). The other side of the diagram indicates that if the individual had maintained normal body fat he might have retained normal glucose tolerance. There is a query in this pathway, because

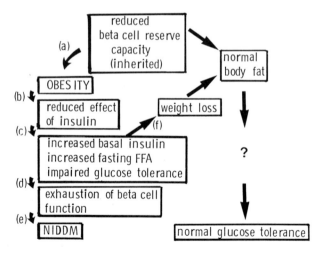

Fig. 13.4 Scheme showing the sequence of events which may cause an individual with liability to diabetes to develop the disease (left side) or retain normal glucose tolerance (right side). Maintenance of normal body fat is crucial step

the ability to retain normal glucose tolerance obviously depends on the original inherited deficit in beta cell function.

A point about which there is controversy concerns step (a) in Figure 13.4. Does the inheritance of a diabetic tendency in some way predispose to obesity? A possible link is the observed reduced thermic effect of glucose in glucose-tolerant Pima Indians (Bogardus et al 1985b). This has been reported also in obese subjects both before and after weight loss (Schutz et al 1984). However both obese and diabetic subjects have higher than normal RMRs, so if total energy expenditure is calculated the reduced thermic response cannot explain the tendency to obesity (Nair et al 1986). A similar comment may be made about the recent study by Devlin & Horton (1986) on the thermic effects of exercise and insulin infusions in normal, obese and diabetic subjects. There was some diminution in the thermogenic response of obese and diabetic subjects ater exercise, but their total energy expenditure was still greater than that of the normal controls.

Clinically the most important step in Figure 13.4 is (f), which indicates that the obese person with impaired glucose tolerance can escape from NIDDM and achieve normal glucose tolerance by weight loss if that step is taken before the beta cells have become exhausted. Henry et al (1986) review many studies which have shown improved glucose tolerance in obese diabetics after weight loss, and provide information about the mechanisms involved. They studied 8 obese diabetics on weight-maintenance diet when they weighed 103 kg, and again after 3 weeks on weight-maintenance diet some 60–380 days later when they had reduced to 86 kg. The loss of 17 kg was associated with a 55% decrease in fasting plasma glucose concentration, a 37% decrease in hepatic glucose output, and an increase of 135% to 165% in peripheral glucose disposal during eugylycaemic glucose clamp studies. They conclude that in obese diabetics

'weight loss results in improved glucose homeostasis with 1) reduced basal hepatic glucose output predominantly responsible for lowering fasting glucose levels, 2) improved postprandial glucose excursions with marked amelioration of peripheral insulin resistance due to improved post-receptor insulin action, which is at least partly due to enhanced glucose transport system activity; and 3) unchanged absolute insulin levels in the face of markedly reduced glycaemia, indicative of enhanced beta-cell sensitivity to insulinogenic stimuli.'

They point out that these changes are attributable to the weight loss, not the low-energy diet, because both sets of tests were performed in a weight-stable state.

Obese diabetics cannot necessarily expect to be cured by weight loss, because a person who has progressed too far towards beta cell exhaustion cannot expect to regain normal glucose tolerance. Probably the report of Modan et al (1986) provides the best indication of how changes in obesity status affect the risk of subsequent glucose intolerance and diabetes. This was a study of a representative sample of 2140 Israelis aged 40–70, whose W/H^2 had been measured on 2 occasions 10 years apart. They were assigned to low (W/H^2 <23), medium (W/H^2 23–26.9) and high (W/H^2 >27) groups. Those individuals who were in the low, medium and high W/H^2 group at the time of both examinations had prevalences of impaired glucose tolerance (IGT) of 22.4%, 27.4% and 47.0% respectively. The 92 individuals who were in the 'low' group ten years previously, but in the 'medium' group at the second examination had a prevalence of IGT of 21.2%, which was very similar to the currently 'low' individuals. However the 90 present 'medium' people who had been formerly 'high' had a prevalence of 40.0%, which is intermediate between those who were constantly high (47.0%) and those who were constantly 'medium' (27.4%).

The message therefore seems to be that although weight reduction in overweight people reduces the proportion who will develop impaired glucose tolerance, the past record still leaves its legacy. If the idea of beta cell exhaustion is valid, then the sooner weight is reduced the greater will be the remaining capacity to secrete insulin and the greater the chance of living without clinically significantly impaired glucose tolerance.

MANAGEMENT OF THE OBESE DIABETIC

Newburgh (1938) published a startling paper entitled: 'A new interpretation of diabetes mellitus in obese middle-aged persons: recovery through reduction of weight.' The recorded discussion after the paper indicates that the diabetes experts of the day did not really understand the significance of his message, which was summarised in his concluding remarks: 'I look upon the hyperglycaemia and glycosuria in the middle-aged, obese group as a complication of obesity. To my mind the primary condition is overweight and the lessened ability to lay down glycogen is a complication of the obesity.

In these persons the slowed glycogenesis can be corrected by reducing weight to normal.'

Many workers in the last half-century have confirmed Newburgh's opinion (Genuth 1979, Liu et al 1985), but still the dietary treatment of NIDDM in obese people is given little emphasis. For example a recent paper from the Mayo Clinic in a prestigious journal reported a comparison of treatment of NIDDM by sulphonylureas or exogenous insulin (Firth et al 1986). The patients were grade II obese, and during the study they were on a weight-maintaining diet. The authors conclude that sulphonylureas and exogenous insulin result in equal improvement in insulin action in these patients, so 'the choice between these agents should be based on considerations other than their ability to ameliorate insulin resistance.'

In an editorial comment in the same issue Martin (1986) begins by asking: 'What is one to do for patients with non-insulin-dependent diabetes whose blood sugar levels do not fall into a satisfactory range after an appropriate trial of diet?' He goes on to discuss oral agents and insulin, each of which has problems, but does not define what is 'an appropriate trial of diet'. If patients with NIDDM are given half-hearted dietary advice, and put on medication at the next visit if their blood glucose is still raised, many cases will miss the opportunity to escape down the right-hand pathway in Figure 13.4.

The problem with obese patients with NIDDM is insulin resistance. When insulin is synthesised it is a long curled molecule (proinsulin) which is later chopped at two points to form the double-stranded biologically active insulin molecule, and a waste length of connecting peptide (C-peptide). From the rate of urinary excretion of C-peptide it is possible to calculate the rate of insulin secretion. In a normal person this will be about 30 U/day, in an insulin-dependent diabetic it may be virtually nil, while in an obese diabetic it will be perhaps 50 U/day (Genuth 1973). An obese non-diabetic may secrete over 100 U/day. Therefore,the logical approach to the treatment of an obese diabetic is to try to reduce insulin resistance, not to try to increase insulin production yet further by giving sulphonylurea drugs, thus flogging the failing pancreas. It is still less logical to give exogenous insulin unless this is absolutely necessary, since this further complicates rational dietary therapy. In either case the drug treatment puts the patient at risk of hypoglycaemia, which is very unlikely to occur with dietary treatment. Biguanide drugs are regarded with suspicion in the USA, but metformin is probably the best drug to use as an oral hypoglycaemic in obese diabetics.

If the objective in treating obese patients with NIDDM is to reduce insulin resistance, there are two tools available with which this may be achieved — diet and exercise — and if at all possible they should both be used.

Until recently, teaching about diabetic diets has been very confused and contradictory: the permitted amount of carbohydrate in the diet was finely judged to steer the diabetic between the perils of hyperglycaemia and hypoglycaemia. Certainly the dietary management of thin insulin-dependent diabetics may be a tricky problem, but the dietary management of obese diabetics is delightfully simple: it is simply a vigorous version of the treatment of obesity. Genuth (1979) comments that when put on a 'protein-sparing fast' diet untreated NIDDM patients become normoglycaemic in 3 weeks, and patients who have been taken off sulphonylurea drugs show a steady decline of blood sugar to normal levels over a period of several months. The mechanism by which this transformation occurs has been documented: when energy intake is restricted there is an increase in insulin sensitivity even before there is any significant weight loss. Both fasting and post-prandial glucose decreases with little change in insulin concentration, insulin-stimulated glucose disposal improves, and plasma cholesterol and triglyceride concentrations decrease (Liu et al 1985). These changes can reliably be shown in virtually any patient with NIDDM in a metabolic ward, where the diet can be strictly controlled, but the results cited above by Liu et al (1985) were in fact achieved in a series of obese NIDDM outpatients.

It is not suggested that the 'protein-sparing fast' is the ideal diet for NIDDM patients: Genuth's experience was quoted to show that we need no longer be so concerned about the diabetes of the obese diabetic — if we effectively treat his or her obesity the diabetes will automatically improve. Policy statements on dietary management of diabetes have been issued by the American Diabetes Association (1979) and the British Diabetic Association (1982) which are essentially similar. They agree in stating 'Ultimately, total energy intake is probably the key to diabetic control'. In the case of the obese diabetic, energy balance is not an objective: a daily energy deficit of 500–800 kcal (2.0–3.4 MJ) will simplify diabetic control and provide a rate of weight loss in the range shown in Figure 9.1. Although insulin resistance develops rather early in the development of obesity, and does not greatly increase with progression to massive obesity (Bogardus et al 1985a), the regain of insulin sensitivity occurs at an early stage of weight loss.

Within the limits of desired energy intake the main source of calories should be complex carbohydrate. The old-fashioned restrictions on carbohydrate in the diabetic diet were based on the belief that a high-carbohydrate diet caused large post-prandial increases in blood glucose, and that these should be avoided. In fact a diet high in complex carbohydrate gives better control of blood sugar than an iso-energetic high fat diet (Hockaday et al 1978), but simple sugars (glucose, sucrose, etc.) should be restricted in the diet of the obese diabetic. Fat should not provide more than 35% of the diet energy and protein about 12%.

It is also recommended that diabetic diets should be high in dietary fibre, in order to delay the digestion and absorption of associated dietary carbohydrates, and thus to avoid uncontrolled post-prandial peaks in blood glucose. However, there was no significant difference in glucose or lipid metabolism in NIDDM patients when high-carbohydrate diets were compared which contained either high (27 g/1000 kcal) or normal (11 g/1000 kcal) amounts of fibre (Hollenbeck et al 1986).

Physical training also increases insulin sensitivity in NIDDM, although the mechanism by which this occurs is not entirely clear (Krotkiewski & Bjorntorp 1986). The study of Krotkiewski et al (1984) showed that the effect did not depend on fat loss. In that study 10 obese women (weight 96.3 ± 4.1 kg) undertook 3 exercise sessions per week for 3 months, while eating ad libitum. Neither body weight nor body fat decreased at all, but fitness increased as measured by heart rate and blood pressure during graded exercises. There was no significant change in glucose tolerance after a 100 g oral glucose load, but both insulin and C-peptide concentrations decreased, indicating an enhanced insulin sensitivity. A similar increase in insulin sensitivity was reported by Trovati et al (1984) after a 6-week programme of exercise for 1 h daily, 7 days/week at 50–60% of maximal oxygen uptake. Annuzzi et al (1985) report that glucose intolerant subjects were less physically fit, and took less leisure-time exercise, than normal subject of similar age, sex and degree of obesity.

In their review of the effect of exercise treatment in diabetes mellitus Krotkiewski & Bjorntorp (1986) observe that some studies have shown very little improvement in the glucose tolerance of patients with NIDDM after physical training, and that these benefits are seen only in those subjects who also show objective signs of increasing fitness, such as a higher maximal oxygen uptake or lower heart rate. Some of the improved glucose tolerance is associated with the depletion and repletion of muscle glycogen which occurs during and after fairly strenuous exercise. The response to exercise also varies with the pattern of fat distribution (Krotkiewski & Bjorntorp 1986).

This chapter has concentrated on glucose tolerance in non-insulin-dependent diabetes, and the relation to obesity. However, this field overlaps with the topic of the next chapter: hypertension, hyperlipidaemia and coronary heart disease. It is not just a coincidence that obesity and glucose intolerance combine to increase the risk of death from coronary heart disease as shown in Figure 1.10 (Fuller et al 1980). There is a strong association between glucose intolerance and hypertension. Modan et al (1985) and Christleib et al (1985) suggest that hyperinsulinaemia may be the link between these two conditions, both of which are also independently associated with increasing age and obesity.

14

Management of obesity with hypertension or hyperlipidaemia

Epidemiological evidence about the contribution of obesity to cardio-vascular disease appears paradoxical to the initiated. Life insurance data show that mortality among overweight people is increased, and a large proportion of the excess mortality is due to deaths from cardiovascular disease (see Figure 1.7). This is not just a peculiarity of those who take out life insurance, because the same trend is seen in other types of survey not using insured people (Lew & Garfinkel 1979). However large surveys, set up especially to investigate the causes of cardiovascular disease and other causes of death in middle-aged men (Keys et al 1972a, 1984, Paffenberger et al 1986) report that increased weight-for-height makes no contribution to excess mortality, or even has a protective effect in some instances.

These paradoxical results arise for several reasons, of which confounding variables are probably the most important. It is very difficult to analyse the results of large surveys in a manner which gives the correct weight to each variable when many variables are related to each other and interact with each other. Two experts may arrive at different conclusions from the same data. For example, Hubert (1984) interprets the results of Keys et al to show an inde-pendent association between obesity and coronary heart disease and myocardial infarction, while the investigators who collected the data do not. The difficulty arises in the calculation of 'independent' risk, which can be illustrated by following example.

Noah, we are told (*Genesis* 7:19) was instructed to take into his ark a pair of each animal species. Assuming that among the animals who were competing for the available space there were elephants and mammoths (both very large, trunk-bearing animals) he may have noted that the ark-sinking propensity of a group of animals could be predicted by the proportion of trunk-bearing animals in the group. If some of the elephants were of the small Cretan form he might further discover (when suitable correction had been made for trunk-prevalence), that if he included a high proportion of Cretan elephants in his cargo this actually increased the buoyancy of his ark. Since we have the benefit of the insights provided by Archimedes we can easily see that Noah in the above example was misled by the confounding variables of trunk-bearing and weight.

Of course all this is very well known to epidemiologists, and they try very hard not to be misled by confounding variables. However, in analysing the contribution of obesity to cardiovascular disease the problem is that so many of the risk factors for heart disease are themselves associated with changes in body weight: cigarette smoking is associated with decreased body weight, but age, hypertension, hyperlipidaemia and impaired glucose tolerance are associated with increased body weight. Whether an 'independent' effect of obesity on cardiovascular disease is found depends on the loading used to 'correct' for these risk factors.

Obesity and incidence of cardiovascular disease

It is probably best to start with data on incidence of cardiovascular disease by age, sex and degree of obesity, such as that shown in Figure 14.1, taken from the Framingham study (Hubert 1984). It is obvious that, in both sexes, and in both age groups, the individuals who were more than 130% of desirable weight suffered a greater incidence of cardiovascular disease than those who were less than 110% of desirable weight. But is the obesity contributing to the disease, or is it (like the elephant's trunk) a confounding variable attached to true risk factors such as hypertension and high blood cholesterol? In other words, if an obese person happens to have normal blood pressure and blood lipids would weight loss confer any protection against cardiovascular disease? Hubert (1984) concludes that it would:

> We were able to observe the 'independent' role of obesity in predicting long-term risk by adjusting for the influence of the coexisting levels of the major cardiovascular disease risk factors, including age, systolic blood pressure, serum cholesterol, cigarettes smoked per day, glucose tolerance, and electrocardiographic left ventricular hypertrophy. Results showed that the percent of desirable weight on initial examination was a significant, independent predictor of the 26-year incidence of coronary disease (both angina and coronary disease other than angina), coronary death and congestive failure in men. The

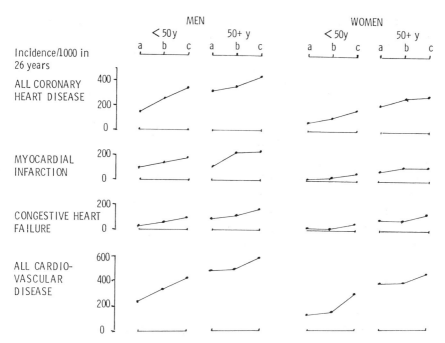

Fig. 14.1 Incidence of cardiovascular disease by age, sex and obesity status in Framingham cohort: (a) less than 110% of desirable weight, (b) 110–130% of desirable weight, (c) more than 130% of desirable weight (Data of Hubert 1984)

degree of obesity in women was also positively and independently associated with coronary disease, atherothrombotic stroke, congestive failure and coronary and cardiovascular disease death. In fact obesity among women was one of the best predictors of cardiovascular disease, following only age and blood pressure in relative importance. Similar 'multivariate' results were evident when body mass, calculated as weight divided by height squared, was used as the index of obesity.

Others disagree (Keys et al 1984):

The risk of all-causes or CHD death did not increase with increasing relative body weight in any of the regions of the study. The only region in which relative weight was significant was southern Europe where the probability of all-causes death was *decreased* with increasing body mass index. . . . This is not to say, however, that relative weight is unimportant at the extremes of the population distribution. It appears that both extreme obesity and extreme emaciation carry excessive risks of premature death.

Perhaps this contradiction will be resolved when we have a better understanding of the significance of the pattern of fat distribution in the body. Coronary heart disease is a particularly male disease, to which pre-menopausal women are remarkably immune (see Figure 14.1). New light has been thrown on the relation of fat distribution to cardiovascular disease and death in middle-aged men by the report of Larsson et al (1984) on their 13-year follow-up study of a random sample of 792 men born in Gotenberg in 1913, and first examined in 1967, at age 54 years. Their W/H^2 was 25 ± 3.3, and more than half smoked cigarettes. During 13 years of follow-up, 33 cases of stroke, 91 cases of ischaemic heart disease and 109 deaths were recorded among men without previous evidence of myocardial infarction. The incidence of stroke was positively associated with the waist : hip circumference ratio (W/H), but ischaemic heart disease and total mortality was negatively associated with W/H^2, but positively associated with smoking, in this sample. Stroke, ischaemic heart disease and total deaths were all positively associated with waist : hip circumference ratio, but not independently when serum cholesterol and blood pressure were included in the multivariate analysis. Data for women aged 38–60 also show a significant association between waist:hip circumference ratio and myocardial infarction and death in the following 12 years (Lapidus et al 1984). In Paris, Ducimetiere et al (1986) studied 6718 men aged 42–53 years, with 6.6 years follow-up, during which there were 212 coronary heart disease events. These were positively associated with fatness (judged by skinfolds) and particularly truncal fatness.

These studies suggest a special role in heart disease for intra-abdominal fat, which discharges its lipid directly into the portal circulation and thus exposes the liver to high fatty acid concentrations. A high rate of fat oxidation itself inhibits glucose utilization, since factors common to the Krebs cycle and glycolytic pathways become limiting (DeFronzo et al 1985). Similarly, Weinsier et al (1985) report a significant association between hypertension and central fat distribution. It may turn out, therefore, that intra-abdominal fat, rather than total body fat, is the important factor in determining liability to cardiovascular disease, and since typically middle-aged men show an increase in intra-abdominal fat this may in part explain the difference in incidence of heart disease between men and women.

BODY WEIGHT AND HYPERTENSION

Although there is room for debate about the independent role of weight in the aetiology of cardiovascular disease there can be no doubt that obesity is associated with hypertension, which is certainly a risk factor. Many studies which confirm this association have recently been reviewed by Hubert (1986). The association does not continue into extreme values, i.e. very obese people are not very hypertensive, but with increasing obesity there is an increasing proportion of subjects with diastolic pressures of 90–104 mmHg (Velasquez & Hoffmann 1985).

The association between obesity and hypertension is seen in both black and white populations, and in adolescents as well as adults (Buzina et al 1986). A study of black physicians with measurements at medical school, and again 22 years later, confirmed the association of hypertension with concurrent obesity, and showed that moderate obesity as students, and increase in body weight since leaving medical school, both significantly predicted hypertension in later adult life (Neser et al 1986). They conclude: 'Weight control would appear to be a potentially important nonpharmacologic hypertension risk reduction measure.' However, the association between age and blood pressure is independent of weight, so even normal-weight people will develop increasing blood pressure with increasing age (Pan et al 1986).

There is impressive and increasing evidence that hyperinsulinaemia is a factor linking hypertension and obesity. Studies in Israel (Modan et al 1985) and the USA (Lucas et al 1985, Christlieb et al 1985) have shown a highly significant association between hypertension and glucose intolerance, or serum insulin concentration, when other variables such as age, weight and serum glucose were controlled. This association is of great clinical importance, since it links the liability of obese people to develop non-insulin-dependent diabetes (discussed in the last chapter) with their liability to develop cardiovascular diseases. If it is true that high insulin levels predispose to hypertension this is another reason for trying to treat NIDDM by reducing insulin resistance, rather than by seeking to raise serum insulin levels still further to achieve normoglycaemia. It also suggests that the strategies which improve insulin sensitivity in obese diabetics, namely a restricted energy diet, weight loss and increased exercise, should be beneficial in the management of obese hypertensive patients also.

WEIGHT LOSS AND HYPERTENSION

The efficacy of dietary treatment in preventing coronary heart disease is a perennial subject for debate: for some commentators the evidence is strong that the consumption of saturated fats should be reduced throughout the population (Keys 1986), while others point to weak links in the chain of logic (Mitchell 1984). The argument cannot easily be settled, because it is impossible to show that an individual has suffered, or been saved from, coronary heart disease by virtue of his diet. In the case of weight loss and hypertension the evidence is clearer, since the effect of weight loss can be seen immediately in obese hypertensive subjects.

Borkan et al (1986) report on the effect of weight change over a period of 15 years on 8 putative coronary disease risk factors in 1396 men participating in the Veterans Administration Normative Ageing Study. The men were screened at entry to provide an initially healthy population: the mean age at entry was 42 years. Seventy-five men lost more than 10% body weight in the 15-year follow-up period, 168 gained more than 10%, and the remainder showed smaller weight changes. Weight change was significantly related to all the risk factors (increasing weight made the risk worse in each case) but the correlation between weight change and blood pressure (systolic 0.15, diastolic 0.22, both $P<0.01$) was greater than for the other 6 risk factors (cholesterol, triglycerides, fasting glucose, post-prandial glucose, uric acid and forced vital capacity). The magnitude of the observed change in systolic/diastolic pressure (mmHg) was $-6.5/-6.9$ among the men who lost more than 10% of body weight, and $+7.4/+3.0$ among those who gained more than 10% body weight, with intermediate values for intermediate weight changes. Borkan et al (1986) conclude: 'After controlling for initial levels of the risk factor, weight, age, and smoking status, change in weight remained a significant predictor of long-term change in each of the risk factors studied.' This is a very important conclusion, because it shows that these risk factors associated with obesity are reversible by weight loss in a normal population.

Rissanen et al (1985) report the results of 12-month counselling programmes designed to cause weight loss, decrease in salt intake, or both, in a series of 64 obese (Grade II) hypertensive patients aged about 45 years. The results at the start, after 3 months and after 12 months were for the weight-loss group: weight 96.8, 89.9 and 90.6 kg, and for blood pressure 159.0/101.0, 143.5/91.0, and 147.5/94.0 mmHg. The weight loss and salt restricted group had the following results: weight 87.0, 82.0 and 82.0 kg, and blood pressure 150.0/98.0, 139.5/87.5 and 143.5/93.0 mmHg. The salt restricted only group results were: weight 90.2, 88.6 and 90.8 kg, and blood pressure 154.0/100.0, 149.0/98.0 and 150.0/97.5 mmHg. The authors conclude: 'Improved BP control was strongly related to weight loss but not to reduced sodium excretion. Weight reduction programmes with even modest success help most obese patients with established hypertension, whereas moderate salt restriction gives little added benefit.'

MacMahon et al (1985) compared a 21-week course of weight reduction with the drug metoprolol (100 mg b.d.) in a randomised placebo-controlled trial on 56 young overweight patients. Two subject in the placebo group withdrew from the trial, 2 in the metoprolol group, and 3 in the weight reduction group. All results were analysed on the basis of 'intention to treat'. The change in weight and systolic/diastolic bloodpressure in the weight reduction group was −7.4 kg and −13.3/−9.8 mmHg. The change in the metropolol group was +2.0 kg and −9.9/−6.2 mmHg, and in the placebo group +0.5 kg and −7.4/−3.1 mmHg. In the weight reduction group the ratio of total cholesterol to HDL-cholesterol changed favourably from 5.2 to 4.6, but in the drug-treated group the ratio worsened from 5.4 to 6.4. The authors conclude: 'The results suggest that in the first step of treatment for hypertension in overweight patients, modest weight reduction produces significant and clinically important reductions in blood pressure, without incurring the adverse effects on plasma lipids and lipoproteins often associated with the first step of drug therapy.'

Croft et al (1986) note that obese hypertensive patients in general practice are better at losing weight than obese normotensive patients (8.0 kg vs 6.1 kg at 6 months). They conclude: 'Weight reduction appears to be an effective first-line therapy for approximately 50% of obese patients with mild to moderate hypertension, and raised blood pressure appears to provide motivation for such patients to attend a dietitians clinic and lose weight.'

Cohen & Flamenbaum (1986) report the effect of a VLCD for 10.6 ± 5.4 weeks on the blood pressure of severely obese hypertensive subjects. Thirty subjects who were previously not on medication for hypertension reduced in weight from 108.2 kg to 88.1 kg, and in blood pressure from 143.1/95.2 mmHg to 123.3/77.2 mmHg. Subjects who were on medication reduced from 102.5 kg to 84.5 kg, and in blood pressure from 139.6/88.6 mmHg to 127.2/81.5 mmHg, and also reduced their medication significantly. The authors comment: 'Given the large weight losses in the majority of subjects, there appears to be a degree of weight loss beyond which further decrements of blood pressure will not occur.' However, since the decrease in blood pressure was maintained at follow-up 8 weeks after the end of the dieting period they conclude that the decrease was due to weight loss, not just a direct effect of the diet. At the other extreme, small weight losses do not necessarily affect blood pressure either: Haynes et al (1984) report no decrease in blood pressure in mildly hypertensive obese subjects who lost 4.1 kg in a 6-month behaviourally-orientated weight loss programme.

In summary: most obese patients are moderately hypertensive, and probably the mechanism accounting to this is related to the insulin insensitivity which goes with obesity. Most trials which have achieved weight reduction, or which have observed spontaneous weight change, have found corresponding changes in blood pressure which are small, but clinically significant. Drug treatment of hypertension often has adverse effects (Editorial 1986), so first step treatment by weight reduction is logical with reference to hypertension itself, as well as to diminish the other health hazards associated with obesity.

SERUM CHOLESTEROL AND HEART DISEASE

One of the few points on which epidemiologists are virtually agreed is that middle-aged men with high serum cholesterol concentrations tend to die young. Any quibbling on the matter must surely be silenced by the publication by Martin et al (1986) of the 6-year mortality figures from 361 622 men aged 35–57 years, who were screened for the Multiple Risk Factor Intervention Trial (MRFIT). The relation of serum cholesterol concentration to age-adjusted 6-year total mortality, and coronary heart disease mortality is shown in Figure 14.2. These results leave no room for doubt that coronary mortality increases steadily from concentrations of 181 mg/dl (4.68 mmol/l), and rather more steeply above concentrations of 246 mg/dl (6.36 mmol/l), so men in this upper band have a risk of dying of coronary heart disease which is 3.4 times greater than that of men in the lowest band of cholesterol concentrations.

The increase in total and coronary heart disease mortality with increasing centiles of serum cholesterol is almost exactly superimposable on the curves for mortality related to centiles of diastolic blood pressure (Martin et al 1986). The significance of this finding

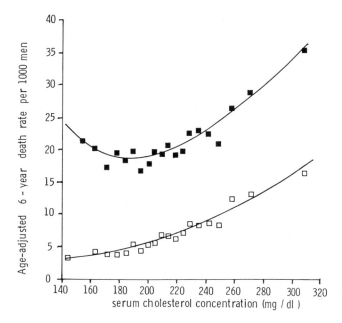

Fig. 14.2 Relation of serum cholesterol concentration to 6-year age-adjusted mortality from all causes (solid squares) and from coronary heart disease (open squares) among 361 622 men aged 35–57 years screened for the MRFIT trial (Data of Martin et al 1986)

is that the influence of cholesterol concentrations, or of diastolic blood pressure, on mortality in these men is not restricted to those with very high levels of either variable: it is a continuous spectrum, with each higher decile above the 20th having a significantly higher mortality than the decile below.

A similar conclusion comes from the 10-year mortality data from the Whitehall Study of 17 718 civil servants aged 40–64 years at entry (Rose & Shipley 1986). In that study 26% of deaths from coronary heart disease occurred in men with the highest decile of cholesterol concentration, but 54% occurred in the middle three-fifths of the distribution.

INFLUENCE OF OBESITY, CIGARETTE SMOKING, PHYSICAL ACTIVITY, ALCOHOL AND DIETARY FAT ON BLOOD LIPIDS AND LIPOPROTEINS

Lipids are transported in the blood attached to lipoproteins which make them water soluble: these complexes contain varying propor-tions of triglyceride, cholesterol, cholesteryl ester and phospholipids.

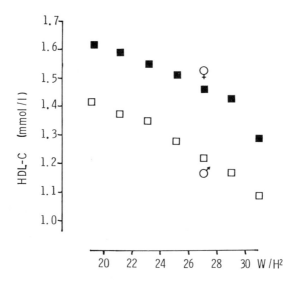

Fig. 14.3 Relation of HDL-C concentration to W/H² among 14 106 healthy Norwegian men and women. HDL-C values have been corrected for influence of age, physical activity and cigarette smoking (Data of Forde et al 1986)

Various classifications are used, but for this discussion we will be concerned mainly with HDL-C, which appears to be protective against coronary atheroma, total cholesterol (TC) which is associated with increased liability to coronary disease, and triglyceride (TG).

The association between HDL-C concentrations and QI is shown in Figure 14.3. These data were obtained from a sample of 7338 healthy men and 6768 healthy women aged 20–53 years living in Finnmark County, in north Norway (Forde et al 1986). HDL-C was lower in smokers than non-smokers, and increased with increasing age and increasing leisuretime physical activity. The values in Figure 14.3 are adjusted to allow for the effects of age, physical activity and cigarette smoking. Obesity is the strongest influence on HDL-C cholesterol values in this study.

There is a tendency for obese subjects to have raised concentrations of triglycerides and cholesterol, but this is not true of every obese person, nor is there any relation between the severity of obesity and the degree of hyperlipidaemia (see Figures 1.8 and 1.9). The perceived disadvantage of high blood lipid levels is the enhanced risk of coronary heart disease, so large-scale trials of lipid-lowering have been conducted on middle-aged men in order to reduce coronary heart disease incidence. In the Normative Ageing Study (Borkan et al 1986) the men who lost 10% of body weight in 15 years showed a decrease in serum triglyceride concentration of 22.5 mg/dl and an increase in cholesterol of 2.6 mg/dl, while those who gained 10% in body weight showed an increase of 42.7 mg/dl in triglycerides and of 41.8 mg/dl in cholesterol, with intermediate results for intermediate weight changes. The change in blood lipids with weight change is statistically significant (P<0.01) but less marked that the corresponding change in blood pressure.

There have recently been reports on the results of three large intervention trials, designed to reduce the multiple risk factors associated with coronary heart disease: the MRFIT intervention trial, directed at a sample of the population shown in Figure 14.2 who had the highest cholesterol concentration, the Lipid Research Clinics Coronary Primary Prevention Trial (LRC-CPPT) involving 3806 men aged 35–59 years (Glueck et al 1986), and the 6-year results of the WHO European Collaborative Group (1986) trial on coronary prevention. None of these trials used weight reduction as a primary strategy, but adopted a multiple intervention approach including advice on cholesterol-lowering diets, control of smoking, overweight and blood pressure, encouragement of exercise and, in the case of part of the LRC-CPPT trial, treatment with cholestyramine. The results were moderately successful in achieving the desired behaviour change, which in turn was moderately successful in reducing coronary disease incidence. It is difficult to extract the contribution made by weight reduction to this result, but Kuller et al (1983) calculate that, when other factors affecting cholesterol concentrations are allowed for, each 3 kg weight loss was associated with an increase of about 1.2 mg/dl of high-density lipoprotein cholesterol (HDL-C).

There are several studies relating factors other than obesity or weight loss to subsequent longevity and freedom from coronary heart disease. They may or may not act by influencing HDL-C. Among 16 936 Harvard alumni aged 35–74 years there is a remarkably strong association between longevity and physical activity, which is not explained by differences in blood pressure, cigarette smoking, body weight or body weight change since leaving college, or history of early parental death (Paffenberger et al 1986). In the Minnesota Heart Study (Folsom et al 1985) leisuretime physical activity among a sample of 3488 participants aged 25–74 years was significantly associated with higher levels of HDL-C, lower QI, and lower systolic blood pressure.

In a study of 1630 subjects in Quebec city, Leclerc et al (1985) did not find a significant relationship between energy expenditure computed from a 3-day activity record and blood lipid concentrations, but they did find a significant increase in HDL-C and decrease in triglyceride concentrations among those with the highest measured work power output. They interpret this to indicate that exercise of fairly high intensity is needed to cause desirable changes in blood lipids. However, Salonen et al (1985) studied military recruits in Finland, and conclude that quite modest physical activity increases HDL-C, which is also increased by alcohol intake.

Any inference that alcohol and exercise are alternative strategies to achieve coronary protection is firmly rejected by Eichner (1985) who also reviews the literature on this point. He points out that with respect to body weight, blood pressure and glucose tolerance alcohol and exercise have opposite effects: that of exercise is beneficial, and that of alcohol detrimental. All investigators seem agreed that cigarette smoking decreases HDL-C, and tends to negate any beneficial effects of physical activity in this respect (Stamford et al 1984).

While the HDL-C component of cholesterol is influenced by the factors discussed above, serum total cholesterol and triglyceride is affected mainly by dietary intake. Formulae have been proposed by which the atherogenic potential of various types oif food can be predicted, based on the content of saturated fatty acids and cholesterol (Connor et al 1986). However most expert committees have advised that, within reasonable limits, dietary cholesterol has relatively little influence on serum cholesterol concentration. There is agreement, however that to reduce the risk of cardiovascular disease it is desirable to maintain body weight within the desirable range, to encourage exercise, and to limit the intake of fat to a maximum of 35% of energy intake.

To calculate total energy intake for this purpose alcohol should be excluded (COMA 1984). Since fat contributes over 40% of the non-alcohol energy in the average British diet (see Table 8.3) fat intake needs to be reduced and replaced by complex carbohydrates, not by simple sugars or alcohol. There is a striking similarity between the advice given to the population in order to reduce serum cholesterol concentrations (and hence probably coronary heart disease) and the advice given to obese people to reduce the risk of developing insulin resistance and hence non-insulin-dependent diabetes (see Ch. 13).

All this is generally agreed, but debate rumbles on about the extent to which the fatty acid composition of dietary fat can usefully be manipulated. The generally held view is that reduction of saturated fat is the most important factor, but there are those who remain unconvinced that this is necessary (Gorringe 1986), or that the proportions of dietary fatty acids have much effect on plasma lipid levels (Berry et al 1986). There is intriguing evidence from analyses of fat biopsies from patients with and without conorary heart disease that fatty acids of the n-6 series, especially linoleic acid, may be particularly important in protecting against coronary heart disease (Riemersma et al 1986). The n-3 fatty acids found mainly in fish are potent in lowering cholesterol, but they are also potentially immunosuppresive, so it is not yet known if they are on balance benficial.

The other debate concerns the acceptability of a diet along the lines suggested by the NACNE (1983). The NACNE diet recommended fat reduced to 30%, saturated fat to 10%, sugar to 10%, alcohol to 8% of total energy, salt limited to 3600 mg/day and fibre increased to 30 g/day. Interpretations of these guidelines, and the extent to which they can be achieved, are given by Black et al (1984), Nelson (1985) and Cole-Hamilton et al (1986). Certainly it is possible to follow these guidelines if people are convinced that it is necessary. Pacy et al (1986) report a 3-month trial of such a diet with 17 diabetic patients with intermittent claudication, and they showed a significant decrease in body weight, blood pressure, cholesterol, triglyceride and glycosylated haemoglobin. However such a diet represents a considerable change from the average Western diet. It is suggested that it is the diet natural to primitive man, but the nature of that diet is open to speculation.

A careful study was reported by Milton (1984) of the diet of the Maku Indians in Nortwestern Amazonia, who are perhaps the most remote and un-urbanised people whom it is possible to study. The striking feature was that these people were obliged to spend 8 h per day in food gathering, and the product of this labour was a varied diet of fish, mammals, birds, insects, reptiles, manioc and fruit with about 50 g protein but a total energy content of about 1600–1800 kcal/day. The feature which is most different in a modern Western diet is the high total energy intake.

15

Other diseases associated with obesity

The excess mortality associated with obesity is mainly explained by diabetes and cardiovascular diseases, which were discussed in the two previous chapters. However other diseases related to obesity contribute significantly to the morbidity of this condition. They may be grouped under four headings: (a) social and psychological; (b) gallbladder and liver disease; (c) mechanical (which includes osteoarthritis of weight-bearing joints, gout, and problems with wound closure and pulmonary function); (d) disorders of the reproductive system, which includes certain cancers which are more common in obese people.

This grouping is used as a way of organising discussion of these diverse diseases, but the classification should not be taken to imply any thorough understanding of their aetiology.

a. SOCIAL AND PSYCHOLOGICAL CONSEQUENCES OF OBESITY

A review with this title by Wadden & Stunkard (1985) reveals the level of hostility which exist between American society and some obese Americans. The prejudice against fatness extends even to schoolchildren, who reject outline drawings of obese children as even less likeable than those who have physical handicaps such as missing hands. Some obese Americans have found it necessary to found a National Association to Aid Fat Americans (Allon 1975) to fight back against what they see as a tyranny of fashion designers and the slimming industry. There may be rather less animosity towards, and by, obese people in other societies; for example, in some North African countries fatness is considered evidence of health, prosperity, social status and even sexual attractiveness.

Probably there is discrimination against employing obese people, because they are considered to be lazy, slow and greedy. People disabled by obesity tend to be less generously regarded than those suffering equivalent disability from alcoholism. Many obese patients share this unflattering view of themselves: they are ashamed of their inability to lose weight at will, which they believe to be an attribute possessed by any normal person. In fact the feat of self-denial by dieting being asked of an obese person who has to lose 30 kg is probably beyond the capacity of most lean people; fortunately for the 'normal' people they are not being asked to do it.

Wadden & Stunkard (1985) comment that, considering the social prejudice against them, obese people show remarkably little psychopathology. Gilbert & Garrow (1983) found that patients attending a hospital obesity clinic showed normal scores for extroversion on the Eysenck Personality Inventory, and male patients scored within the normal range for neuroticism (10.5 ± 4.7), but the score for women was 14.0 ± 0.5, which is similar to Eysenck's group of mixed neurotics (14.9 ± 5.5). However, response to this questionnaire did not predict the outcome of treatment. There may be a bias in the hospital sample because the more disturbed obese patients apply sufficient pressure to the general practitioner to achieve hospital referral. Generally the psychological status of severely obese patients improves with massive weight loss, but it is not uncommon for the husband of a formerly obese women to become anxious about the consequences of his wife's liberation from the 'safety' of her former obesity.

Obese patients often offer a history of binge eating as evidence that they are psychologically deranged. Certainly it is irrational for a person who is trying to lose weight by dieting to eat massive amounts of food in secret, the eating bout continuing long after hunger is satisfied, and eventually being limited by physical discomfort. However, Keys et al (1950) point out that overeating to an extent which may endanger life has often been reported in non-obese people who were given access to unlimited food after prolonged energy restriction; for example, in released prisoners of war, or castaways who were rescued. It is therefore not clear if the tendency to binge is a personality characteristic of some obese people, or merely an extreme response to prolonged energy restriction.

Obese people who feel socially isolated and discriminated against clearly need support and reassurance, but it is irresponsible to give wholehearted endorsement to the slogans of the fat liberation movement, such as 'Whatever you weigh is right' (Louderback 1970). Ample evidence has been presented in this book that if what you weigh places you in grade III you are inviting medical problems which have nothing to do with your acceptability by society. I do not see much difficulty in being courteous, sympathetic and constructively encouraging to severely obese in their efforts to lose weight, without consenting to the view that obesity really does not matter. It is easy to gain approval for liberal views by playing down the medical importance of obesity, but if the patient then becomes diabetic, or develops one of the other obesity-related diseases, both patient and doctor may come to wish that you had been less enlightened, and more determined to achieve normal weight. With grade 0 obesity the situation is quite different, and reassurance is a main line of management, as it may be in grade I (see Table 9.1).

Certainly everyone concerned with the treatment of obesity has a duty to oppose any tendency to ridicule or humiliate obese people. Our civilisation has advanced to a point at which it is no longer considered appropriate to make fun of hunchbacks, on which the marionette figure of Punch is based, and mental defect is not a suitable subject for comedy. We must work to achieve a normal level of dignity and social acceptance for obese people in our societies, but that need not involve pretending that obesity does not matter.

b. GALLBLADDER AND LIVER DISEASE

The epidemiological evidence linking gallbladder disease and obesity has been reviewed by Bray (1985b). It is the commonest form of digestive disease in obese people, and the mortality from digestive diseases is more than twice as high among grade II obese people as among grade 0 people.

The mechanism relates to the excretion of excessive amounts of cholesterol in the bile. Normally bile is rendered soluble by the presence of bile salts, but if the ratio of cholesterol to bile salt become too high the cholesterol is liable to precipitate and form gallstones. This process can be quantified by calculating a saturation index (SI) (Thomas & Hofmann 1973). In the case of obese people the rate of secretion of lipid into the bile is increased above normal, and the SI is particularly high (Whiting et al 1984). However, the SI decreases with a low energy intake (Reuben et al 1985b). During weight reduction cholesterol is released from the adipose tissue which is being mobilised, so the effect of weight reduction on the SI in bile depends on the balance between reduced secretion and increased mobilisation of cholesterol. Obese patients with gallstones are generally resistant to treatment with chenodeoxycholic acid (CDCA), which normally desaturates duodenal bile in non-obese gallstone patients, and may eventually lead to the dissolution of the gallstone. This is probably because in obese subjects with gallstones the bile has a SI much higher than that of non-obese subjects with gallstones. However, with weight loss the ability on CDCA to desaturate bile in obese patients is enhanced (Reuben et al 1985b).

The increased cholesterol flux in obese people is a consequence of the large fat stores, not the characteristics of their diet. The Pima Indians have a very high prevalence of gallbladder disease, which increases with age, and is higher among women. Among Pima women aged 15–24 years the prevalence is 13%, and by age 25–34 years it is 73%. Among Pima men the prevalence at 25–34 years is 4%, and over 65 years it is 68%. However, no differences have been found between the diet of Pima Indians who do, or do not, have gallstones (Reid et al 1971).

Severe fatty infiltration of the liver occurs rarely in non-alcoholic obese people, and is reversible with weight reduction (Eriksson et al 1986). Abnormal liver function tests occur frequently in moderately obese people (Nomura et al 1986).

c. MECHANICAL DISORDERS RELATED TO OBESITY

Some of the diseases associated with obesity are plausibly explained by the mechanical stress imposed by excess weight. A good example of this class is osteoarthritis of weight-bearing joints. Hartz et al (1986) reviewed the literature on this subject and found that 14 out of 16 studies showed an association between overweight and osteoarthritis of weight-bearing joints and two failed to find any such association. Seidel et al (1986a) reported a significantly increased morbidity from arthrosis among overweight men and women aged 30–39 years, but not in older or younger people. Hartz et al (1986) analysed data on 4225 subjects aged 40–69 years from the National Health and Nutrition Examination Survey (HANES) conducted in 1971–74. There was a statistically significant association between overweight and osteoarthritis of the knees in both men and women, in both blacks and whites, and in each decade of age. The association was stronger in women than in men. Weight reduction does not reverse the destructive lesion, but may be more effective in relieving the pain of osteoarthritic knees than any form of drug treatment (Dixon & Henderson 1973). Gout is also significantly associated with obesity (Bray 1985b, Seidell et al 1986b). It is not clear why this should be so.

Respiratory insufficiency in obese subjects is at least partly due to mechanical problems. Very obese subjects are liable to sleep-apnoea, as depicted in the fat boy in *Pickwick Papers*. This is a form of self-narcosis associated with very low blood oxygen concentrations, and it is considerably helped by weight loss, presumably because this improves pulmonary ventilation (Harman & Block 1986).

Severely obese patients present the surgeon with problems concerning the closure of abdominal wounds. In very fat patients the incision has to be bigger than normal to give the surgeon access to the abdominal contents. Closing the incision is made difficult by the weight of tissue tending to pull the wound open, and by the difficulty of preventing blood oozing from the fat layer which will not hold sutures. These problems are reviewed by Kozol et al (1986).

d. DISORDERS OF REPRODUCTIVE FUNCTION

The special problems of obese women during menstruation and pregnancy are discussed in the next chapter. However, there are also disorders of reproductive function associated with obesity in non-pregnant women and in men. The excess of cancers in overweight subjects occur in breast, endometrium and ovary in women and in prostate in men. These are all tissues sensitive to sex hormones. However, in the American Cancer Society study overweight men also had an excess of colorectal cancers, and overweight women a significant excess mortality from cancer of the gallbladder and biliary passages (Garfinkel 1985). Biliary cancer may be related to the trauma and infection associated with gallstones, which were discussed above.

Obesity affects the metabolism of both androgens and oestrogens, since adipose tissue contains aromatase, an enzyme involved in the interconversion of testosterone and oestradiol (Longcope et al 1986). There is some evidence that a high concentration of non-protein-bound oestradiol is involved in the development of breast cancer, and this hormone is present in higher concentrations in overweight women than in normal-weight women (Ota et al 1986). Polycystic disease of the ovaries is often associated with obesity, and treatment with anti-androgens is more effective after weight loss (Pasquali et al 1986). The endocrine disorder associated with polycystic disease of the ovaries is very complex, but in general there is a trend towards normal hormone levels, and normal ovarian function, with loss of the excess weight (Friedman & Kim 1985). Disorders of reproductive function are also seen in severely obese men, but there is little evidence about the effects of weight loss on these endocrine abnormalities (Friedman & Kim 1985).

16

Management of obesity in pregnant women

The dietary management of pregnant women is a subject on which many obstetricians have strong views. There is good epidemiological evidence that fetal growth is impaired in women of lower socio-economic groups. One of the respects in which these women differ from more affluent women is a lower plane of nutrition. There is ample evidence from, for example, pig farmers that very well-fed sows produce heavier and healthier piglets. On this basis Brewer (1967) says that it is mandatory that pregnant women should be given truly heroic quantities of food, especially protein. He ascribes growth failure in the fetus largely to maternal malnutrition. If we adopt this view there can be no question of attempting to treat obesity during pregnancy.

Craddock (1973) adopts a different attitude: 'The six month period during which a pregnant woman attends for antenatal supervision affords the physician the chance of practising true preventive medicine, the like of which is hard to equal in the whole field of patient/doctor contact in the western world.'

He feels that if the pregnant woman is obese this is an opportunity to control the situation, at least by limiting weight gain during pregnancy. Hytten (1979) takes a characteristically cool view. He notes that attempts to control pre-eclamptic toxaemia by dietary restriction have failed, and does not expect attempts to control obesity to do much better. He concedes that there may be a case for intervention in grossly obese women, but 'to attempt reduction of food intake when the woman is having a surge of appetite is swimming against the tide. . . .' It may be quite sensible to try to swim against the tide if the alternative — drifting with the tide — is very likely to land you in trouble.

The weight gain during a normal pregnancy averages about 12.5 kg. In their classic review Hytten & Leitch (1964) calculate that

7 kg of this is water, about 0.9 kg is protein of which half is in the fetus, and about 4 kg of fat are added to the mother's energy stores, as a reserve to support lactation.

The measurements of Pipe et al (1979) agree with these estimates: they found that of a weight gain of 10.4 kg between 12 and 37 weeks of pregnancy 7.2 kg could be accounted for as water. The increase in fat stores occurs mainly during the first trimester of pregnancy, and a modest increase in the lean tissues of the mother — about 0.9 kg — occurs in the last two trimesters. In the patients studied by Pipe et al (1979) body weight and composition returned almost exactly to the values at 10–14 weeks gestation within 6–15 weeks of delivery of the baby.

This return to pre-pregnancy weight is the crucial point concerning the importance of pregnancy to subsequent obesity. Hytten (1979) says that there is a trend for women to become heavier with increasing age, but that parity makes a negligible contribution to this weight increase. This view is supported by the data of Billewicz & Thomson (1970). They compared the weight at 20 weeks gestation in a first pregnancy with the weight at 20 weeks gestation in subsequent pregnancies in a large series of women in Aberdeen. On average, having allowed for the expected increase in weight with time, the weight increase from first to second pregnancies was 1 kg, from first to third was 1.5 kg, and from first to fourth 1.9 kg. These weight increases are indeed small on average, but a minority of women gained an unusually large amount of weight with parity. The mean weight gain among women who were initially overweight gained an average of 2.4 kg. Furthermore, those women who gained most weight between pregnancies tended to gain most during pregnancies.

Similar conclusions can be derived from the data of Beazley & Swinhoe (1979), which are illustrated in Figure 16.1. They followed the weight change of 50 women in Liverpool through five successive pregnancies. For the first three pregnancies, weight 6 weeks post-partum had fallen below weight at the 20th week of pregnancy, but for the fourth and fifth pregnancies this was no longer so. Weight gain tended to be greatest among those who were heaviest: the average weight of the whole series increased by 5.1 kg between the 20th week of the first and fifth pregnancy (from 59.1 kg to 64.2 kg), but the heaviest quartile of mothers increased 7.83 kg (from 73.02 kg to 80.85 kg).

The stepwise increase in body weight shown in Figure 16.1 is the

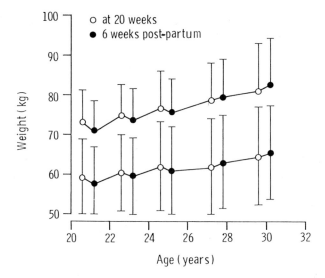

Fig. 16.1 Weight change between 20 weeks gestation and 6 weeks post partum in 50 women followed through 5 successive pregnancies (Data of Beazley & Swinhoe 1979). Lower line shows mean ± s.e.m. for whole series; upper line shows data for the heaviest quartile of mothers at start of study. The more obese mothers become even more obese with successive pregnancies

result of a rather complex interaction between parity and age. This relationship is further illustrated in Figure 16.2 which is constructed from the data of the Cardiff Birth Survey (Newcombe 1982) on the pre-pregnant weight of 35 556 women having 4 or fewer previous deliveries. The weight of each woman has been adjusted to that which she would have had if her height had been 1.6 m. The figure shows that by the age of 40–44 years the number of previous deliveries has very little influence on body weight (namely about 61.5 kg) except in those women having 4 previous deliveries, who had an average weight of 62.7 kg. However, among women aged 20–24 years the number of previous deliveries had a striking influence on body weight: the expected age-related weight gain occurred very much more rapidly among women who had several previous pregnancies.

So the answer to the question: 'does pregnancy predispose to obesity?' is that it appears to do so in a section of the population who are disposed to obesity anyway, and it appears to accelerate age-related weight gain, but it does not necessarily lead to a higher body weight at the end of the child-bearing period.

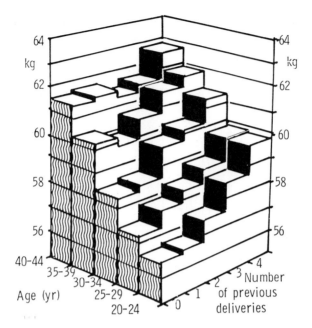

Fig. 16.2 Interaction of age and parity among 35 556 pregnant women (Data of Newcombe 1982). Multiple pregnancies in young women accelerate age-related weight gain

EFFECT OF FAMINE ON HUMAN PREGNANCY

It is less easy to obtain hard evidence about the possible effects of dietary restriction during pregnancy on the subsequent development of the child. Obviously development is influenced by many factors other than intra-uterine nutrition, so it is difficult to attribute developmental handicap in later life to any particular perinatal factor. One piece of evidence which was thought to indicate that intra-uterine nutrition affected mental development was derived by intelligence testing of twins. Twins have a lower birth weight than singleton babies, and they tend to score lower in intelligence tests than singleton babies matched for social class. This might indicate that the twin, who had to share the intra-uterine nutrition, suffered a permanent setback to mental development. The fallacy of this conclusion was shown by McKeown (1970). He compared the score of twins with singleton children in the '11-plus' examination, dsesigned to select children for academic secondary schooling, and found that they scored lower, as expected. However when children were chosen who were single survivors of twin pregnancies the difference from singleton pregnancies vanished. This strongly suggests that the poorer score of twins was largely due to post-natal factors, and not to the level of intrauterine nutrition.

There is much epidemiological evidence of mental impairment in children living in poor social circumstances, but it is impossible to dissect away nutritional factors from those connected with genetic endowment and environmental factors such as the level of intellectual stimulation of the child. From the scientific viewpoint we need a randomly selected sample of population who were subjected to severe dietary restriction in an otherwise affluent community. This is obviously ethically impossible as a scientific experiment, but something very near to this experiment happened inadvertently in Holland during the winter of 1944–45. The Allied forces entered the Netherlands on 14 September 1944, and planned to sieze the bridges of Arnhem and Nijmegen, which were the key to the cities of the north-west — The Hague, Amsterdam and Rotterdam. To hamper the German defence of this territory the Dutch government-in-exile in London broadcast an appeal to resistance workers to sabotage the transport system, while an airborne unit tried to take the bridges. The transport strike was successful, but the paratroop raid was not, so by mid-November 1944 the Allied forces had liberated the Netherlands south of the Rhine, but the north-west coastal cities were completely cut off from their sources of food supply. That winter was exceptionally severe, and there were no stocks of food, so until 7 May 1945 there was famine in north-west Holland, but relatively normal food supply in the south of the country.

The effect of this famine on the development of children born before, during and after the hungry winter has been carefully documented by Stein et al (1975) in one of the classic studies of human undernutrition. The average quarterly rations distributed in the Western Netherlands are shown in Figure 16.3. Until November 1943 the diet had contained about 1800 kcal with about 60 g protein, and a high proportion of the energy coming from carbohydrate — what would now be called a 'prudent' diet. With the start of the blockade food supplies decreased rapidly to reach a minimum in the first quarter of 1944, which was less than half the previous ration. With the arrival of Allied troops in May the situation improved, and supplies were back to normal by mid-summer. Thus there was a period of about 6 months of severe undernutrition, with everyone, including pregnant women, having an energy intake less than half requirements. The effect on birth rate 9 months later is shown in

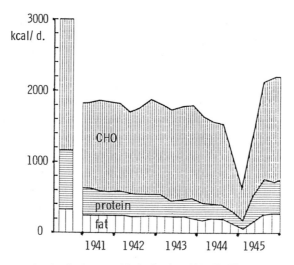

Fig. 16.3 Dietary ration in the western Netherlands, 1941–45. The transport strike in November 1944 caused famine during that winter, which was relieved on arrival of Allied troops in May 1945 (From Stein et al 1975)

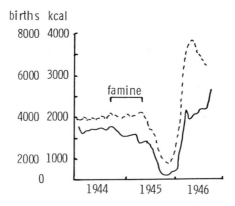

Fig. 16.4 Effect of famine winter in western Netherlands (see Figure 16.3) on birth rate 9 months later. Dietary ration indicated by continuous line, and birth rate by broken line. Curve for diet has been displaced 9 months later, to indicate calorie ration at time of conception (Data of Stein et al 1975)

Figure 16.4, in which the birth rate has been related to the dietary conditions at conception. It can be seen that the famine caused a virtual cessation of new pregnancies, which was not seen in the regions in the Netherlands not affected by the famine.

It was possible to compare children born in the blockaded zone with those born at the same time in parts of the country where there was adequate food. If, as Brewer (1967) suggests, maternal malnutrition leads to fetal malnutrition, there should have been no difficulty in demonstrating the fact in the children born in the famine area, but the only striking finding was that the starved women ceased to menstruate. This seems to be the defence of the human species against famine: women become infertile — but once a pregnancy is established in a reasonably well-nourished mother the fetus does not go short. Compared with the young of other species the human baby is unusually small and slow-growing, so it presents a far smaller nutritional burden on the mother. As Hytten (1980) puts it: 'The point to be made here is that, within wide limits, the fetus of a reasonably healthy, pregnant woman is remarkably unaffected by dietary inadequacy during pregnancy and is difficult to damage by overall restriction of food.'

The relative immunity of an established pregnancy to undernutrition in the mother is remarkable in view of the recommendations of expert committees that the cost of pregnancy is about 80 000 kcal, requiring an increased energy intake of about 200 kcal/day above non-pregnant requirements. These estimates were based on measurements of well-nourished women (Blackburn & Calloway 1976). However, it is becoming evident that in populations on marginal energy intakes energy expenditure rises very little during pregnancy, but there seems to be a greater efficiency of energy utilisation (Lawrence et al 1985).

MATERNAL OBESITY, WEIGHT GAIN, AND THE OUTCOME OF PREGNANCY

Obese women have a significantly increased incidence of complications in pregnancy (Peckham and Christianson 1971, Efiong 1975, Maeder et al 1975, Edwards et al 1978). Garbaciak et al (1985) analysed the records of 9667 deliveries and report that the incidence of antepartum complications in women <85% of ideal weight, 85–120%, 120–150% and >150% of ideal weight were 28%, 25%, 33% and 48% respectively. Thus both underweight and overweight is associated with an increased risk of complications, but the rate is very high in very overweight women. However, the very obese women without complications had an increased caesarean section rate, but no increase in pre-natal mortality. These investigators conclude that it is the complications associated with obesity, rather than obesity itself, which affects the outcome of pregnancy.

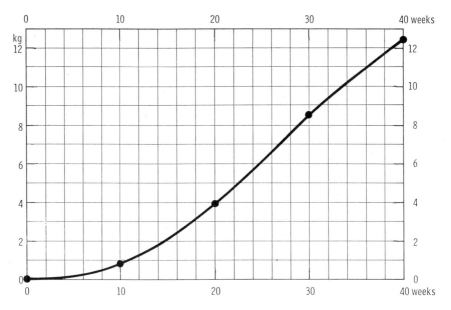

Fig. 16.5 Desirable weight gain in normal-weight women, related to stage of pregnancy (Data of Hytten & Leitch 1964)

It is well established that the pattern of weight gain shown in Figure 16.5 is optimum for pregnancies in well-nourished normal-weight women (Hytten & Leitch 1964). However, an analysis of 53, 518 pregnancies by Naeye (1979) showed that this rule did not hold for women whose QI was over 28, in whom a weight gain of about 4 kg was associated with a lower perinatal mortality than the 'normal' 12 kg weight gain at term. This conclusion is supported by the report of Abrams & Laros (1986) who analysed the relation of maternal pregnancy weight gain to the infants' birth weight in a series of 2946 live births. There was the expected association between maternal weight gain and infant birth weight (20.1 g gain by the baby for each 1 kg gain by the mother) for mothers whose QI was under 28. However, among obese mothers ($W/H^2 >28$) there was no significant increase in birth weight with increasing weight gain in the mother. These authors conclude that recommendations for a minimum weight gain are not required for obese pregnant women over that limit.

A recent editorial interprets these data cautiously (Drife 1986): 'Recommendations for a minimum weight gain in pregnancy should take account of the weight before pregnancy: underweight women need to gain more weight than overweight women.' How much weight overweight women should optimally gain we do not know, but probably 6 kg is nearer the mark than the 'normal' 12 kg. The evidence does not justify trying to reduce the weight of obese women during pregnancy: 'It is probably better to try to reduce the obese woman's weight either before or after the pregnancy' (Campbell 1983). This is probably a good policy, but it is doubtful if obstetricians are likely to carry it out.

17

Management and prevention of obesity in children

Reviews on obesity in childhood tend to be rather pessimistic; it is agreed that the problem is an important one, but results are often poor: 'Obesity is a relatively common problem in childhood and is often very difficult to manage' (Brooke & Abernethy 1985), and 'The therapy of childhood obesity has been notably unsuccessful' (Dietz 1986). There are three reasons why it is more difficult to treat obese children than obese adults, which will be discussed in turn. First, it is more difficult to diagnose obesity in children than in adults. Second, treatment must be negotiated through other people (parents, school meals organisers, etc.) who may view the problem quite differently from either the child or the therapist. Third, negative energy balance required to treat the obesity must be moderated by the need to ensure that the growth and development of the child is not impaired.

DIAGNOSIS OF OBESITY IN CHILDREN

The physician who is used to dealing with obese adults may forget that obesity in children may be part of an inborn error of metabolism. It is beyond the scope of this book to discuss these disorders, but a useful rule-of-thumb is that genetic disorders which cause fatness in children almost always are also associated with short stature, so a fat child who is tall for his or her age (as most children with 'simple' obesity are) is unlikely to have one of these genetic disorders. An exception to this rule is the syndrome associated with acanthosis nigricans (Richards et al 1985). Babies of diabetic parents tend to be large, and continue to be large children (Pettit et al 1985), and there is a general tendency for high birth weight to be associated with high weight gain in the first 5 years of life (Garn 1985), so birth weight and parents' stature should be considered when assessing the fatness of a young child.

The simple scheme shown in Figure 1.1, based on the ranges of QI, will not serve to classify obesity in children, since during the period of growth they increase in height and weight at different rates. Two alternative schemes are therefore available. The first is to use triceps skinfold thickness. The technique for measuring skinfold thickness is decribed in section 3.e. The centiles for male and female subjects are shown in Figures 17.1 and 17.2. For boys the 50th centile is about 10 mm throughout life, but for girls it increases from infancy to the age of about 50 and then declines. An alternative system is to use QI related to age-specific standards. Figures 17.3 and 17.4 show the centiles lines for French children born in 1953 (Rolland-Cachera et al 1982), with the values for British children born in 1958 at age 7. 11 and 16 years superimposed (Stark et al 1986). It is evident that the British children are a little heavier than French children of the same height.

It is therefore possible to estimate how a child of a given age and sex rates in fatness compares with the general population. However, we cannot say what level of fatness is excessive, because there are no prospective studies relating the triceps skinfold, or QI, of children to their subsequent mortality or morbidity. In the absence of an objective criterion of obesity in children discussions about the prevalence of childhood obesity are somewhat fruitless, since the

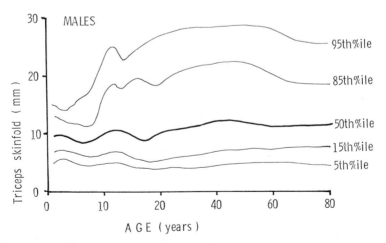

Fig. 17.1 Centile values for triceps skinfold thickness in white American males (Data of Garn & Clark 1976)

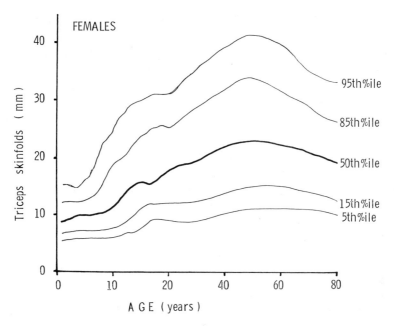

Fig. 17.2 Centile values for triceps skinfold thickness in white American females (Data of Garn & Clark 1976).

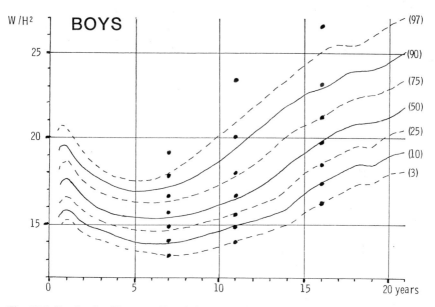

Fig. 17.3 Centiles for QI among French boys born in 1953 (data of Rolland-Cachera et al 1982), with superimposed points for British boys born in 1958, at ages 7, 11 and 16 years (data of Stark et al 1986)

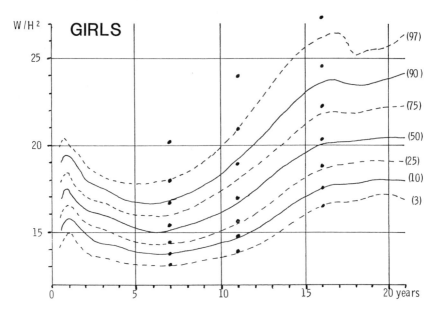

Fig. 17.4 Data for girls corresponding to that for boys in Figure 17.3.

observed prevalence will depend entirely on the arbitrary criteria for diagnosis which the author happens to choose.

If we knew that (say) the fattest 10% of children became the fattest 10% of adults we could reasonably ascribe risk to fatness in children as we do in adults. However many surveys have shown that during the first two or three years of life children change weight categories quite freely. Asher (1966) reviewed her experience in a clinic in Birmingham, England, and noted that 44% of the obese schoolchildren she saw had been obese before the age of 5 years. She found that the results of treatment of those who had been obese in infancy were particularly bad. Obesity was defined by the child's weight relative to the standard centile charts: those more than 25% above their expected weight were classified as obese. She concluded that better treatment of obesity in infancy would help to prevent intractable obesity later in life.

Eid (1970) studied the rate of weight gain of children in Sheffield, England, and related this to their weight at age 6–8 years. He concluded that rapid weight gain in the first 6 months of life was related to subsequent obesity, and associated this with the early introduction of cereals into the babies' feed. However, when his data are examined in the light of subsequent experience the evidence for this conclusion is not very strong. Among 138 infants who gained weight rapidly (faster than the 90th centile) in the first 6 months there were 28 (20.3%) who were at least 10% overweight at age 6–8 years. This is statistically a significant association, but it must be remembered that nearly 80% of the infants with rapid weight gain were not 10% overweight at age 6–8 years. Furthermore among the 86 infants who did not show rapid weight gain, 6 (6.9%) were at least 10% overweight at age 6–8 years. These two studies therefore showed that there was a significant tendency for fat babies to be over-represented subsequently among the obese population of schoolchildren, but that by no means all fat school children had been fat babies, nor would all fat babies remain fat.

The surveys of Abraham et al (1971) in Hagerstown, USA, and of Sohar et al (1973) in Tel Aviv, Israel, started with rather older children. The Hagerstown survey showed that by age 9–13 years the weight pattern for later life had been largely set. Sohar et al (1973) state: 'The relative weight of both obese and non-obese subjects seems to be determined in early infancy, and tends to remain constant during childhood, adolescence and usually during adult life.' However, this conclusion goes beyond their data, which concern the children's weight, as a percentage of ideal weight, at age 6–7 years and at age 13–14 years. The results are shown in Figure 17.5. At age 6–7 years there were 17 children in the heaviest group (131–150% of ideal weight) and all of these were in the same weight category at age 13–14 years. However, the less overweight children did not keep within their weight categories on follow-up, although the majority did.

It can be seen from Figure 17.5 that of the 39 most-overweight children at age 13–14 years 17 came from the most-overweight group of 6–7-year-olds, but 6 came from those previously 111–130% of ideal weight, 12 from those previously 91–110%, and 4 from those previously 71–90% of ideal weight. Clearly there is a tendency for children to keep within their relative weight groups during their schooldays, but less than half of the most over-weight children at 13–14 years had been in the most-overweight group at 6–7years.

The report of Fisch et al (1975) is particularly valuable, because a large series of babies were studied prospectively at birth, age 4 years and age 7 years. The ratio of weight to height was taken as a measure of obesity. The 96 children who were heaviest at birth provided a significantly larger than expected proportion of the children who were heaviest at age 4 years and 7 years ($P < 0.05$).

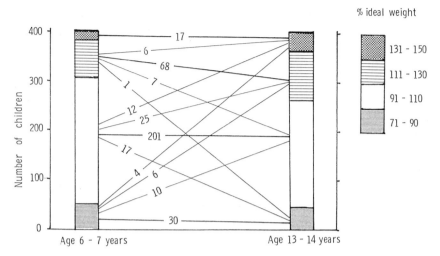

Fig. 17.5 Change in weight-for-height among 404 children studied by Sohar et al (1973) at age 6–7 years, and again at age 13–14 years. Numerals on lines indicate number of children travelling between weight-for-height groups over 7-year interval. Most-overweight category at age 13–14 years recruited children from each weight group at age 6–7 years, so proportion of overweight children increased. However, this age interval is probably the best one at which to *decrease* the proportion of overweight children (see text)

However, when the heaviest 5% of children at age 7 years were traced back to their birth weight there were no more than might happen by chance among the heaviest at birth. Between 4 years and 7 years there was little change in ranking order for weight. Charney et al (1976) traced the adult weight of children who had been either fat, average, or thin in the first 6 months of life. Of the 32 adults who were over 120% of average weight-for-height 17 had been in the group of fattest babies, 6 had been average-weight babies, and 9 had been thin babies.

The publications reviewed so far emphasise the fact that fat children are more likely to be fat later in life than thin children. However the important question is: can the weight, or rate of weight gain, early in life be used to predict obesity later? If this is possible then children who are particularly at risk to become severely obese could be identified, and some preventive measures could be concentrated on this high-risk group.

Mellbin & Vuille (1973) analysed data on 972 children in Uppsala, Sweden, to see if it was possible to predict weight for height at age 7 years from data about birth weight, birth length, monthly gain in weight during the first year, maximum monthly weight gain, or the ratio of maximum monthly gain to mean monthly gain. For both boys and girls the best single factor to predict weight-for-height at age 7 was weight gain during the first 12 months, but the correlation coefficients were low: r = 0.056 for girls, and r = 0.082 for boys. Even with the other factors added in a multiple regression analysis the data on growth in the first year could only explain 9% of the variation in weight for height at age 7 years among girls, and only 18% of the variation among boys. This is useless for effective prevention.

To take one of the more promising predictive models, it might be supposed that boys who gained more than 7.5 kg in the first year would be at high risk for future obesity. There were 140 out of 465 boys who exceeded this rate of weight gain. If 10% overweight at age 7 is taken as the criterion of obesity the rapidly gaining infants were divided 33 : 104 between the overweight and normal weight classes at age 7, while the infants who did not have rapid weight gain in the first year were divided 27 : 298 between overweight and normal weight at age 7 years.

Prediction of overweight with girls was still less successful. Thus if the criteria used to predict obesity are set in such a way that one third of babies are thought to be potentially obese, this group will contain only about half of the children who eventually are found to be overweight. This is too small a catch for so wide a net.

The results of Poskett & Cole (1977) support a similar conclusion. They traced 203 children who had been surveyed at about 5 months of age, and assessed their weight-for-height and skinfold thickness. Most of the previously obese infants had returned to normal weight by the age of 5 years. Sveger (1978) also found that obese infants were no longer obese by the age of 4 years. Dine et al (1979) traced back the weight history of the heaviest 10% children at age 5 years, and found that whatever measure of obesity was used these children could not have been identified by their weight during the first year of life. Durnin & McKillop (1978) also found a low correlation between measures of fatness (weight-for-height or skinfolds) at age 0–2 years and 14 years later.

The children studied by Hawk & Brook (1979) were rather older at the time of the first survey: between 2 and 15 years of age. When they were examined 15 years later the correlation between the ranking of the skinfold measurements at first and second examination was 0.56 for male and 0.45 for female subjects. This is a rather better level of prediction than that achieved from measurements in the first year of life but still not very impressive. Better correlations were obtained by Zack et al (1979) from the data of the US Health Examination surveys of 2177 children at 6–11 years and again at age 12–17 years. Of the children who were in the 20% most obese at the time of the first survey about 70% were in the correspondingly obese group at the time of the second survey, and about 20% were in the next-most-obese category.

Shapiro et al (1984) measured weight, height and skinfold thicknesses prospectively on 450 babies aged 6 months to 9 years. Of the observed variation in skinfold thickness at 9 years the proportion explained by the skinfold thickness at 6 months was 5%, at 1 year 8%, at 2 years 29%, at 3 years 38%, at 4 years 42% and at 6 years 72%. They conclude that 'impending or actual obesity begins at ages 6 to 9 years . . .'.

In summary, therefore, attempts to predict adult obesity from the fatness of children before the age of 5 years have had very poor success. By the age of 11 years the correlation with adult fatness is becoming stronger. This is predictable, since by the age of 7 years a normal child has fat stores which are more than half the normal adult fat stores, and an obese child at 11 years may well have fat stores greater than that of a normal adult. This means that the obese 11-year-old child would have to lose fat in order to become a normal adult, and it is unlikely that this will happen.

It can be seen from Figures 17.3 and 17.4 that among the fattest children QI is at a minimum value at age 5 years, while in the thinnest children it is at a minimum at 7 years. It seems that primary school age (about 5–12 years) is a good period during which to try to prevent obesity by steering those children in the upper centiles of skinfold thickness, or QI, back towards the 50th centile. The teenager will be increasingly resistant to coercion in the matter of diet (or anything else), so the next opportunity to treat obesity does not occur until about the age of 18 years, when the young person may have decided to do something about his or her obesity, without reference to any adult authority. However by 18 years the fattest children are already into Grade I obesity by adult standards, so the chance has already been lost to attain normal weight as an adult by not gaining fat, rather than having to lose fat.

MANAGEMENT OF OBESITY IN CHILDREN

It is almost always fair to say that the cause of obesity in a teenager is the failure of his or her parents, schoolteachers etc. to prevent that obesity. An exception can be made for the unfortunate children with the Prader–Willi syndrome, whose drive to eat will defeat the most vigilant parent, and even well-trained nurses in a hospital ward. However, 'simple' obesity in children arises because the child was allowed to eat too much and exercise too little. Of course it is difficult to restrict the food intake of a fat child if the siblings can afford to eat ad libitum, but just as different children have different educational and emotional requirements, so they have different energy requirements also. Ideally, therefore, childhood obesity should be prevented, so the need to treat it does not arise.

One of the important tasks of a school doctor, along with detecting defects in sight and hearing among the children, is to check that the children are not becoming too fat. If a child is creeping upwards across centile lines it is necessary to mobilise support from the parents and school catering authorities to provide food of a lower energy density which will supply all the necessary nutrients. One obvious target for reducing energy intake with negligible loss of nutrients is to restrict the number of sweets the child eats. This need not be seen as a punishment, because a child who cannot afford to eat the high-energy foods which other children eat is entitled to some compensating treat of a non-nutritive variety, just as a child with some physical handicap might be compensated. The important point is that if the child is never allowed to become very overweight it will never be necessary to impose very severe restrictions, so the problem will not get out of hand. However, this requires co-operation and vigilance on the part of those responsible for caring for the child, and unfortunately this is not always forthcoming. It is astonishing how often severely obese parents watch their children becoming obese in a spirit of resignation, rather than acting to save their offspring from the trouble they have themselves encountered.

The principle of treatment is to restrict energy intake so as to reduce increase in weight while permitting normal increase in height. The required small decrease in energy intake can usually be achieved by reducing consumption of sweets, and substituting fruit and low-energy soft drinks and snacks for the usual potato crisps, biscuits and ice cream. Dietz & Hartung (1985) report that reduction of energy intake to about two-thirds of the usual daily intake caused a mean weight loss of 4.5 ± 5.3 kg in 9.7 months in a group of obese children aged 8.5 ± 2.7 years, but those who lost more than the average amount of weight showed a significant slowing of height velocity. If the problem of obesity is skilfully tackled between the age of 5 years and 11 years it should be possible for the obese 5-year-old child to become a normal-weight 11-year-old child without at any stage losing weight.

Exercise programmes are excellent if they can be presented in such a way that the child regards the activity as a treat rather than a penalty. Unfortunately, obese children tend to have rather a negative view of physical activity (Worsley et al 1984), which is another reason for establishing an active lifestyle in children susceptible to obesity before their obesity becomes established. The success of the programme depends on the level of parental co-operation, which in turn depends on the extent to which the parents realise that they are performing an important service for their children by preventing them from becoming obese teenagers. The results obtained by Brownell & Stunkard (1978b) and by Epstein et al (1985) are very encouraging. These programmes used a combination of behaviour therapy and exercise, and involved monetary deposits which the participating parents had refunded contingent on attending the course and following the prescribed programme. This procedure must have had the effect of selecting the more highly motivated parents, and it is not applicable to parents who do not know, or care, about the obesity status of their children. That problem can only be tackled by an effective programme of health education, which is the topic of the next chapter.

18

Obesity and health education

It might be supposed that the prevention of obesity would be high on the agenda of professional health educators. It has been declared by various expert committees to be one of the most important public health problems of our time, and the evidence on which that judgement was made has been presented earlier in this book. It is an avoidable cause of ill-health, since any well-informed person in the less severe grades of obesity can adopt the treatment strategies which have been suggested in previous chapters. The evidence is quite strong that the health risks of obesity are largely reversible by weight loss, but it is obviously better still to avoid obesity. In the case of children the avoidance of obesity depends on teaching their parents the importance of avoiding excessive weight gain, for reasons discussed in Chapter 17. Despite all this the avoidance of obesity receives rather scanty attention in health education campaigns, at least in the UK.

There are several reasons which may explain why obesity gets less publicity than, for example, cigarette smoking. It is proper to give to the public the advice 'do not smoke', since anyone who smokes cigarettes should stop doing so, and people who do not smoke cigarettes recognise that it is advice which they are already following. The message about obesity must be more cautiously worded, since an exhortation to the third of the population who are overweight to lose weight will be siezed upon by some potential cases of anorexia nervosa (who are, by their own standards, overweight) as justification for still further weight loss. For this reason the health education message about obesity must be a two-stage process: '1. Are you overweight?', and then to the subsection who reply 'yes', '2. Then this is what to do.' This is not a uniquely difficult problem among health education messages: advice to take more exercise needs to be related to the individual's present level of activity and physical fitness, and advice to reduce intake of saturated fat needs to be related to the individual's current diet. However, the two-stage approach presents a genuine difficulty in trying to transmit effective information about obesity: health educators soon learn that only simple messages make any impact. (So I will keep this chapter short.)

Another view which may have reduced the enthusiasm for propaganda about obesity is that obesity is not itself a health hazard, and, even if it were, not much can be done about it. Anyone who reads this book will know that there is a substantial body of evidence against this view, but it is possible to see a basis for it. The media are full of advertisements urging women to lose weight and become more glamorous. Fashion models are often emaciated, and seldom above the middle of the grade 0 range of QI. Any ordinary person who tries to emulate this level of thinness will indeed find it difficult to achieve, and, if achieved, will gain no advantage from the viewpoint of health. It is not to be expected that the slimming industry will aim to limit its advertising to those who are really overweight, since they would thereby deprive themselves of access to many potential customers. The health educator who wishes to tell the public that obesity is unhealthy may find that this transmission is jammed by much more powerful signals which tell the public that thin is beautiful. The legitimate weight-loss message is discredited by association with the commercial pressure groups. Well-intentioned reporters expose the fallacy of weight-loss claims, but neglect to make the important point that the benefits of weight loss depend (among other things) on your starting weight.

These problems will not go away. Progress will not be easy even when the majority of health educators are clear in their own minds about what constitutes overweight, and are convinced that something can and should be done to combat this avoidable cause of ill-heath. It would be gratifying if the evidence presented in this book helped to clarify the issues about obesity, and to indicate what can be done about it.

19

Summary and conclusions

Obesity is one of the most important medical and public health problems of our time, whether we judge importance by a shorter expectation of life, increased morbidity, or cost to the community in terms of both money and anxiety.

DEFINITION OF OBESITY

Quetelet's index W/H^2 (kg/m^2) is a satisfactory basis on which to classify obesity in adult men and women. The range of QI between 20 and 25 is associated with minimum mortality and morbidity in young adults, and is therefore termed 'grade 0'. Health hazards arising from obesity are increasingly severe above this range. Three grades of obesity are described in this book depending on the QI: grade I from 25 to 29.9, grade II from 30 to 40, and grade III over 40. It is not possible to provide an objective definition of obesity in children.

PREVALENCE OF OBESITY

In the UK the proportion of men aged 16–64 years in grades I, II and III are 34%, 6% and 0.1%. The corresponding figures for women are 24%, 8% and 0.3%. Reports from other European countries, Australia, Canada and the USA indicate similar prevalences of obesity. The more severe grades of obesity are more prevalent in women than in men.

MORTALITY AND MORBIDITY OF OBESITY AND RELATED DISEASES

The mortality ratio (compared with grade 0 = 100) of grade I obesity is about 115, at the middle of grade II it is about 200, and in grade III it is very high, but the numbers of people affected are too small to yield reliable statistics. The curve of mortality ratio related to QI is similar in men and women, and in smokers and non-smokers, but smokers have a generally higher mortality risk. The excess mortality associated with obesity is more marked among young people than among those over the age of 50 years. The increased mortality among obese men and women is mainly explained by increased risk of death from cardiovascular diseases and non-insulin-dependent diabetes.

Obesity contributes to 'risk factors' such as hypertension, hyper-lipidaemia and impaired glucose tolerance, but has now also been shown to be an independent risk factor for several forms of cardio-vascular disease, including coronary heart disease, myocardial infarc-tion and congestive heart failure. Obesity is also associated with an increased risk of gallbladder disease, gout, some cancers, impaired lung and liver function, osteoarthritis of weight-bearing joints, and some social and psychological disabilities. There is good evidence that the excess mortality and morbidity associated with obesity is reversible with weight loss.

ENERGY BALANCE AND THE AETIOLOGY OF OBESITY

Obesity occurs when, and only when, energy intake exceeds energy expenditure over a long period of time. The excess energy is stored as about 75% fat and 25% non-fat tissue. There are three compo-nents of the energy balance equation: energy stores, energy intake and energy output.

Of these three, habitual energy intake is by far the most difficult to measure accurately, because intake fluctuates widely from day to day and is very likely to be influenced by the techniques used to measure it. Much of the mystery about the aetiology of obesity arises from inaccurate data about energy intake. Fortunately, by accurate measurements of energy expenditure and energy stores it is possible to make a reliable estimate of average energy intake over a long period. The regulation of energy intake in man is the result of a complex interaction between physiological and cognitive influences. Man is very much less competent than the laboratory rat at adjusting intake to changes in requirement, and lean human subjects are not much better at this in the short term than obese human subjects.

Energy expenditure in developed countries is mainly determined by resting metabolic rate (RMR), which accounts for about 73% of total energy expenditure. The thermic effect of food accounts for about another 10% of expenditure among subjects who are in energy balance, leaving only 17% for physical activity and all other forms of thermogenesis. Resting metabolic rate is closely related to fat-free mass (FFM), and since obese people have a larger FFM than lean people they also have a higher RMR. It is unlikely that pre-obese people had a low RMR before becoming obese, because in the obese state their RMR/kg FFM is still slightly greater than normal. However, the coefficient of variation in RMR among people of the same age, sex, weight and FFM is about 10%, so *some* obese individuals will have lower energy expenditures than *some* lean individuals. A reduced thermogenic response of obese subjects to various stimuli has been reported by some, but not all, investigators. Physical activity usually makes a fairly small contribution to energy expenditure in both lean and obese people, and there is little evidence to suggest that the energy expended in physical activity is reduced in obesity.

In general, therefore, obesity is associated with a significantly increased RMR and increased total energy expenditure, so to maintain body weight obese opeople need an increased energy intake. After obese patients reduce weight their metabolic rate and energy expenditure is reduced relative to their obese state, but should not be less than that of individuals of similar age, sex, weight and FFM who were never obese.

The aetiology of obesity in man has genetic, social, cultural and psychological components in different proportions in different people. Obesity is associated with important endocrine changes, notably affecting the action of insulin and sex hormones, but these hormonal changes are probably secondary rather than causal, since they can be induced by experimentally overfeeding normal volunteers. There is evidence that obesity associated with a central fat distribution, indicated by a high waist : hip circumference ratio, is particularly associated with metabolic disorders. This fat distribution is also associated with male hormones. The hormonal abnormalities in obesity revert towards normal with weight reduction. Any undiscovered 'inborn error of metabolism' which causes obesity must ultimately increase energy intake or reduce energy output: there is no evidence of an increased metabolic efficiency in obese people. It is a plausible hypothesis that long-term regulation of energy balance in man is achieved mainly by cognitive means, and the essential defect in obesity is that in obese people this cognitive control is ineffective.

OPTIMUM RATE OF WEIGHT LOSS

If energy intake is less than energy output then the energy stores in the body must be burned. The most labile energy store is a mixture of glycogen and water with an energy value of 1000 kcal/kg, so this component of body weight is quite rapidly lost. The magnitude of the glycogen : water store depends on the previous diet, but it is rarely more than 6 kg. Once the glycogen in exhausted weight loss should be at the expense of excess tissue which is 75% fat and 25% non-fat, and has an energy value of 7000 kcal/kg. However during total starvation roughly 50 : 50 fat : FFM is lost, which has an energy value of 5000 kcal/kg.

It has been empirically determined that, after the initial rapid phase of weight loss, a rate of weight loss between 0.5 and 1.0 kg/week is optimum. The lower rate is applicable to older, shorter patients, and the upper rate to younger taller patients. At this rate of weight loss the correct 75% fat: 25% FFM loss is observed.

TREATMENT OF OBESITY

The general objective is to attain, and sustain, the optimum rate of weight loss described above until the obese patient enters grade 0, but this plan may be modified in certain circumstances. The cornerstone of treatment is a conventional reducing diet (800–1200 kcal), but treatment strategies will vary according to the grade of obesity and other factors. These variations are set out in Chapters 9, 10 and 11, and cannot conveniently be summarised here. Advice and support for people who worry about their weight, although they are not actually obese, is discussed in Chapter 12.

OBESITY, IMPAIRED GLUCOSE TOLERANCE AND CARDIOVASCULAR DISEASE

There are striking similarities between the metabolic derangements in these two diseases associated with obesity. Hyperinsulinaemia may be the link between them. Exercise has a special role in increasing insulin sensitivity by some means not yet fully understood. There is good evidence that the avoidance of obesity, or weight loss in those who are obese, will reduce the risk of non-insulin-dependent diabetes and many forms of cardiovascular disease.

OBESITY IN PREGNANCY

The interests of the obese pregnant woman and her baby are best served if weight gain in pregnancy is limited to about 6 kg, instead of the average 12 kg. It is probably unwise to try to reduce the weight of obese pregnant women.

OBESITY IN CHILDREN

Children change weight-for-height categories quite freely during the first 5 years of life, but by the time they enter their teens it is possible to predict those who will become obese adults. The optimum time to treat or prevent obesity in children is probably between 5 years and 12 years. This can usually be achieved by substituting fruit and low-energy drinks for biscuits, crisps and high-energy soft drinks. The objective is to retard weight gain while height growth continues. This strategy requires the active co-operation of parents and school staff.

HEALTH EDUCATION TO PREVENT OBESITY

Publicity aimed at preventing obesity has been rather ineffective and muted, due to understandable anxiety not to provoke inappropriate weight loss in potential cases of anorexia nervosa. Also, health educators have not been entirely convinced that obesity is an independent risk to health about which something can and should be done. It is hoped that this book may do something to remove inhibitions on this latter point.

Appendix 1
Weight-reducing diet

The diet below is used by the Dietetic Department, Harrow Health District. The number of slices of bread per day is adjusted to provide the required energy content. With 2 large slices of bread (3 oz, or 80 g) or equivalent in exchanges, this diet provides about 1000 kcal (4 MJ) per day.

Suggested meal pattern
Use milk from your allowance for tea, coffee and cereal.

Early morning	Tea or coffee — no sugar.
Breakfast	Grapefruit or juice or fruit from allowance. Egg or small portion of bacon, ham or fish or cheese if desired. Tomatoes or mushrooms if desired (NO FAT) . . . . slices of bread with butter or margarine from allowance OR . . . . cereal. Tea or coffee — no sugar.
Mid morning	Tea or coffee — no sugar. or low calorie squash or Bovril or Oxo.
Mid day or evening	Clear Soup. Lean meat, fish, cheese, egg or liver. Salad or green vegetable as desired or root vegetable. . . . . slices bread OR . . . . potatoes. Fruit from allowance.
Mid afternoon	Tea or coffee — no sugar. or low calorie drink, e.g. squash, or Bovril, Oxo.
Evening or mid day	Clear Soup. Lean meat, fish, cheese, egg or liver. Salad or green vegetables. . . . . slices bread OR . . . . potatoes. Fruit from allowance.
Bedtime	Tea or coffee OR rest of milk from allowance. OR low calorie squash or Bovril or Oxo.

Food portion guide

Lean meat	50 g (2 oz) per cooked portion. This includes beef, lamb, pork, poultry, ham, bacon, liver. BUT you must not fry or use thickened gravies.
Fish	100 g (4 oz) per cooked portion. You may take all kinds of fish. BUT no fried fish or thickened sauces. Drain the oil off tinned fish.
Cheese	25 g (1 oz) per portion of hard cheese, e.g. Cheddar, 100 g (4 oz) per portion cottage cheese. Avoid cream cheese, cheese spread.
Egg	Boiled or poached only. 1 or 2 eggs per portion.
Milk	Keep to 250 ml ($\frac{1}{2}$ pint) a day or 500 ml (1 pint) skimmed milk or 4 tbls skimmed milk powder. Alternatively 150 ml ($\frac{1}{4}$ pint) milk + carton plain unsweetened yoghurt.
Fruit	3 helpings. These can be fresh, frozen, cooked, or tinned in water and includes oranges, apples, pears, peaches, plums, strawberries, blackberries, etc. If sweetening is necessary, use saccharin. In cooking, it should be added at the end just before serving, otherwise a bitter taste will develop. A glass of unsweetened pineapple, orange, tomato or grapefruit juice counts as a helping of fruit.
Root & pulse vegetables	Not more than one tablespoon per day of carrots, parsnips, beetroot, peas, broad beans, sweetcorn, turnips.
Butter or Margarine	Not more than 10 g ($\frac{1}{3}$ oz) per day (or 20 g $-\frac{2}{3}$ oz low fat spread). 75 g (3 oz) should last you a week.
Bread	. . . . slices from large medium cut loaf.
Exchanges	1 slice large loaf (40 g) can be exchanged for the following: 2 small thin cut slices bread 75 g boiled rice — 2 heaped tablespoons 2 Potatoes, size of an egg 75 g boiled spaghetti (15 strands raw) 25 g unsweetened breakfast cereal — 5 tablespoons, preferably wholewheat 3 crispbread 2 Pieces of fruit 2 semi-sweet biscuits or cream crackers

You may eat the following foods freely

Green vegetables	Cabbage, greens, sprouts, cauliflower, green beans, spinach, brocolli, marrow, mushrooms, onions, aubergines
Salads	Lettuce, tomato, cucumber, radishes, celery, spring onions, chicory, cress
Soups	Clear Soups, stock cubes, Bovril, Marmite, Oxo.
Pickles	Pickles in vinegar, e.g. gherkins, Worcester sauce, salt, mustard, pepper, herbs and spices.

Other	Tea, coffee, sodawater, low calorie squashes, sugar-free fizzy drinks, natural P.L.J. etc., saccharin tablet or liquid.

Foods to avoid

Sugary foods	Sugar, glucose, jam, honey, marmalade, syrup, treacle. Chocolates, peppermints and confectionery Ice cream, ice lollies, jellies, fruit yoghurts, instant desserts and mousses.
Fatty foods	Fried foods, dripping, oil, lard, cream, tinned milk, salad cream, mayonnaise and salad dressing.
Drinks	Sweet fruit Squashes, soft drinks, sweetened fizzy drinks, e.g. Lucozade and lemonade. Cocoa and malted milk drinks.
Alcohol	Beer, stout, ale, cider, spirits, wine and sherry.
Cereals	Sugar-coated breakfast cereals, muesli, semolina, sago, tapioca, rice in puddings, cakes, pastry, pies, scones, tinned spaghetti.
Fruit	Tinned fruit in syrup or sorbitol, bananas, grapes, nuts, dried fruit.
Proprietary foods	Slimming foods and diabetic foods (except squashes), powdered sweeteners.
Vegetables	Butter beans, baked beans, barley, lentils, crisps.

It is advisable to eat foods rich in iron such as liver, kidney and corned beef regularly.

Appendix 2
Energy and protein content of common foods

The energy and protein content of some common foods are listed in the following sequence:
Meat and meat products
Eggs
Fish
Milk and cream
Cheese
Bread
Cereals, cakes and biscuits
Fats and oils
Sugar and preserves
Vegetables
Fruit and nuts
Beverages and soft drinks.
Values have been taken from Paul and Southgate (1978) and refer to 100 g portions of food as normally eaten, (eg. meat, cooked, without bone).

Estimates of average consumption of each food group are derived from the National Food Survey for 1978.

Energy value of common foods, and their chief nutritional significance

Meat and meat products
Source of about 16% of energy and 35% of protein intake by average household. Average consumption 140 g/day. Important source of Fe, P and B vitamins, but expensive.

	Energy		*Protein*
	kcal	MJ	g
Bacon, fried, average	480	1.9	24
grilled, average	410	1.7	25
Beef, sirloin, roast	280	1.2	24
Lamb, roast	410	1.7	19

	Energy		Protein
	kcal	MJ	g
Pork, chops, grilled	330	1.4	28
Veal, fillet, roast	230	1.0	32
Chicken, roast	210	0.9	23
Duck, roast	340	1.4	20
	Energy		Protein
	kcal	MJ	g
Turkey, roast	170	0.7	28
Rabbit, stewed	180	0.7	27
Kidney, ox, stewed	170	0.7	26
Liver, calf, fried	250	1.0	27
Tongue, ox, boiled	290	1.2	19
Beef, corned	210	0.9	27
Sausages, pork, fried	320	1.3	14
pork, grilled	320	1.3	14

Eggs
Source of about 2% of energy and 5% of protein intake by average household. High cholesterol content.

	Energy		Protein
	kcal	MJ	g
Eggs, boiled	150	0.6	12
fried	230	1.0	14
scrambled	250	1.0	11

Fish
Source of about 1% of energy and 5% of protein intake by average household. Average consumption 17 g/day. Fatty fishes have higher energy content. Fish oils rich in vitamins A and D. Seafood has high iodine content.

	Energy		Protein
	kcal	MJ	g
Cod, grilled	90	0.4	21
fried in batter	200	0.8	20
Haddock, fried	170	0.7	21
Lemon sole, fried	220	0.9	16
Mackerel, fried	190	0.8	22
Salmon, steamed	200	0.8	20
smoked	140	0.6	25
Lobster, boiled	120	0.5	22
Scampi, fried	320	1.3	12

Milk and cream
Source of about 15% of energy and 17% of protein intake of average household. Average consumption 375 g/day. Sole food for infants: important source of many nutrients, especially Ca and P, but not of Fe or vitamins C or D.

	Energy		Protein
	kcal	MG	g
Milk, cows', fresh, whole	65	0.3	3.3
fresh, skimmed	33	0.14	3.4
Cream, single	210	0.9	2.4
double	450	1.8	1.5

Cheese
Source of about 2% of energy and 7% of protein intake of average household.
Average consumption 17 g/day. Important source of Ca, vitamin A and riboflavin.

	Energy		Protein
	kcal	MJ	g
Camembert	300	1.2	23
Cheddar	400	1.7	26

	Energy		Protein
	kcal	MJ	g
Danish blue	350	1.5	23
Stilton	460	1.9	26
Cottage cheese	100	0.4	14

Bread
Source of about 15% of energy and 16% of protein intake of average households.
Average consumption 140 g/day. Nutrient content affected by milling of grain:
wholemeal flour (100% extraction) contains more fibre than white flour (70% extraction). Wheat bran contains B vitamins, Ca, Fe and Zn, but also phytate which
inhibits absorption of these minerals.

	Energy		Protein
	kcal	MJ	g
Bread, wholemeal	220	0.9	8.8
white	230	1.0	7.8
malt	248	1.1	8.3
Rolls, crusty	290	1.2	11.6

Cereals, cakes, biscuits
Source of about 12% of energy and 6% of protein intake of average household.
Average consumption 80 g/day. Nutritional significance similar to that of bread.

	Energy		Protein
	kcal	MJ	g
Bran, wheat	210	0.9	14
Oatmeal, raw	400	1.7	12
Spaghetti, boiled	120	0.5	4.2
Cornflakes	370	1.6	8.6
Cream crackers	440	1.9	9.5
Crispbread, rye	320	1.4	9.4
Biscuit, digestive, plain	470	2.0	9.8
chocolate	490	2.1	6.8
shortbread	500	2.1	6.2
Cake, fruit, rich	330	1.4	3.7
gingerbread	370	1.6	6.1
sponge, without fat	300	1.3	10.0
Doughnuts	350	1.5	6.0
Pastry, shortcrust	530	2.2	6.9
Pancakes	310	1.3	6.1
Treacle tart	370	1.6	3.8

Fats and oils
Provides 15% of energy intake, and negligible protein. Vitamin content of butter
is variable: margarine is fortified with vitamin A and D. Average consumption
40 g/day.

	Energy		Protein
	kcal	MJ	g
Butter, margarine	740	3.0	—
Vegetable oil, lard, dripping	900	3.7	—

Sugar and preserves
Source of about 10% of energy intake of average household. Negligible contribution to nutrition otherwise. Average consumption about 60 g/day.

	Energy		Protein
	kcal	MJ	g
Sugar, white or Demerara	400	1.7	—
Syrup, golden	300	1.3	—
Honey, comb	280	1.2	—
Jam, fruit with edible seeds	260	1.1	0.6
Marmalade	260	1.1	—
Chocolate, milk	530	2.2	8.4
plain	520	2.2	4.7
Toffee	430	1.8	2.1

Vegetables
Source of about 7% of energy intake and 8% of protein intake of average household. Potato (180 g/day) accounts for the major part of vegetable consumption (340 g/day) and for an even higher proportion of nutrient intake from this group. Food values are affected by freshness of vegetables, processing and cooking.

	Energy		Protein
	kcal	MJ	g
Potatoes, boiled	80	0.34	1.4
baked, with skin	85	0.36	2.1
roast	160	0.66	2.8
chips	250	1.06	3.8
crisps	530	2.22	6.3
Beans, runner, boiled	20	0.08	1.9
broad, boiled	50	0.2	4.1
Beetroot, boiled	40	0.2	1.8
Brussels, sprouts, boiled	20	0.08	2.8
Cabbage, white, raw	20	0.09	1.9
Carrots, boiled	20	0.08	0.6
Celery, raw	8	0.04	0.9
Lettuce, raw	10	0.05	1.0
Mushrooms, raw	10	0.5	1.8
fried	210	0.9	2.2
Mustard and cress, raw	10	0.05	1.6
Onions, boiled	10	0.5	0.6
fried	350	1.4	1.8
Parsnips, boiled	60	0.2	1.3
Peas, fresh, boiled	50	220	5.0
Tomatoes, raw	10	0.06	0.9
fried	70	0.3	1.0

Fruit and nuts
Source of about 2% of energy intake and 1% of protein intake of average household.

Average consumption 90 g/day. Important source of vitamin C, especially from raw and citrus fruit. Generally low energy concentration, since weight is mostly water and cellulose.

	Energy		Protein
	kcal	MJ	g
Apples, eating, raw	50	0.2	0.3
Avocado pear	220	0.9	4.2
Banana, raw	80	0.3	1.1
	Energy		Protein
	kcal	MJ	g
Cherries, raw	50	0.2	0.6
Damson, raw	40	0.2	0.5
Dates, dried	250	1.1	2.0
Gooseberries, raw	20	0.07	1.1
stewed with sugar	50	0.2	0.9
Grapes, raw	60	0.3	0.6
Grapefruit, raw	50	0.2	0.8
Melon, Honeydew, raw	20	0.1	0.6
Oranges, raw	40	0.2	0.8
Peaches, raw	40	0.2	0.6
Pears, raw	40	0.2	0.3
Raspberries, raw	30	0.1	0.9
Strawberries, raw	30	0.1	0.6
Sultanas, dried	250	1.1	1.8
Almonds	560	2.4	16.9
Coconut, fresh	350	1.4	3.2
Peanuts, roasted and salted	570	2.4	24.3
Walnuts	530	2.2	10.6

Beverages
Infusions of coffee and tea (without added milk or sugar) have negligible nutritional value except as vehicles for water. They contain the stimulant caffeine.

Soft drinks and alcoholic beverages
Contribution to average energy intake not known, since they are often consumed outside the home and are not monitored in the National Food Survey. Beer, spirits and wines provided about 160 kcal (0.7 MJ) per head of population per day in 1975. Soft drinks may contribute significant energy to the diet, especially for people on reducing diets.

	Energy		Protein
	kcal	MJ	g
Coca-cola	40	0.2	—
Grapefruit juice, sweetened	40	0.2	—
Lucozade	70	0.3	—
Orange juice, unsweetened	30	0.1	—
sweetened	50	0.2	—
Tomato juice, canned	20	0.07	0.7
Beer (most types)	30	0.15	—
strong ale	70	0.3	—
Cider, sweet or dry	40	0.16	—
vintage	100	0.4	—

	Energy		Protein
	kcal	MJ	g
Wine, dry	70	0.3	—
sweet	90	0.4	—
Port	160	0.6	—
Sherry	120	0.5	—
Spirits, 70% proof	220	0.9	—

References

Abraham S, Carroll M D, Najjar M F, Robinson F (1983) Obese and overweight adults in the United States. Vital and Health Statistics USDHHS, publ. no (PHS)83–1680, PHS NCHS series 11, No 230.

Abraham S, Collins G, Nordseik M (1971) Relationship of childhood weight status to morbidity in adults. Health Services and Mental Health Administration Health Reports. 86: 273–284.

Abrams B F, Laros R K (1986) Prepregnancy weight, weight gain, and birthweight. American Journal of Obstetrics and Gynecology 154: 503–509.

Acheson K J, Campbell I T, Edholm O G, Miller D S, Stock M J (1980) Measurement of food and energy intake in man — an evaluation of some techniques. American Journal of Clinical Nutrition 33: 1147–1154.

Agarwal N, Lee B Y, Del Guercio L R M (1985) Energy expenditure in spinal cord injured patients. American Journal of Clinical Nutrition 41:861.

Alexander M K (1964). The postmortem estimation of total body fat, muscle and bone. Clinical Science 26: 193–202.

Allan M (1974) The Joy of Slimming. London, Wolfe Publishing, 353pp.

Allen D W, Quigley B M (1977) The role of physical activity in the control of obesity. Medical Journal of Australia 2:434–438.

Allen T H, Krzywicki H J, Roberts J E (1959) Density, fat, water and solids in freshly isolated tissues. Journal of Applied Physiology 14: 1005–1008.

Allon N (1975) The stigma of overweight in everyday life. In: Bray G, ed. Obesity in Perspective. U.S. Government Printing Office, Washington, 83–102.

Alpert M A, Terry B E, Kelly D L (1985) Effect of weight loss on cardiac chamber size, wall thickness and left ventricular function in morbid obesity. American Journal of Cardiology 55: 783–786.

Amaral J F, Thompson W R (1985) Gallbladder disease in the morbidly obese. American Journal of Surgery 149: 551–557.

American Diabetes Association (1979) Principles of nutrition and dietary recommendations for individuals with diabetes mellitus. Diabetes 28:1027.

Andersen T, Backer O G, Stokholm K H, Quaade F (1984) Randomised trial of diet and gastroplasty compared with diet alone in morbid obesity. New England Journal of Medicine 310: 352–356.

Andersen T, Pedersen B H (1984) Pouch volume, stoma diameter and clinical outcome after gastroplasty for morbid obesity. Scandinavian Journal of Gastroenterology 19: 643–649.

Andres R, Elahi D, Tobin J D, Muller D C, Brant L (1985) Impact of age on weight goals. Annals of Internal Medicine 103: 1030–1033.

Annuzzi G, Vaccaro O, Caprio S, DiBonito P, Caso G, Riccardi G, Rivellese A.

(1985) Association between low habitual physical activity and impaired glucose tolerance. Clinical Physiology 5: 63–70.

Apfelbaum M (1987) A review of the development of VLCD and new experience. In: Eliahou H, ed. Recent Advances in Obesity Research: V. London : John Libbey (in press).

Aschoff J, Pohl H (1970) Rhythmic variations in energy metabolism. Federation Proceedings 29: 1541–1552.

Asher P (1966) Fat babies and fat children. The prognosis for obesity in the very young. Archives of Disease in Childhood 41: 672–673.

Ashwell M A (1973) A survey investigating patients' views on doctors' treatment of obesity. Practitioner 211: 653–658.

Ashwell M (1978) Commercial weight loss groups. In: Bray G, ed. Recent Advances in Obesity Research : II. London, Newman Publishing, 266–276.

Ashwell M, Chinn S, Stalley S, Garrow J S (1982) Female fat distribution — a simple classification based on two circumference measurements. International Journal of Obesity 6: 143–152.

Ashwell M, Cole T J, Dixon A K (1985) Obesity: new insight into the anthropometric classification of fat distribution shown by computed tomography. British Medical Journal 290: 1692–1694.

Ashwell M A, Etchell L (1974) Attitude of the individual to his own body weight. British Journal of Preventive and Social Medicine 28: 127–132.

Ashwell M, McCall S A, Cole T J, Dixon A K (1987) Fat distribution and its metabolic complications: interpretation. Euro-Nut Workshop on Body Composition and Fat Distribution (in press).

Ashwell M, Priest P, Bondoux M, Sowter C, McPherson C K (1976) Human fat cell sizing — a quick, simple method. Journal of Lipid Research 17: 190–192.

Ashworth A, Wolff H S (1969) A simple method for measuring calorie expenditure during sleep. Pflugers Archives: European Journal of Physiology 306: 191–194.

Astrup A (1986) Thermogenesis in human brown adipose tissue and skeletal muscle induced by sympathomimetic stimulation. Acta Endocrinologica 112, suppl. 278:32pp.

Astrup A, Lundsgaard C, Madsen J, Christensen N J (1985) Enhanced thermogenic responsiveness during chronic ephedrine treatment in man. American Journal of Clinical Nutrition 42: 83–94.

Atwater W O, Benedict F G (1899) Experiments in the metabolism of matter and energy in the human body. Bulletin U S partment of Agriculture 69: 112pp.

Atwater W O, Benedict F G (1905) A respiration calorimeter with appliances for the direct determination of oxygen. Carnegie Institution of Washington, Publication 42, 4pp .

Avons P, James W P T (1986) Energy expenditure of young men from obese and non-obese families. Human Nutrition: Clinical Nutrition 40C: 259–270

Bachynsky N (1987) A reassessment of the potential of 2, 4-dinitrophenol in weight reduction. In: Eliahou H, ed. Recent Advances in Obesity Research: V. London, John Libbey (in press).

Baecke J A H, Burema J, Frijters J E R, Hautvast J G A J, van der Weil-Wetzels W A M (1983) Obesity in young Dutch adults: 1. sociodemographic variables and body mass index. International Journal of Obesity 7: 1–12.

Baird I M (1981) Low-calorie-formula diets — are they safe? International Journal of Obesity 5: 249–256.

Baird I M, Parsons R L, Howard A N (1974) Clinical and metabolic studies of chemically defined diets in the management of obesity. Metabolism 23: 645–657.

Baird J D (1973) The role of obesity in the development of clinical diabetes. In: Robertson R F, Proudfoot A T, eds. Anorexia nervosa and obesity. Edinburgh, Royal College of Physicians, 83–99.

Baron J A, Schori A, Crow B, Carter R, Mann J I (1986) A randomised controlled trial of low carbohydrate and low fat/high fibre diets for weight loss. American Journal of Public Health 76: 1293–1296.

Beazley J M, Swinhoe J R (1979) Body weight in parous women: is there any alteration between successive pregnancies? Acta Obstetrica et Gynecologica Scandinavica 58: 45–47.

Beeston J W U (1965) Determinations of specific gravity of live sheep and its correlation with fat percentage. In: Brozek J, ed. Human Body Composition, Pergamon Press, Oxford, 49–55.

Behnke A R, Feen B G, Welham W C (1942) The specific gravity of healthy men; body weight and volume as an index of obesity. Journal of the American Medical Association. 118: 495–498.

Benedict F G (1930) A helmet for use in clinical studies of gaseous metabolism. New England Journal of Medicine 203: 150–158.

Benedict F G, Benedict C G (1933) Mental effort in relation to gaseous exchanges, heart rate and the mechanics of respiration. Carnegie Institute of Washington, Publ 446, 83pp.

Benedict F G, Miles W R, Roth P, Smith M (1919) Human vitality and efficiency under prolonged restricted diet. Washington, DC: Carnegie Institution publ. 280, 83pp.

Bennett P, Rushforth N B, Miller M, LeCompte P M (1976) Epidemiologic studies of diabetes in the Pima Indians. Recent Progress in Hormone Research 32: 333–376.

Benzinger T H, Huebscher R G, Minard D, Kitzinger C (1958) Human calorimetry by means of the gradient principle. Journal of Applied Physiology 12, Suppl 1: 1–28.

Berchtold P, Jorgens V, Finke C, Berger M (1981) Epidemiology of obesity and hypertension. International Journal of Obesity 5: 1–7.

Berchtold P, Sims E A H (1981) Obesity and hypertension: conclusions and recommendations. International Journal of Obesity 5: 183–184.

Berry E M, Hirsch J, Most J, McNamara D J, Thornton J (1986) The relationship of dietary fat to plasma lipid levels as studied by factor analysis of adipose tissue fatty acid composition in a free-living population of middle-aged American man. American Journal of Clinical Nutrition 44: 220–231.

Bielinski R, Schutz Y, Jequier E (1985) Energy metabolism during the post-exercise recovery in man. American Journal of Clinical Nutrition 42: 69–82.

Billewicz W Z, Thomson A M (1970) Body weight in parous women. British Journal of Social and Preventive Medicine 24: 97–104.

Bingham S A, Cummings J H (1985) Urine nitrogen as an independent validatory measure of dietary intake: a study of nitrogen balance in individuals consuming their normal diet. American Journal of Clinical Nutrition 42: 1276–1289.

Bistrian B R (1978) Clinical use of a protein-sparing modified fast. Journal of the American Medical Association 240: 2299–2302.

Bjorntorp P (1985) Regional patterns of fat distribution. Annals of Internal Medicine 103: 994–995.

Bjorntorp P, Carlgren G, Isaksson B, Krotkiewski M, Larsson B, Sjostrom L (1975) Effect of an energy-reduced dietary regimen in relation to adipose tissue cellularity in obese women. American Journal of Clinical Nutrition 28: 445–452.

Bjorvell H, Rossner S (1985) Long-term treatment of severe obesity: four year follow up of results of combined behavioural modification programme. British Medical Journal 291: 379–382.

Black A E, Ravenscroft C, Sims A J (1984) The NACNE report: are dietary goals realistic? Comparisons with the dietary patterns of dietitians. Human Nutrition: Applied Nutrition 38A: 165–179.

Blackburn M W, Calloway D H (1976) Energy expenditure and consumption of mature, pregnant and lactating women. Journal of the American Dietetic Association 69: 29–37.

Blair S N, Haskell W L, Ho P, Paffenbarger R S, Vranizan K M, Farquhar J W, Wood P D (1985) Assessment of habitual physical activity by a seven-day recall in a community survey and controlled experiments. American Journal of Epidemiology 122: 794–804.

Blaza S E (1980) Thermogenesis in lean and obese individuals. PhD thesis, CNAA.

Blaza S E, Garrow J S (1980) The effect of anxiety on metabolic rate. Proceedings of the Nutrition Society 39:13A.

Blaza S, Garrow J S (1983) Thermogenic response to temperature, exercise and food stimuli in lean and obese women, studied by 24 h direct calorimetry. British Journal of Nutrition 49: 171–180.

Bloom W L (1959) Fasting as an introduction to the treatment of obesity. Metabolism 8: 214–220.

Blundell J E, Hill A H (1986) Paradoxical effects of an intense sweetener (Aspartame) on appetite. Lancet i: 1092–1093.

Boddy K, Hume R, White C, Pack A, King P C, Weyers E, Rowan T, Mills E (1976) The relation between potassium in body fluids and total body potassium in healthy and diabetic subjects. Clinical Science and Molecular Medicine 50: 455–461.

Bogardus C, Lillioja S, Mott D M, Hollenbeck C, Reaven G (1985a) Relationship between degree of obesity and in vivo insulin action in man. American Journal of Physiology 248: E286–E291.

Bogardus C, Lillioja S, Mott D, Zawadzki J, Young A, Abbott W (1985b) Evidence for reduced thermic effect of insulin and glucose infusions in Pima Indians. Journal of Clinical Investigation 75: 1264–1269.

Bogardus C, Lillioja S, Ravussin E, Abbott W, Zawadzki J K, Young A, Knowler W C, Jacobwitz R, Moll P P (1986) Familial dependence of the resting metabolic rate. New England Journal of Medicine 315:96-100.

Bogle S, Burkinshaw L, Kent J T (1985) Estimating the composition of tissue gained or lost from measurements of elementary body composition. Physics in Medicine and Biology 30: 369–384.

Bolden K J (1975) Against the active treatment of obesity in general practice. Update 2: 339–348.

Bo-Linn C W, Carol A S A, Morawski S G, Fordtran J S (1982) Starch blockers — their effect on calorie absorption from a high starch meal. New England Journal of Medicine 307:1413.

Bonham G S, Brock D B (1985) The relationship of diabetes with race, sex, and obesity. American Journal of Clinical Nutrition 41: 776–783.

Booth D A (1977) Satiety and appetite are conditioned reactions. Psychosomatic Medicine 39: 76–81.

Booth D A, Lee M, McAleavey C (1976) Acquired sensory control of satiation in man. British Journal of Psychology 67: 137–147.

Booth R A D, Goddard B A, Paton A (1966) Measurement of fat thickness in man: a comparison of ultrasound,Harpenden calipers and electrical conductivity. British Journal of Nutrition 20: 719–725.

Boothby W M, Sandiford I (1929) Normal values for standard metabolism.
American Journal of Physiology 90: 290–291.

Boothby W M, Berkson J, Dunn H L (1936) Studies of the energy metabolism
of normal individuals: a standard for basal metabolism with a nomogram for
clinical application. American Journal of Physiology 116:468–4484.

Borjeson M (1976) The aetiology of obesity in children. Acta Paediatrica
Scandinavica 65: 279–287.

Borkan G A, Gerzof S G, Robbins A H, Hults D E, Silbert C K, Silbert J E
(1982) Assessment of abdominal fat content by computed tomography.
American Journal of Clinical Nutrition 36: 172–177.

Borkan G A, Sparrow D, Wisniewski C, Vokonas P S (1986) Body weight and
coronary heart disease risk: patterns of risk factor change associated with long-
term weight change. American Journal of Epidemiology 124: 410–419.

Bouchard C (1987) Genetics of body fat, energy expenditure and adipose tissue
metabolism. In: Eliahou H, ed. Recent Advances in Obesity Research: V.
London,John Libbey (in press)

Bouchard C, Savard R, Despres J-P, Tremblay A, Leblanc C (1985) Body
composition in adopted and biological siblings. Human Biology 57: 61–75.

Braddon F E M (1985) Exercise and obesity in a national birth cohort.
Proceedings of the Nutrition Society 44:25A.

Braitman L E, Adlin E V, Stanton J L (1985) Obesity and caloric intake: the
national health and nutrition examination survey of 1971–1975 (HANES I).
Journal of Chronic Diseases 38: 727–732.

Bray G A (ed.) (1979) Obesity in America. National Institute of Health
Publication No 79–358: US Department of Health Education and Welfare,
Washington, 285pp

Bray G A (1985a) Obesity: definition, diagnosis and disadvantages Medical
Journal of Australia 142: S2–S8.

Bray G A (1985b) Complications of obesity. Annals of Internal Medicine
103: 1052–1061.

Bray G A, Gallagher T F (1975) Manifestation of hypothalamic obesity in man.
Medicine (Baltimore) 54: 301–330.

Brewer T (1967) Human pregnancy nutrition: a clinical view. Obstetrics and
Gynecology 30: 605–607.

British Diabetic Association (1982) Dietary recommendations for diabetics in the
1980s. Human Nutrition: Applied Nutrition 36A: 378–394.

Brook C G D, Huntley R M C, Slack J (1975) Influence of heredity and
environment in determination of skinfold thickness in children. British Medical
Journal ii: 719–721.

Brooke O G, Abernethy E (1985) Obesity in children. Human Nutrition: Applied
Nutrition 39A: 304–314.

Brownell K D, Stunkard A J (1978) Behavioural treatment of obesity in children.
American Journal of Disease of Children 132: 403–412.

Bruch H (1974) Eating disorders: obesity, anorexia nervosa, and the person
within. London, Routledge & Kegan Paul. pp396.

Bryson E, Dore C, Garrow J S (1979) Wholemeal bread and satiety. Lancet
ii: 260–261.

Burch P R J, Spiers F W (1953) Measurement of the gamma radiation from the
human body. Nature (London) 172: 519–521.

Burkinshaw L, Cotes J E, Jones P R M, Knibbs A V (1971) Prediction of total
body potassium from anthropometric measurements. Human Biology 43: 344–355.

Buzina R, Suboticanec K, Stavljenic A (1986) Adolescent obesity and risk factors
of coronary heart disease. Bibliotheca Nutritia et Dieta 37: 18–26.

Cairns S R, Kark A E, Peters T J (1986) Raised hepatic free fatty acids in a patient with acute fatty liver after gastric surgery for morbid obesity. Journal of Clinical Pathology 39: 647–649.

Campbell D M (1983) Dietary restriction in obesity and its effect on neonatal outcome. In:

Campbell D M, Gilmer M D G, eds.Nutrition in pregnancy: proceedings of the tenth study group of the Royal College of Obstetricians and Gynaecologists. London:RCOG. 243–250.

Campbell R G, Hashim S A, van Itallie T B (1971) Nutritive density and food intake in man. New England Journal of Medicine 285: 1402–1407.

Cardus D, Wesley G, McTaggart B S (1985) Body composition in spinal cord injury. Archives of Physical Medicine and Rehabilitation 66: 257–259.

Cataldo J (1985) Obesity: a new perspective on an old problem Health Education Journal 44: 213–218.

Cauderay M, Tappy L, Temler E, Jequier E, Hillebrand I, Felber J-P (1985) Effect of alpha-glycohydrolase inhibitors (Bay m1099 and Bay01248) on sucrose metabolism in normal men. Metabolism 35: 472–477.

Challis R A J, Arch J R S, Newsholm E A (1985) The rate of substrate cycling between fructose 6-phosphate and fructose 1,6-biphosphate in skeletal muscle from cold-exposed, hyperthyroid or acutely exercised rats. Biochemical Journal 231: 217–220.

Charney E, Goodman H C, McBride M, Lyon B, Pratt R (1976) Childhood antecedents of adult obesity. New England Journal of Medicine 295: 6–9.

Christlieb A R, Krolewski A S, Warram J H, Soeldner J S (1985) Is insulin the link between hypertension and obesity? Hypertension 7, suppl II: II–54–II–57.

Cochrane G, Friesen J (1986) Hypnotherapy in weight loss treatment. Journal of Consulting and Clinical Psychology 54: 489–492.

Cohen N, Flamenbaum W (1986) Obesity and hypertension: demonstration of a floor effect. American Journal of Medicine 80: 177–181.

Cohn S H, Ellis K J, Wallach S (1974) In vivo neutron activation analysis: clinical potential in body composition studies. American Journal of Medicine 57: 683–686.

Cohn S H, Vaswani A N, Vartsky D, Yasumura S, Sawitsky A, Gartenhaus W, Ellis K J (1982) In vivo quatification of body nitrogen for nutritional assessment. American Journal of Clinical Nutrition 35: 1186–1191.

Cohn S H, Vaswani A N, Yasumura S, Yuen K, Ellis K J (1984) Improved models for determination of body fat by in vivo neutron activation. American Journal of Clinical Nutrition 40: 255–259.

Cole-Hamilton I, Gunner K, Leverkus C, Starr J (1986) A study among dietitians and adult members of their households of the practicalities and implications of folowing proposed dietary guidelines in the UK. Human Nutrition: Applied Nutrition 40A: 365–389.

Colt E W D, Wang J, Stallone F, Van Itallie T B, Pierson R N (1981) A possible low intracellular potassium in obesity. American Journal of Clinical Nutrition 34: 367–372.

COMA (1984) Diet and cardiovascular disease. DHSS Report on Health and Social Subjects No 28, Committee on Medical Aspects of Food Policy, HMSO, London, 32pp

Connor S L, Gustafson J R, Artaud-Wild S M, Flavell D P, Classick-Kohn C J, Hatcher L F, Connor W E (1986) The cholesterol/saturated-fat index: an indication of the hypercholesterolaemic and atherogenic potential of food. Lancet i: 1229–1232.

Conway J M, Norris K H, Bodwell C E (1984) A new approach for the estimation of body compositiomn: infrared interactance. American Journal of Clinical Nutrition 40: 1123–1130.

Coupar A M, Kennedy T (1980) Running a weight control group: experiences of a psychologist and a general practitioner. Journal of the Royal College of General Practitioners 30: 41–48.

Coward W A, Prentice A M, Murgatroyd P R, Davies H L, Cole T J, Sawyer M, Goldberg G R, Halliday D, Macnamara J P (1985) Measurement of CO_2 and water production rates in man using $^2H_2{}^{18}O$-labelled H_2O; comparisons between calorimeter and isotope values. In: van Es AJH, ed. Human energy metabolism: physical activity and energy expenditure measurements in epidemiological research based on direct and indirect calorimetry. EUR-NUT Report No 5, Wageningen, Netherlands. 126–128.

Craddock D (1973) Obesity and Its Management. Edinburgh, Churchill Livingstone, 205pp

Crisp A H (1973) The nature of primary anorexia nervosa. In: Robertson R F, ed. Anorexia Nervosa and Obesity. Edinburgh, Royal College of Physicians, 18–30.

Croft P R, Brigg D, Smith S, Harrison C B, Branthwaite A, Collins M F (1986) How useful is weight reduction in the management of hypertension? Journal of the Royal College of General Practitioners 36: 445–448.

Culebras J M, Fitzpatrick G F, Brennan M F, Boyden C M, Moore F D (1977) Total body water and exchangeable hydrogen. II. A review of comparative data from animals based on isotope dilution and desiccation, with a report of new data from the rat. American Journal of Physiology 232: R60–R65.

Cunningham S, Leslie P, Hopwood D, Illingworth P, Jung R T, Nicholls D G, Peden N, Rafael J, Rial E (1985) The characterisation and energetic potential of brown adipose tissue in man. Clinical Science 69: 343–348.

Dallosso H M, James W P T (1984) The role of smoking in the regulation of energy balance. International Journal of Obesity 8: 365–375.

Daly J M, Heymsfield S B, Head C A, Harvey L P, Nixon D W, Katzeff H, Grossman G D (1985) Human energy requirements: overestimation by widely used prediction equation. American Journal of Clinical Nutrition 42: 1170–1174.

Daniels R J, Katzeff H L, Ravussin E, Garrow J S, Danforth E Jr. (1982) Obesity in the Pima Indians: is there a thrifty gene? Clinical Research 30:244A.

Dauncey M J (1981) Influence of mild cold on 24h energy expenditure, resting metabolism and diet-induced thermogenesis. British Journal of Nutrition 45: 257–267.

Dauncey M J, Murgatroyd P R, Cole T J (1978) A human calorimeter for the direct and indirect measurement of 24 h energy expenditure. British Journal of Nutrition 39: 557–566.

Davidson S, Passmore R, Brock J F, Truswell A S (1979) Human Nutrition and Dietetics (7th edition) Edinburgh, Churchill Livingstone. p 246.

Dawes M G (1984) Obesity in a Somerset town: prevalence and relationship to morbidity. Journal of the Royal College of General Practitioners 34: 328–330.

DeFronzo R A (1981) Insulin and renal sodium handling : clinical implications. International Journal of Obesity 5: 93–104.

DeFronzo, R A, Golay A, Felber J-P (1985) Glucose and lipid metabolism in obesity and diabetes mellitus. In: Garrow J S, Halliday D, eds. Substrate and Energy Metabolism in Man. Third Clinical Research Centre Symposium, 17–19 September 1984. London, Libbey, 70–81.

De Garine I (1972) The sociocultural aspects of nutrition. Ecology Food and Nutrition 1: 143–163.

Dempsey D T, Crosby L O, Lusk E, Oberlander J L, Pertsschuck M J, Mullen J L (1984) Total body water and total body potassium in anorexia nervosa. American Journal of Clinical Nutrition 40: 260–269.

Devlin J T, Horton E S (1986) Potentiation of the thermic effect of insulin by exercise: differences between lean, obese and non-insulin-dependent diabetic men. American Journal of Clinical Nutrition 43: 884–890.

Dickerson J W T, Widdowson E M (1960) Chemical changes in skeletal muscle during development. Biochemical Journal, 74: 247–257.

Diethelm R, Garrow J S, Stalley S F (1977) An apparatus for measuring the density of obese patients. Journal of Physiology (London) 267: 14P–15P.

Dietz W H (1986) Preventions of childhood obesity. Pediatric Clinics of North America 33: 823–833.

Dietz W H, Hartung R (1985) Changes in height velocity of obese preadolescents during weight reduction. American Journal of Diseases of Childhood 139: 705–707.

Dine M S, Gartside P S, Glueck C J, Rheines L, Greene G, Khoury P (1979) Where do the heaviest children come from? A prospective study of white children from birth to 5 years of age. Pediatrics 63: 1–7.

Dixon A S, Henderson D (1973) Prescribing for osteoarthritis. Prescribers' Journal 13: 41–49.

Dore C, Hesp R, Wilkins D, Garrow J S (1982) Prediction of energy requirements of obese patients after massive weight loss. Human Nutrition: Clinical Nutrition 36C: 41–48.

Drenick E J, Hargis H W (1978) Jaw wiring for weight reduction. Obesity and Bariatric Medicine 7: 210–213.

Drenick E J, Swenseid M E, Tuttle S G , Blahd W H (1964) Prolonged starvation as a treatment for obesity. Journal of the American Medical Association 187: 100–105.

Drife J O (1986) Weight gain in pregnancy: eating for two or just getting fat? British Medical Journal 293: 903–904.

Dublin L I (1953) Relation of obesity to longevity. New England Journal of Medicine 248: 971–974.

Ducimetiere P, Richard J, Cambien F (1986) The pattern of subcutaneous fat distribution in middle-aged men and the risk of coronary heart disease: the Paris prospective study. International Journal of Obesity 10: 229–240.

Durnin J V G A (1959) The use of surface area and of body weight as standards of reference in studies on human energy expenditure. British Journal of Nutrition 13: 68–71.

Durnin J V G A, Armstrong W H, Womersley J (1971) An experimental study on the variability of measurement of skinfold thickness by three observers on twenty-three young women and twenty-seven young men. Proceedings of the Nutrition Society 30: 9A–10A.

Durnin J V G A, McKillop F M (1978) The relationship between body build in infancy and percentage body fat in adolescence: a 14 year follow-up of 102 infants. Proceedings of the Nutrition Society 37:81A.

Durnin J V G A, Passmore R (1967) Energy Work and Leisure. London, Heinemann, 165pp

Durnin J V G A, Rahaman M M (1967) The assessment of the amount of fat in the human body from measurement of skinfold thickness. British Journal of Nutrition. 21: 681–689.

Durnin J V G A, Satwanti (1982) Variations in the assessment of the fat content of the human body due to experimental technique in measuring body density. Annals of Human Biology 9: 221–225.

Durnin J V G A, Womersley J (1974) Body fat assessed from body density and its estimation from skinfold thickness: measurement on 481 men and women from 16–72 years. British Journal of Nutrition 32: 77–97.

Durrant M L, Garrow J S, Royston P, Stalley S F, Sunkin S, Warwick P M (1980) Factors influencing the composition of the weight lost by obese patients on a reducing diet. British Journal of Nutrition 44: 275–285.

Durrant M, Wloch R (1979) The effect of palatability on energy intake in two obese women. Proceedings of the Nutrition Society 38:37A.

Dustan H P (1985) Obesity and hypertension. Annals of Internal Medicine 103: 1047–1049.

Dwyer J T, Berman E M (1978) Battling the bulge: a continuing struggle. Two-year follow-up of successful losers in a commercial dieting concern. In: Bray G, ed. Recent Advances in Obesity Research:II. London, Newman Publishing, 277–294.

Editorial (1986) Risks of antihypertensive therapy. Lancet ii: 1075–1076.

Edwards D A W (1950) Observations of the distribution of subcutaneous fat. Clinical Science 9: 259–270.

Edwards L E, Dickes W F, Alton I R, Hakanson E Y (1978) Pregnancy in the massively obese: course outcome and obesity prognosis for the infant. American Journal of Obstetrics and Gynecology 131: 479–483.

Efiong E I (1975) Pregnancy in the overweight Nigerian. British Journal of Obstretrics and Gynaecology 82: 903–906.

Eichner E R (1985) Alcohol versus exercise for coronary protection. American Journal of Medicine 79: 231–240.

Eid E E (1970) Follow-up study of physical growth of children who had excessive weight gain in first six months of life. British Medical Journal ii: 74–76.

Eliahou H E, Iaina A, Gaon T, Shochat J, Modan M (1981) Body weight reduction necessary to attain normotension in the overweight hypertensive patient. International Journal of Obesity 5: 157--63.

Ellis K J, Shukla K K, Cohn S H, Pierson R N (1974) A predictor of total body potassium on man based on height, weight, sex and age: applications to metabolic disorders. Journal of Laboratory and Clinical Medicine 83: 716–727.

Englyst H N, Cummings J H (1986) Digestion of the carbohydrates of banana (Musa paradisiaca sapientum) in the human small intestine. American Journal of Clinical Nutrition 44: 42–50.

Epstein L H, Wing R R, Penner B C, Kress M J (1985) Effect of diet and controlled exercise on weight loss in obese children. Journal of Pediatrics 107: 358–361.

Eriksson S, Erikssson K-F, Bondesson L (1986) Nonalcoholic steatohepatitis in obesity: a reversible condition. Acta Medica Scandinavica 220: 83–88.

Fanger P O (1970) Thermal Comfort. New York, McGraw-Hill, 244pp.

Feigin R D, Beisel W R, Wannemacher R W (1971) Rhythmicity of plasma amino acids and relation to dietary intake. American Journal of Clinical Nutrition 24: 329–341.

Fentem P H (1985) Exercise and the promotion of health, Proceedings of the Nutrition Society 44: 297–302.

Finer N, Swan P C, Mitchell F T. (1986) Metabolic rate after massive weight loss in human obesity. Clinical Science 70: 395–401.

Firth R G, Bell P M, Rizza R A (1986) Effects of tolazamide and exogenous insulin on insulin action in patients with non-insulin-dependent diabetes mellitus. New England Journal of Medicine 314: 1280–1286.

Fisch R, Bilek M K, Ulstrom R (1975) Obesity and leanness at birth and their relationship to body habitus in later childhood. Pediatrics 56: 521–528.

Flatt J-P (1985) Energetics of intermediary metabolism. In: Garrow J S, Halliday D, eds. Substrate and Energy Metabolism in Man. Third Clinical Research Centre Symposium, 17–19 September 1984. London, Libbey, 58–69.

Folsom A R, Castersen C J, Taylor H L, Jacobs D R, Luepker R V, Gomez-Marin O, Gillum R F, Blackburn H (1985) Leisure time physical activity and its relationship to coronary risk factors in a population-based sample. American Journal of Epidemiology 121: 570–579.

Forbes G B, Bruining G J (1976) Urinary creatinine excretion and lean body mass. American Journal of Clinical Nutrition 29: 1359–1366.

Forbes G B, Drenick E J (1979) Loss of body nitrogen on fasting. American Journal of Clinical Nutrition 32: 1570–1574.

Forbes G B, Lewis A M (1956) Total sodium, potassium and chloride in adult man. Journal of Clinical Investigation 35: 596–600.

Forbes G B, Welle S L (1983) Lean body mass in obesity. International Journal of Obesity 7: 99–107.

Forbes R M, Cooper A R, Mitchell H H (1953) The composition of the adult human body as determined by chemical analysis, Journal of Biological Chemistry 203: 359–366.

Forbes R M, Mitchell H H, Cooper A R (1956) Further studies on the gross composition and mineral elements of the adult human body, Journal of Biological Chemistry 223: 969–975.

Forde O H, Thelle D S, Arnesen E, Mjos O D (1986) Distribution of high density lipoprotein cholesterol according to relative body weight, cigarette smoking and leisure time physical activity. Acta Medica Scandinavica 219: 167–171.

Fordyce G L, Garrow J S, Kark A E, Stalley S F (1979) Jaw wiring and gastric bypass in the treatment of severe obesity. Obesity and Bariatric Medicine 8: 14–17.

Fournier P F, Otteni F M (1983) Lipodissection in body sculpturing: the dry procedure. Plastic and Reconstructive Surgery 72: 598–609.

Freedman-Akabas S, Colt E, Kissilef H R, Pi-Sunyer F X (1985) Lack of sustained increase in metabolic rate following exercise in fit and unfit subjects. American Journal of Clinical Nutrition 41: 545–549.

Friedman C I, Kim M H (1985) Obesity and its effect on reproductive function. Clinical Obstetrics and Gynecology 28: 645–663.

Fuller J H, Shipley M J, Rose G, Jarrett R J, Keen H (1980) Coronary-heart-diesease risk and impaired glucose tolerance: the Whitehall study. Lancet i: 1373–1376.

Garbaciak J A, Richter M, Miller S, Barton J J (1985) Maternal weight and pregnancy complications. American Journal of Obstetrics and Gynecology 152: 238–245.

Garfinkel L (1985) Overweight and cancer. Annals of Internal Medicine 103: 1034–1036.

Garn S M (1961) Radiographic analysis of body composition. In: Brozek J, Henschel A, eds. Techniques for Measuring Body Composition, Nat. Acad. Sci. — Nat. Res. Council, Washington D.C., 36–58.

Garn S M (1985) Relationship between birthweight and subsequent weight gain. American Journal of Clinical Nutrition 42: 57–60.

Garn S M, Clark D C. (1976) Trends in fatnesss and the origins of obesity. Pediatrics 57: 443–456.

Garnett E S, Barnard D L, Ford J, Goodbody R A, Woodhouse M A (1969) Gross fragmentation of cardiac myofibrils after therapeutic starvation for obesity. Lancet i: 914–916.

Garren L, Garren M, Plotzker R, Werbitt W, Giordano F (1987) The Garren gastric bubble: an aid for weight loss in the obese. In: Eliahou H, ed. Recent Advances in Obesity Research: V. London, John Libbey (in press).

Garrow J S (1974a) Dental splinting in the treatment of hyperphagic obesity. Proceedings of the Nutrition Society 33:29A.

Garrow J S (1974b) Energy Balance and Obesity in Man. Amsterdam, Elsevier/North-Holland Biomedical Press, 335pp

Garrow J S (1975) A survey of three slimming and weight control organisations in the U.K. In: Howard A, ed. Recent Advances in Obesity Research:I. London, Newman Publishing, 301–304.

Garrow J S (1981) Treat Obesity Seriously: A Clinical Manual. London: Churchill Livingstone, 246pp

Garrow J S, Durrant M L, Mann S, Stalley S F, Warwick P M (1978) Factors determining weight loss in obese patients in a metabolic ward. International Journal of Obesity 2: 441–447.

Garrow J S, Durrant M L, Blaza S, Wilkins D, Royston P, Sunkin S. (1981) The effect of meal frequency and protein concentration on the composition of the weight lost by obese subjects. British Journal of Nutrition 45: 5–16.

Garrow J S, Gardiner G T (1981) Maintenance of weight loss in obese patients after jaw wiring. British Medical Journal 282: 858–860.

Garrow J S, Hawes S. (1972) The role of amino acid oxidation in causing specific dynamic action in man. British Journal of Nutrition 27: 211–219.

Garrow J S, Scott P F, Heels S, Nair K S, Halliday D (1983) A study of 'starch blockers' in man using ^{13}C-enriched starch as a tracer. Human Nutrition: Clinical Nutrition 37C: 301–305.

Garrow J S, Stalley S F (1975) Is there a set point for human body weight? Proceedings of the Nutrition Society 34:84A.

Garrow J S, Stalley S, Diethelm R, Pittet Ph, Hesp R, Halliday D (1979) A new method for measuring the body density of obese adults. British Journal of Nutrition 42: 173–183.

Garrow J S, Webster J (1985a) Quetelet's index (W/H^2) as a measure of fatness. International Journal of Obesity 9: 147–153.

Garrow J S, Webster J. (1985b) Are pre-obese people energy-thrifty? Lancet i: 670–671.

Garrow J S, Webster J D. (1986a) A computer-controlled indirect calorimeter for the measurement of energy expenditure in one or two subjects simultaneously. Human Nutrition: Clinical Nutrition 40C: 315–321.

Garrow J S, Webster J D (1986b) Long-term results of treatment of severe obesity with jaw wiring and waist cord. Proceedings of the Nutrition Society 45:119A.

Garrow J S, Wright D (1980) Burning off unwanted energy, Lancet i:377.

Geleibster A, Westreich S, Pierson R N, Van Itallie T B (1986) Extra-abdominal pressure alters food intake, intragastric pressure, and gastric emptying rate. American Journal of Physiology 250: R549–R552.

Genuth S M (1973) Plasma insulin and glucose profiles in normal, obese, and diabetic persons. Annals of Internal Medicine 79: 812–822.

Genuth S (1979) Supplemented fasting in the treatment of obesity and diabetes. American Journal of Clinical Nutrition 32: 2579–2586.

Gilbert S, Garrow J S (1983) A prospective controlled trial of outpatient treatment for obesity. Human Nutrition: Clinical Nutrition 37C: 21–29.

Glueck C J, Gordon D J, Nelson J J, Davis C E, Tyroler H A (1986) Dietary and other correlates of changes in total and low density lipoprotein cholesterol in hypercholesterolemic men: the lipid research clinics coronary primary prevention trial. American Journal of Clinical Nutrition 44: 489–500.

Goldblatt P E, Moore M E, Stunkard A J (1965) Social factors in obesity. Journal of the American Medical Association 192: 2039–1044.

Goldman R F, Buskirk E R (1961) Body volume measurement by underwater weighing: description of a method. In: Brozek J, Henschel A, eds. Techniques for Measuring Body Composition, National Academy of Sciences, Washington, D.C. 78–89.

Goranzon H, Forsum E (1985) Effect of reduced energy intake versus increased physical activity on the outcome of nitrogen balance experiments in man. American Journal of Clinical Nutrition 41: 919–928.

Goranzon H, Forsum E, Thilen M (1983) Calculation and determination of metabolisable energy in mixed diets to humans. American Journal of Clinical Nutrition 38: 954–963.

Gordon T, Kannel W B. (1973) The effects of overweight on cardiovascular disease. Geriatrics 28: 80–88.

Gorringe J A L (1986) Why blame butter?: discussion paper. Journal of the Royal Society of Medicine 79: 661–663.

Gour K N, Gupta M C (1968) Social aspects of overweight and obesity. Journal of the Association of Physicians of India 16: 257–261.

Grauer W O, Moss A A, Cann C E, Goldberg H I (1984) Quantification of body fat distribution in the abdomen using computed tomography. American Journal of Clinical Nutrition 39: 631–637.

Grazer F M (1983) Suction-assisted lipectomy, suction lipectomy, lipolysis. Plastic and Reconstructive Surgery 72: 620–623

Greenway R M, Houser H B, Lindan O, Weir D R (1969) Long-term changes in gross body composition of paraplegic and quadriplegic patients. Paraplegia 7: 301–318.

Griffiths M, Payne P (1976) Energy expenditure in small children of obese and non-obese parents. Nature 260: 698–700.

Grimes D S, Goddard J (1977) Gastric emptying of wholemeal and white bread. Gut 18: 725–729.

Grimes F, Franzini L R (1977) Skinfold measurement techniques for estimating percentage body fat. Journal of Behavior Therapy and Experimental Psychiatry 8, 65–69.

Halliday D, Miller A G (1977) Precise measurement of total body water using trace quantities of deuterium oxide. Biomedical Mass Spectrometry 4: 82–87.

Halverson J D, Printen K J (1986) Perspective: gastric restriction for morbid obesity. Surgery 100: 126–128.

Hanssen M (1982) Much interest in new 'starch blockers'. Pharmacy Journal 229:124.

Harding P E (1980) Jaw wiring for obesity. Lancet i: 534–535.

Harju E, Pernu H (1984) Weight changes after jaw fixation due to sagittal split ramus osteotomy for correction of prognathous. Resuscitation 12: 187–191.

Harman E M, Block A J (1986) Why does weight loss improve the respiratory insufficiency of obesity? Chest 90: 153–154.

Hartz A J, Fischer M E, Bril G, Kelber S, Rupley D, Oken B, Rimm A A (1986) The association of obesity with joint pain and osteoarthritis in the HANES data. Journal of Chronic Diseases 39: 311–319.

Haskell W L (1985) Physical activity and health: need to define the required stimulus. American Journal of Cardiology 55: 4D–9D.

Haslett C, Douglas J G, Chalmers S R, Weighhill A, Munro J F (1983) A double-blind evaluation of Evening Primrose Oil as an anti-obesity agent. International Journal of Obesity 7: 549–554.

Hawes S F, Albert A, Healy M J R, Garrow J S (1972) A comparison of soft-tissue radiography, reflected ultrasound, skinfold calipers and thigh circumference for estimating the thickness of fat overlying the iliac crest and greater trochanter. Proceedings of the Nutrition Society 31:91A.

Hawk L J, Brook C G D (1979) Influence of body fatness in childhood on fatness in adult life. British Medical Journal i: 151–152.

Haymes E M, Lundegren H M, Loomis J L, Buskirk E R (1976) Validity of the ultrasonic technique as a method of measuring subcutaneous adipose tissue. Annals of Human Biology 3: 245–251.

Haynes R B, Harper A C, Costley S R, Johnston M, Logan A G, Flanagan P T (1984) Failure of weight reduction to reduce mildly elevated blood pressure: a randomised trial. Journal of Hypertension 2: 535–539.

Head C A, McManus C B, Seitz S, Grossman G D, Staton G W, Heymsfield S B. (1984) A simple and accurate indirect calorimetry system for assessment of resting energy ependiture. Journal of Parenteral and Enteral Nutrition 8: 45–48.

Heaton K W (1973) Food fibre as an obstacle to energy intake. Lancet ii: 1418–1421.

Henry C J K, Rivers J P W, Payne P R (1986) Does the pattern of tissue mobilization dictate protein requirements? Human Nutrition: Clinical Nutrition 40C: 87–92.

Hepner G, Fried R, St Jeor S, Fusetti L, Morin R (1979) Hypocholesterolemic effect of yoghurt and milk. American Journal of Clinical Nutrition 32: 19–24.

Herman C P, Mack D (1975) Restrained and unrestrained eating. Journal of Personality 43: 647–660.

Herman C P, Polivy J (1980) Stress-induced eating and eating-induced stress (reduction?): a response to Robbins and Fray. Appetite 1: 135–140.

Hermansen L, Grandmontagne M, Moehlum S, Ingnes I. (1984) Post-exercise elevation of resting oxygen uptake: possible mechanisms and physiological significance. Medicine and Sports Science 17: 119–129.

Hermansen L, Von Dobeln W (1971) Body fat and skinfold measurements. Scandinavian Journal Clinical and Laboratory Investigation 27: 315–319.

Hervey G R, Tobin G (1983) Luxuskonsumption, diet-induced thermogenesis and brown fat: a critical review. Clinical Science 64: 7–18.

Heymsfield S B, Arteaga C, McManus C, Smith J, Moffitt S (1983) Measurement of muscle mass in humans: validity of the 24-hour urinary creatinine method. Americal Journal of Clinical Nutrition 37: 478–494.

Hill G L, Bradley J A, Collins J P, McCarthy I, Oxby C B, Burkinshaw L (1978) Fat-free body mass from skinfold thickness: a close relationship with total body nitrogen. British Journal of Nutrition 39: 403–405.

Himes J H, Bouchard C (1985) Do the new Metropolitan Life insurance weight-height tables correctly assess body frame and body fat relationships? American Journal of Public Health 75: 1076–1079.

Himms-Hagen J (1984) Thrermogenesis in brown adipose tissue as an energy buffer: implcations for obesity. New England Journal of Medicine 311: 1549–1558.

Hirsch J (1975) Cell number and size as a determinant of subsequent obesity. In: Winick M, ed. Childhood Obesity. New York, John Wiley, 15–21.

Hirsch J, Gallian E (1968) Methods for the determination of adipose cell size in man and animals. Journal of Lipid Research, 9, 110–119.

Hockaday T D R, Hockaday J M, Mann J I, Turner R C (1978) Prospective comparison of modified-fat-high-carbohydrate with standard low-carbohydrate dietary advice in the treatment of diabetes: one year follow-up study. British Journal of Nutrition 39: 357–362.

Hofstetter A, Schutz Y, Jequier E, Wahren J (1986) Increased 24-hour energy expenditure in cigarette smokers. New England Journal of Medicine 314: 79–82.

Hollenbeck C B, Coulston A M, Reaven G M (1986) To what extent does increased dietary fiber improve glucose and lipid metabolism in patients with noninsulin-dependent diabetes mellitus (NIDDM)? American Journal of Clinical Nutrition 43: 16–24.

Howard A N (1984) The Cambridge Diet. Journal of the American Medical Association 252:897.

Howard A N, Marks J (1977) Hypocholesterolaemic effect of milk. Lancet ii: 255–256.

Hubert H B (1984) The nature of the relationship between obesity and cardiovascular disease. International Journal of Cardiology 6: 268–274.

Hubert H B (1986) The importance of obesity in the development of coronary risk factors and disease: the epidemiological evidence. Annual Reviews of Public Health 7: 493–502.

Hubert H B, Feinleib M, McNamara P M, Castelli W P (1983) Obesity as an independent risk factor for cardiovascular disease: a 26-year follow-up of participants in the Framingham heart study. Circulation 67: 968–977.

Hughes J R, Casal D C, Leon A S (1986) Psychological effects of exercise: a randomised cross-over trial. Journal of Psychosomatic Research 30: 355–360.

Humphrey S J E, Wolff H S (1977) The oxylog. Journal of Physiology (Lond) 267:12P.

Hunt J N, Cash R, Newland P (1978) Energy density of food, gastric emptying, and obesity. American Journal of Clinical Nutrition 31: (10 Suppl) S259–S260.

Hytten F E (1979) Restriction of weight gain in pregnancy: is it justified? Journal of Human Nutrition 33: 461–463.

Hytten F E (1980) Nutrition. In: Hytten F, Chamberlain G, eds. Clinical Physiology in Obstetrics. Oxford, Blackwell Scientific, 163–192.

Hytten F E, Leitch I (1964) The Physiology of Human Pregnancy. Oxford, Blackwell, 463pp

Hytten F E, Taylor K, Taggart N (1966) Measurement of total body fat in man by absorption of 85Kr. Clinical Science 31: 111–119.

Irsigler K, Heitkamp H, Schlick W, Schmid P (1975) Diet and energy balance in obesity. In: Jequier E, ed. Regulation of Energy Balance in Man. Geneva, Editions Medicine et Hygiene, 72–83.

Isaacs A J, Parry P S (1984) A clinical assessment of Modifast in U.K. general practice. Postgraduate Medical Journal 60: (suppl 3) 74–82.

Jacobsen S, Johansen O, Garby L (1985) A 24-m^3 direct heat sink calorimeter with on-line data acquisition, processing and control. American Journal of Physiology 249: E416–E432.

James W P T (1976) Research on obesity: a report of a DHSS/MRC Group. London, HMSO, 94pp

James W P T (1983) Obesity: a report of the Royal College of Physicians. London, Royal College of Physicians, 58pp James W P T (1985) Is there a thermogenic abnormality in obesity? In: Garrow J S, Halliday D, eds. Substrate and Energy Metabolism in Man. Third Clinical Research Centre Symposium, 17–19 September 1984. London, Libbey, 108–118.

James W P T, Trayhurn P (1981) Thermogenesis and obesity. British Medical Bulletin 37: 43–48.

Jeffery R W, Thompson P D, Wing R R (1978) Effects on weight reduction of strong monetary contracts for calorie restriction or weight loss. Behaviour Research and Therapy 16: 363–369.

Jequier E, Schutz Y (1981) The contribution of BMR and physical activity to energy expenditure. In: Cioffi L A, James W P T, Van Itallie T B, eds. The Body Weight Regulatory System: Normal and Disturbed Mechanisms. New York, Raven Press, 89–96.

Jequier E, Schutz Y (1983) Long-term measurements of energy expenditure in humans using a respiration chamber. American Journal of Clinical Nutrition 38: 989–998.

Johnson P R, Stern J S, Greenwood M R C, Zucker L M, Hirsch J (1973) Effect of early nutrition on adipose cellularity and pancreatic insulin release in the Zucker rat. Journal of Nutrition 103: 738–743.

Jones P R M, Bharadwaj H, Bhatia M R, Malhotra M S (1976) Differences between ethnic groups in the relationship of skinfold thickness to body density. In: Bhatia B, Chhina G S, Singh B, eds. Selected Topics in Environmental Biology. New Delhi, Interprint Publications. 373–376.

Jung R T, James W P T (1986) Obese deceivers? British Medical Journal 293:564.

Jung R T, Shetty P S, James W P T, Barrand M A, Callingham B A (1981) Caffeine: its effect on catecholamines and metabolism in lean and obese humans. Clinical Science 60: 527–535.

Kalkoff R K, Hartz A H, Rupley D, Kissebah A H, Kelber S (1983) Relationship of body fat distribution to blood pressure, carbohydrate tolerance, and plasma lipids in healthy obese women. Journal of Laboratory and Clinical Medicine 102: 621–627.

Keesey R E. (1987) Strategies for changing body weight set point. In: Eliahou H, ed. Recent Advances in Obesity Research V. London, John Libbey, (in press)

Keesey R E. (1986) A set-point theory of obesity. In: Brownell K D, Foreynt J P, eds. Handbook of Eating Disorders. New York, Basic Books, 63–87.

Kesselring U K (1983) Regional fat aspiration for body contouring. Plastic and Reconstructive Surgery 72: 610–619

Keys A (1986) Food items, specific nutrients, and 'dietary' risk. American Journal of Clinical Nutrition 43: 477–479.

Keys A, Aravanis C, Blackburn H, van Buchem F S P, Buzina R, Djordjevic B S, Fidanza F, Karvonen M J, Menotti A, Puddu V, Taylor H L (1972a) Coronary heart disease: overweight and obesity as risk factors. Annals of Internal Medicine 17: 15–27.

Keys A, Brozek J (1953) Body fat in adult man. Physiological Reviews 33: 245–325.

Keys A, Brozek J, Hanschel A, Mickelson O, Taylor H L. (1950) The Biology of Human Starvation. Minneapolis, University of Minnesota Press, 1385pp

Keys A, Fidanza F, Karvonen M J, Kimura N, Taylor H L (1972b) Indices of relative weight and obesity. Journal of Chronic Diseases 25: 329–343.

Keys A, Menotti A, Aravanis C, Blackburn H, Djordevic B S, Buzina R, Dontas A S, Fidanza F, Karvonen M J, Kimura N, Mohacek I, Nedeljkovic S, Puddu V, Punsar S, Taylor H L, Conti S, Kromhout D, Toshima H (1984) The seven countries study: 2289 deaths in 15 years. Preventive Medicine 13: 141–154.

Kihlstrom J E, Lundberg D (1971) Cyclical variations of body temperatures in female rabbits before and after ovariectomy. Acta Physiologica scandinavica 82: 272–276.

Kinney J M (1980) Application of indirect calorimetry to clinical studies. In:

Kinney J M, ed. Assessment of Energy Metabolism in Health and Disease. Columbus, Ohio, Ross Laboratories, 42–48.

Kissileff H R (1982) A quadratic equation adequately describes the cumulative food intake curve in man. Appetite 3: 255–272.

Kissileff H R, Gruss L P, Thornton J, Jordan H A (1984) The satiating efficiency of foods. Physiology and Behavior 32: 319–332.

Kleiber M (1961) The Fire of Life. Huntington, N Y, Robert E Kreiger, 454pp

Knight I (1984) The heights and weights of adults in Great Britain. Office of Population Censuses and Surveys, London, HMSO, 87pp

Knowler W C, Pettit D J, Savage P J, Bennett P H (1981) Diabetes incidence in Pima Indians: contributions of obesity and parental diabetes. American Journal of Epidemiology 113: 144–156.

Kopp W K (1975) Problems with jaw fixation for weight control. Journal of Oral Surgery 33:6.

Kozol R A, Fromm D, Ackerman N B, Chung R (1986) Wound closure in obese patients. Surgery, Gynecology and Obstetrics 162: 442–444.

Krantzler N J, Mullen B J, Schutz H G, Grivetti L E, Holden C A, Meiselman H L (1982) American Journal of Clinical Nutrition 36: 1234–1242.

Krotkiewski M (1984) Effect of guar gum on body-weight, hunger ratings and metabolism in obese subjects. British Journal of Nutrition 52: 97–105.

Krotkiewski M, Bjorntorp P (1986) Muscle tissue in obesity with different distribution of adipose tissue: effects of physical training. International Journal of Obesity 10: 331–341.

Krotkiewski M, Bjorntorp P, Holm G, Marks V, Morgan L, Smith U, Feurle G E (1984) Effects of physical training on insulin, connecting peptide (C-peptide), gastric inhibitory peptide (GIP) and pancreatic polypeptide (PP) levels in obese subjects. International Journal of Obesity 8: 193–19.

Krotkiewski M, Lonnroth P, Mandroukas K, Wroblewski Z, Rebuffe-Scrive M, Holm G, Smith U, Bjorntorp P (1985) The effect of physical training on insulin secretion and effectiveness and on glucose metabolism in obesity and Type II (non-insulin-dependent) diabetes mellitus. Diabetologia 28: 881–890.

Kuller L H, Hulley S B, LaParte R E, Neaton J, Dai W S (1983) Environmental determinants of liver function, and high density lipoprotein cholesterol levels. American Journal of Epidemiology 117: 406–418.

Kvist H, Sjostrom L, Tylen U (1986) Adipose tissue volume determinations in women by computed tomography: technical considerations. International Journal of Obesity 10: 53–67.

Landis C. (1925) Studies of emotional reactions IV. Metabolic rate. American Journal of Physiology 74: 188–203.

Lapidus L, Bengtsson C, Larsson B, Pennert K, Rybo E. Sjostrom L (1984) Distribution of adipose tissue and risk of cardiovascular disease and death: a 12 year follow-up of participants in the population study of women in Gothenburg, Sweden. British Medical Journal 289: 1257–1261.

Larsson B, Svardsudd K, Welin L, Wilhelmsen L, Bjorntorp P, Tibblin G (1984) Abdominal adipose tissue distribution, obesity, and risk of cardiovascular disease and death: 13 year follow up of participants in the study of men born in 1913. British Medical Journal 288: 1401–1404.

Lawrence M, Singh J, Lawrence F, Whitehead R G (1985) The energy cost of common daily activities in African women: increased expenditure in pregnancy? American Journal of Clinical Nutrition 42: 753–763.

Lawson S, Webster J, Pacy P J, Garrow J S (1986) Effect of a 10 week jogging programme on metabolic rate in six lean sedentary females. Proceedings of the Nutrition Society 45:121A.

Leclerc S, Allard C, Talbot J, Gauvin R, Bouchard C (1985) High density lipoprotein cholesterol, habitual physical activity and physical fitness. Atherosclerosis 57: 43–51.

Lennon D, Nagle F, Stratman F, Shrago E, Dennis S (1985) Diet and exercise training effects on resting metabolic rate. International Journal of Obesity 9: 39–48.

Leslie R D G, Pyke D A (1985) Genetics of diabetes. In: Alberti K G M M, Alberti, Krall L P, eds. Diabetes Annual. Amsterdam, Elsevier, 53–66.

Lesser G T, Deutsch S, Markofsky J (1971) Use of independent measurement of body fat to evaluate overweight and underweight. Metabolism 20: 792–804.

Levitz L S, Jordan H A (1973) Manual for the analysis of energy intake and expenditure. In: Bray G A, ed. Obesity in Perspective, Vol 2, Part 1, 94–107.

Lew E A (1985) Mortality and weight: insured lives and the American Cancer Society study. Annals of Internal Medicine 103: 1024–1029.

Lew E A, Garfinkel L (1979) Variations in mortality by weight among 750 000 men and women. Journal of Chronic Diseases 32: 563–576.

Lifson N, McClintock R (1966) Theory of use of the turnover rates of body water for measuring energy and material balance. Journal of Theoretical Biology 12: 46–74.

Linn R, Stuart S L (1976) The Last Chance Diet. Secaucus N J, Lyle Stuart, 206pp

Liu G C, Coulston A M, Lardinois C K, Hollenbeck C B, Moore J G, Reaven G M (1985) Moderate weight loss and sulfonylurea treatment of non-insulin-dependent diabetes mellitus. Archives of Internal Medicine 145: 665–669.

Livingstone S D (1968) Calculation of mean body temperature. Canadian Journal of Physiology and Pharmacology 46: 15–17.

Longcope C, Baker R, Johnston C C (1986) Androgen and estrogen metabolism: relationship to obesity. Metabolism 35: 235–237.

Longini I M, Higgins M W, Hinton P C, Moll P P, Keller J B (1984) Genetic and environmental sources of familial aggregation of body mass in Tecumseh, Michigan. Human Biology 56: 733–757.

Louderback L (1970) Fat Power: Whatever You Weigh Is Right. New York, Hawthorn Books, 208pp

Lucas C P, Estigarribia J A, Darga L L, Reaven G M (1985) Insulin and blood pressure in obesity. Hypertension 7: 702–706.

Lukaski H C, Johnson P E, Bolonchuk W W, Lykken G I (1985) Assessment of fat-free mass using bioelectrical impedance measurements of the human body. American Journal of Clinical Nutrition 41: 810–817.

MacMahon S W, Macdonald G J, Bernstein L, Andrews G, Blacket R B (1985) A randomised controlled trial of weight reduction and metoprolol in the treatment of hypertension in young overweight patients. Clinical and Experimental Pharmacology and Physiology 12: 267–271.

Macnair A L (1979) Burning off unwanted energy. Lancet ii:1300.

Maeder E C, Barno A, Mecklenberg F (1975) Obesity: a maternal high risk factor. Obstetrics and Gynecology 45: 669–671.

Maehlum S, Grandmontagne M, Newsholme E A, Sejersted O M (1986) Magnitude and duration of excess postexercise oxygen consumption in healthy young subjects. Metabolism 35: 425–429.

Martin D B (1986) Type II diabetes: insulin versus oral agents. New England Journal of Medicine 314: 1314–1315.

Martin M J, Hulley S B, Browner W S, Kuller L H, Wentworth D (1986) Serum cholesterol, blood pressure, and mortality: implications from a cohort of 361 662 men. Lancet ii: 933–936.

Mason E (1970) Obesity in pet dogs. Veterinary Record 86: 612–616.

Mattila K, Haavisto M, Rajala S (1986) Body mass index and mortality in the elderly. British Medical Journal 292: 867–868.

Mayer J, Marshall N B, Vitale JJ, Christensen J H, Mashayekhi M B, Stare F J (1954) Exercise, food intake and body weight in normal rats and genetically obese adult mice. American Journal of Physiology 177: 544–548.

Mayer J, Roy P, Mitra K P (1956) Relation between caloric intake, body weight and physical work. American Journal of Clinical Nutrition 4: 169–175.

McFarland R J, Gazet J-C, Pilkington T R E (1985) A 13-year review of jejuno-ileal bypass. British Journal of Surgery 72: 81–87.

McFarland R J, Grundy A, Gazet J C, Pilkington T R E (1987) The intragastric balloon: a novel idea proved ineffective. British Journal of Surgery 74: 137–139.

McGowan C R, Epstein L H, Kupfer D J, Bulik C M, Robertson R J (1986) The effect of exercise on non-restricted caloric intake in male joggers. Appetite 7: 97–105.

McIntosh J F, Moller E, Van Slyke D D (1929) Studies of urea excretion. III. The influence of body size on urea output. Journal of Clinical Investigation 6: 467–483.

McKeown T (1970) Prenatal and early postnatal influences on measured intelligence. British Medical Journal iii: 63–67.

McLean J A (1985) Heat production or oxygen consumption? In: van Es A J H, ed. Human energy metabolism: physical activity and energy expenditure measurements in epidemiological research based on direct and indirect calorimetry. EUR-NUT Report No 5, Wageningen, Netherlands, 187–189.

Mellbin T, Vuille J C (1973) Physical development at 7 years of age in relation to velocity of weight gain in infancy with special reference to incidence of overweight. British Journal of Preventive and Social Medicine 27: 225–235.

Millar W J (1985) Population estimates of overweight and hypertension Canada, 1981. Canadian Journal of Public Health 76: 398–403.

Millar W J, Wigle D T (1986) Socioeconomic disparities in risk factors for cardiovascular disease. Canadian Medical Association Journal 134: 127–132.

Milton K (1984) Protein and carbohydrate resources of the Maku Indians of Northwest Amazonia. American Anthropologist 86: 7–27.

Mitchell H H, Hamilton T S, Steggerda F R, Bean H W (1945) The chemical composition of the adult human body and its bearing on the biochemistry of growth. Journal of Biological Chemistry 158: 625–637.

Mitchell J R A (1984) What constitutes evidence on the dietary prevention of coronary heart disease? Cosy beliefs or harsh facts? International Journal of Cardiology 5: 287–298.

Modan M, Halkin H, Almog S, Lusky A, Eshkol A, Shefi M, Shitrit A, Fuchs Z (1985) Hyperinsulinaemia: a link between hypertension obesity and glucose intolerance. Journal of Clinical Investigation 75: 809–817.

Modan M, Karasik A, Halkin H, Fuchs Z, Lusky A, Shitrit A, Modan B (1986) Effect of past and concurrent body mass index on prevalence of glucose intolerance and type 2 (non-insulin-dependent) diabetes and on insulin response. Diabetologia 29: 82–89.

Montoye H J, Epstein F H, Kjelsberg M O (1965) The measurement of body fatness: a study in a total community. American Journal of Clinical Nutrition 16: 417–427.

Mott T, Roberts J (1979) Obesity and hypnosis — a review of the literature. American Journal of Clinical Hypnosis 22: 3–7.

NACNE (1983) Proposals for nutritional guidelines for health education in Britain. Hational Advisory Council on Nutrition Education. London, Health Education Council, 40pp

Nair K S, Halliday D, Ford G C, Heels S, Garrow J S (1987) Failure of carbohydrate to spare leucine oxidation in obese subjects (in press).

Nair K S, Halliday D, Garrow J S (1983) Thermic response to isoenergetic protein, carbohydrate or fat meals in lean and obese subjects. Clinical Science 65: 307–312.

Nair K S, Webster J, Garrow J S (1986) Effect of impaired glucose tolerance and type II diabetes on resting metabolic rate and thermic response to a glucose meal in obese women. Metabolism 35: 640–644.

National Institutes of Health Consensus Development Panel (1985) Health Implications of Obesity. Annals of Internal Medicine 103: 1073–1077.

Naeye R L (1979) Weight gain and the outcome of pregnancy. American Journal of Obstetrics and Gynecology 135: 3–9.

Neel J V (1962) Diabetes mellitus: a 'thrifty' genotype rendered detrimental by 'progress'? American Journal of Human Genetics 14: 353–362.

Nelson M (1985) Nutritional goals from COMA and NACNE: how can they be achieved? Human Nutrition: Applied Nutrition 39A: 456–464.

Neser W B, Thomas J, Semenya K, Thomas D J, Gillum R F (1986) Obesity and hypertension in a longitudinal study of Black physicians: the Meharry cohort study. Journal of Chronic Diseases 39: 1105–113.

Newburgh L H (1938) A new interpretation of diabetes mellitus in obese, middle-aged persons: recovery through reduction of weight. Transactions of the Association of American Physicians 53: 245–257.

Newcombe R G (1982) Development of obesity in parous women. Journal of Epidemiology and Community Health 36: 306–309.

Nomura F, Ohnishi K, Satomura Y, Ohtsuki T, Fukungaga K, Honda M, Ema M, Tohyama T, Sugita S, Saito M, Iida S, Okuda K (1986) Liver function in moderate obesity — study in 534 moderately obese subjects among 4613 male company employees. International Journal of Obesity 10: 349–354.

Norbury F B (1964) Contraindications to long-term fasting. Journal of the American Medical Association 188:88.

Obarzanek E, Levitsky D A (1985) Eating in the laboratory: is it representative? American Journal of Clinical Nutrition 42: 323–328.

O'Brien C P, Stunkard A J, Ternes J W (1982) Absence of naloxone sensitivity in obese humans. Psychosomatic Medicine 44: 215–218.

Olsson K-E, Saltin B (1970) Variation in total body water with muscle glycogen in man. Acta Physiologica Scandinavica 80: 11–18.

Olsson S-A, Nilsson-Ehle P, Pettersson B G, Sorbris R (1985) Gastroplasty as a treatment for massive obesity: a clinical and biochemical evaluation. Scandinavian Journal of Gastroenterology 20: 215–221.

Orbach S (1978) Fat Is a Feminist Issue. London, Hamlyn, 192pp

Ota D M, Jones L A, Jackson G L, Jackson P M, Kemp K, Bauman D (1986) Obesity, non-protein-bound estradiol levels, and distribution of estradiol in the sera of breast cancer patients. Cancer 57: 558–562.

Pace N, Rathbun E N (1945) Studies on body composition: water and chemically combined nitrogen content in relation to fat content. Journal of Biological Chemistry 158: 685–691.

Pacy P J, Barton N, Webster J D, Garrow J S (1985) The energy cost of aerobic exercise in fed and fasted normal subjects. American Journal of Clinical Nutrition 42: 764–768.

Pacy P J, Dodson P M, Taylor M P (1986) The effect of a high fibre, low fat, low sodium diet on diabetics with intermittent claudication. British Journal of Clinical Practice 40: 313–317.

Paffenberger R S, Hyde R T, Wing A L, Hsieh C-C (1986) Physical activity, all cause mortality, and longevity of college allumni. New England Journal of Medicine 314: 605–613.

Pan W-H, Nanas S, Dyer A, Liu K, McDonald A, Schoenberger J A, Shekelle

R B, Stamler R, Stamler J (1986) The role of weight in the positive assocoation between age and blood pressure. American Journal of Epidemiology 24: 612–623.

Pasquali R, Baraldi G, Casari M P, Melchionda N, Zamboni M, Stefanini C, Raitano A (1985) A controlled trial using ephedrine in the treatment of obesity. International Journal of Obesity 9: 93–98.

Pasquali R, Fabbri R, Venturoli S, Paradisi R, Antenucci D, Melchionda N (1986) Effect of weight loss and antiandrogenic therapy on sex hormone blood levels and insulin resistance in obese patients with polycystic ovaries. American Journal of Obstetrics and Gynecology 154: 139–144.

Passmore R (1967) Energy balances in man. Proceedings of the Nutrition Society 26: 97–101.

Passmore R, Strong J A, Ritchie F J (1958) The chemical composition of the tissue lost by obese patients on a reducing regimen. British Journal of Nutrition 12: 113–122.

Paul A A, Southgate D A T (1978) McCance and Widdowson's The Composition of Foods, 4th edition. Ministry of Agriculture, Fisheries and Food and Medical Research Council, HMSO, London, 418 pp

Peckham C H, Christianson R E (1971) The relationship between pre-pregnancy weight and certain obstetric factors. American Journal of Obstetrics and Gynecology 111: 1–7.

Pettit D J, Bennett P H, Knowler W C, Baird H R, Aleck K A (1985) Gestational diabetes mellitus and impaired glucose tolerance during pregnancy: long-term effects on obesity and glucose tolerance in the offspring. Diabetes 34, Suppl 2: 119–122.

Pflanz M (1962) Medizinisch-soziologische Aspekte der Fettsucht. Psyche 16: 575–591.

Pilkington T R E, Gazet J C, Ang L, Kalucy R S, Crisp A H, Day S (1976) Explanation for weight loss after ileojejunal bypass in gross obesity. British Medical Journal i: 1504–1505.

Pipe N G J, Smith T, Halliday D, Edmonds C J, Williams C, Coltart T M (1979) Changes in fat, fat-free mass and body water in normal human pregnancy. British Journal of Obstetrics and Gynaecology 86: 929–940.

Pi-Sunyer F X, Segal K (1986) After effects of exercise upon resting metabolic rate. American Journal of Clinical Nutrition 43: 174–175.

Pittet P H, Chappius P H, Acheson K, De Techtermann F, Jequier E (1976) Thermic effect of glucose in obese subjects studied by indirect calorimetry. British Journal of Nutrition 35: 281–292.

Pollock M L, Loughridge E E, Coleman B, Limerud A C, Jackson A (1975) Prediction of body density in young and middle-aged women. Journal of Applied Physiology 38: 745–749.

Porikos K P, Booth G, van Itallie T B (1977) Effect of covert nutritive dilution on the spontaneous food intake of obese individuals: a pilot study. American Journal of Clinical Nutrition 30: 1638–1644

Porikos K, Hagamen S (1986) Is fiber satiating? Effects of a high fiber preload on subsequent food intake of normal-weight and obese young men. Appetite 7: 153–162.

Porikos K P, Hesser M F, Van Itallie T B (1982) Caloric regulation in normal-weight men maintained on a palatable diet of conventional foods. Physiology and Behaviour 29: 293–300.

Porikos K P, Pi-Sunyer F X (1984) Regulation of food intake in human obesity: studies with caloric dilution and exercise. Clinical Endocrinology and Metabolism 13: 547–561.

Poskitt E M E, Cole T J (1977) Do fat babies stay fat? British Medical Journal i: 7–9.

Prentice A M, Black A E, Coward W A, Davies H L, Goldberg G R, Murgatroyd P R, Ashford J, Sawyer M, Whitehead R G (1986) High levels of energy expenditure in obese women. British Medical Journal 292: 983–987.

Prentice A M, Coward W A, Davies H L, Murgatroyd P R, Black A E, Goldberg G R, Ashford J, Sawyer M, Whitehead R G (1985) Unexpectedly low levels of energy expenditure in healthy women. Lancet ii: 1419–1422.

Preston T W, Clarke R D (1966) Mortality of impaired lives. Transactions of the Faculty Actuaries 29: 251–315.

Pudel V E, Oetting M (1977) Eating in the laboratory: behavioural aspects of the positive energy balance. International Journal of Obesity 1: 369–386.

Quetelet L A J (1869) Physique Sociale, Vol 2, Brussels, C. Muquardt, 92.

Ravussin E, Acheson K J, Vernet O, Danforth E, Jequier E (1985) Evidence that insulin resistance is responsible for the decreased thermic effect of glucose in human obesity. Journal of Clinical Investigation 76: 1268–1273.

Ravussin E, Burnand B, Schutz Y, Jequier E. (1982) Twenty-four hour energy expenditure and resting metabolic rate in obese, moderately obese, and control subjects. American Journal of Clinical Nutrition 35: 566–573.

Ravussin E, Lillioja S, Christin L, Bogardus C (1987) Determinants of 24-hour energy expenditure in man. In: Eliahou H, ed. Recent Advances in Obesity Research: V. London, John Libbey (in press)

Rebuffe-Scrive M, Enk L, Crona N, Lonnroth P, Abrahamsson L, Smith U, Bjorntorp P (1985) Fat cell metabolism in different regions in women. Journal of Clinical Investigation 75: 1973–1976.

Reid J M, Fullmer S D, Pettigrew K D, Burch T A, Bennett P H, Miller M, Wheldon G D (1971) Nutrient intake of Pima women: relationship to diabetesd mellitus and gallstone disease. American Journal of Clinical Nutrition 24: 1281–1289.

Reuben A, Maton P N, Murphy G M, Dowling R H (1985a) Bile lipid secretion in obese and non-obese individuals with and without gallstones. Clinical Science 69: 71–79.

Reuben A, Qureshi Y, Murphy G M, Dowling R H (1985b) Effect of obesity and weight reduction on biliary cholesterol saturation and the response to chenodeoxycholic acid. European Journal of Clinical Investigation 16: 133–142.

Richards G E, Cavallo A, Meyer W J, Prince M J, Peters E J, Stuart C A, Smith E R (1985) Obesity, acanthosis nigricans, insulin resistance, and hyperandrogenemia: pediatric perspective and natural history. Journal of Pediatrics 107: 893–897.

Riemersma R A, Wood D A, Butler S, Elton R A, Oliver M, Salo M, Nikkari T, Vartiainen E, Puska P, Gey F, Rubba P, Mancini M, Fidanza F (1986) Linoleic acid content in adipose tissue and coronary heart disease. British Medical Journal 292: 1423–1427.

Rissanen A, Pietinen P, Siljamaki-Ojansuu U, Piirainen H, Reissel P (1985) Treatment of hypertension in obese patients: efficacy and feasibility of weight and salt reduction programs. Acta Medica Scandinavica 218: 149–156.

Robbins T W, Fray P J (1980) Stress-induced eating: fact, fiction or misunderstanding? Appetite 1: 103–133.

Robinson S, York D A (1986) Effect of cigarette smoking on the thermic response to feeding. International Journal of Obesity 10: 407–417.

Rodin J, Bray G A, Atkinson R L, Dahms W T, Greenway F L, Hamilton K,

Molitch M (1977) Predictors of successful weight loss in an outpatient obesity clinic. International Journal of Obesity 1: 79–87.

Rodgers S, Burnet R, Goss A, Phillips P, Goldney R, Kimber C, Thomas D, Harding P, Wise P (1977) Jaw wiring in the treatment of obesity. Lancet i: 1221–1223.

Rolland-Cachera M F, Sempe M, Guilloud-Bataille M, Patois E, Pequignot-Guggenbuhl F, Fautrad V (1982) Adiposity indices in children. American Journal of Clinical Nutrition 36: 178–184.

Rolls B J, Van Duijvenvoorde P M, Rolls E T (1984) Pleasantness changes and food intake in a varied four-course meal. Appetite 5: 337–348.

Rookus M A, Burema J, Deurenberg P, Van der Wiel-Wetzels W A M (1985) The impact of adjustment of a weight-height index (W/H^2) for frame size on the prediction of body fatness. British Journal of Nutrition 54: 335–342.

Rookus M A, Deurenberg P, Van Sonsbeek J L A (1986) Obesity in North America and the Netherlands. Lancet i:100.

Rose G, Shipley M (1986) Plasma cholesterol concentration and death from coronary heart disease: 10 year results of the Whitehall study. British Medical Journal 293: 306–307.

Rosen J C, Gross J, Loew D, Sims E A H (1985) Mood and appetite during minimal-carbohydrate and carbohydrate-supplemented hypocaloric diets. American Journal of Clinical Nutrition 42: 371–379.

Rosenbaum S, Skinner R K, Knight I B, Garrow J S (1985) A survey of heights and weights of adults in Great Britain. Annals of Human Biology 12: 115–127.

Rothwell N J, Stock M J (1983) Luxuskonsumption, diet-induced thermogenesis and brown fat: the case in favour. Clinical Science 64: 19–23.

Rozen R, Abraham G, Falcou R, Apfelbaum M (1986) Effects of a 'physiological' dose of triiodothyronine on obese subjects during a protein-sparing diet. International Journal of Obesity 10: 303–312.

Rozin P (1976) Psychobiological and cultural determinants of food choice. In: Silverstone T, ed. Appetite and Food Intake. Berlin, Dahlem Konferenzen. 285–312.

Rudinger E (1978) Which? way to slim. London, Consumer's Association, 205pp

Ruiz L, Colley J R T, Hamilton P J S (1971) Measurement of triceps skinfold thickness. An investigation of sources of variation. British Journal of Preventive and Social Medicine 25: 165–167.

Runcie J, Thomson T J (1970) Prolonged starvation: a dangerous procedure? British Medical Journal 3: 432–435.

Russek M (1976) A conceptual equation of intake control. In: Novin D, Wyrwicka W, Bray G A, eds. Hunger: Basic Mechanisms and Clinical Implications. New York, Raven Press, 327–347.

Russell G (1979) Bulimia Nervosa: an ominous variant of anorexia nervosa. Psychological Medicine 9: 429–488.

Salonen J T, Hamynen H, Leino U, Kostiainen E, Sahi T (1985) Relation of alcohol, physical activity, dietary fat and smoking to serum HDL and total cholesterol in young Finnish men. Scandinavian Journal of Social Medicine 13: 99–102.

Schachter S (1968) Obesity and eating: internal and external cues differentially affect the eating behaviour of obese and normal subjects. Science 161: 751–856.

Schoeller D A, Slater R, Taylor P (1985) Reproducibility of the $^2H_2^{18}O$ method in free-living subjects. In: van Es A J H, ed. Human energy metabolism: physical activity and energy expenditure measurements in epidemiological research based on direct and indirect calorimetry. EUR-NUT Report No 5, Wageningen, Netherlands, 121–125.

Schreiber H, Guyton D P (1986) Gastric bubble therapy of obesity. Ohio State Medical Journal 82: 476–479.

Schutte J E, Townsend E J, Hugg J, Shoup R F, Malina R M, Blomqvist C G (1984) Density of lean body mass is greater in Blacks than in Whites. Journal of Applied Physiology 56: 1647–1649.

Schutz Y (1981) Use of non-calorimetric techniques to assess energy expenditure in man. In: Bjorntorp P, Cairella M, Howard A N, eds. Recent Advances in Obesity Research:III. London, John Libbey, 153–158.

Schutz Y, Golay A, Felber J-P, Jequier E (1984) Decreased glucose-induced thermogenesis after weight loss in obese subjects: a predisposing factor for relapse of obesity? American Journal of Clinical Nutrition 39: 380–387.

Schutz Y, Jequier E. (1986) Energy expenditure. Lancet i: 101–102.

Scott R L, Baroffio J R (1986) An MMPI analysis of similarities and differences in three classifications of eating disorders: anorexia nervosa, bulimia, and morbid obesity. Journal of Clinical Psychology 42: 708–713.

Scrignar C B (1980) Mandatory weight control program for 550 police officers choosing either behaviour modification or 'willpower'. Obesity and Bariatric Medicine 9: 88–92.

Seddon R, Penfound J, Garrow J S (1981) The Harrow Slimming Club: analysis of the results obtained in 249 members of a self-financing, non-profit-making group. Journal of Human Nutrition 35: 128–133.

Segal K R, Gutin B, Nyman A M, Pi-Sunyer F X (1985a) Thermic effect of food at rest, during exercise and after exercise in lean and obese men of similar body weight. Journal of Clinical Investigation 76: 1107–1112.

Segal K R, Gutin B, Presta E, Wang J, Van Itallie T B (1985b) Estimation of human body composition by electrical impedence methods: a comparative study. Journal of Applied Physiology 58: 1565–1571.

Seidell J C, Bakx K C, Deurenberg P, van den Hoogen H J M, Hautvast J G A J, Stijnen T (1986a) Overweight and chronic illness — a retrospective cohort study, with a follow-up of 6–17 years, in men and women initially 20–50 years of age. Journal of Chronic Diseases 39: 585–593.

Seidell J C, de Groot L C P G M, van Sonsbeek J L A, Deurenberg P, Hautvast J G A J (1986b) Associations of moderate and severe overweight with self-reported illness and medical care in Dutch adults. American Journal of Public Health 76: 264–269.

Seltzer C C, Mayer J (1965) A simple criterion of obesity. Postgraduate Medicine 38A: 101–107.

Shapiro L R, Crawford P B, Clark M J, Pearson D L, Raz J, Huenemann R L (1984) Obesity prognosis: a longitudinal study of children from the age of 6 months to 9 years. American Journal of Public Health 74: 968–972.

Shearman C P, Baddeley R M (1986) Which gastroplasty for the correction of massive obesity? Annals of the Royal College of Surgeons of England 68: 139–142.

Sheldahl L M, Buskirk E R, Loomis J L, Hodgson J L, Mendez J (1982) Effects of exercise in cool water on body weight loss. International Journal of Obesity 6: 29–42.

Shetty P S, Jung R T, James W P T, Barrand M A, Callingham B A (1981) Postprandial thermogenesis in obesity. Clinical Science 60: 519–525.

Shizgal M H (1976) Total body potassium and nutritional status. Surgical Clinics of North America 56: 1185–1194.

Silverstone T (1987) Appetite suppressant drugs in the management of obesity. Alimentazione Nutrizione Metabolismo (in press) Silverstone J T, Gordon R P, Stunkard A J (1969) Social factors in obesity in London. Practitioner 202: 682–688.

Simpson G K, Farquhar D L, Carr P, Galloway S McL, Stewart I C, Donald P, Steven F, Munro J F (1986) Intermittent protein-sparing fasting with abdominal belting. International Journal of Obesity 10: 247–254.

Sims E A H, Danforth E Jr, Horton E S, Bray G A, Glennon J A, Salans L B. (1973) Endocrine and metabolic effects of experimental obesity in man. Recent Progress in Hormone Research 29: 457–496.

Siri W E (1961) Body volume measurement by gas dilution. In: Brozek J, Henschel A, eds. Techniques for Measuring Body Composition., National Academy of Sciences, Washington, D.C., 108–117.

Smith T, Hesp R, Mackenzie J (1979) Total body potassium calibrations for normal and obese subjects in two types of whole body counter. Physics in Biology and Medicine 24: 171–175.

Snellen J W, Chang K S, Smith W (1983) Technical description and performance characteristics of a human whole-body calorimeter. Medical and Biological Engineering and Computing 21: 9–20.

Sohar E, Scapa E, Ravid M (1973) Constancy of relative body weight in children. Archives of Disease in Childhood 48: 389–392.

Sorensen T I A, Sonne-Holm S, Christensen U. (1983) Cognitive deficiency in obesity independent of social origin. Lancet i: 1105–1106.

Southgate D A T, Durnin J V G A (1970) Calorie conversion factors: an experimental reassessment of the factors used in the calculation of the energy value of human diets. British Journal of Nutrition 24: 517–535.

Spencer I O B (1968) Death during therapeutic starvation for obesity. Lancet i: 1288–1290.

Spinnler G, Jequier E, Favre R, Dolivo M, Vanotti A (1973) Human calorimnetry with a new type of gradient layer. Journal of Applied Physiology 35: 158–165.

Spitzer L, Rodin J (1981) Human eating behavior: a critical review of studies in normal weight and overweight individuals. Appetite 2: 293–330.

Stalley S, Garrow J S (1975) Photographic and ultrasonic methods for measuring change in subcutaneous fat distribution. In: Howard A N, ed. Recent Advances in Obesity Research : I. London, Newman Publishing, 66–68.

Stamford B A, Matter S, Fell R D, Sady S, Cresanta M K, Papanek P (1984) Cigarette smoking, physical activity, and alcohol consumption: relationship to blood lipids and lipoproteins in premenopausal females. Metabolism 33: 585–590.

Stamler R, Stamler J, Reidlinger W F, Algera G, Roberts R H (1978) Weight and blood pressure. Findings in hypertension screening of 1 million Americans. Journal of the American Medical Association 240: 1607–1610.

Stark O, Peckham C S, Ades A (1986) Weights of British and French children. Lancet 1:862.

Steel J M, Munro J F, Duncan L J P (1973) A comparative trial of different regimens of fenfluramine and phentermine in obesity. Practitioner 211: 232–236.

Stein Z, Susser M, Saenger G, Marolla F (1975) Famine and Human Development: the Dutch winter hunger of 1944–1945. New York, Oxford University Press,. 284pp

Stern J S, Grivetti L, Castonguay T W (1984) Energy intake: uses and misuses. International Journal of Obesity 8: 535–541.

Stitzer M L, Bigelow G E (1984) Contingent reinforcement for carbon monoxide reduction: within-subject effects of pay amounts. Journal of Applied Behavior Analysis 17: 477–483.

Stock M, Rothwell N (1982) Obesity and Leanness: BasicAspects. London, John Libbey, 98pp

Stout R W (1982) Hyperinsulinaemia as an independent risk factor for atherosclerosis. International Journal of Obesity 6: 111–115.

Strakova M, Markova J (1971) Ultrasound used for measuring subcutaneous fat. Reviews in Czechoslovak Medicine 17: 66–73.

Streat S J, Beddoe A H, Hill G L (1985) Measurement of body fat and hydration of the fat-free body in health and disease. Metabolism 34: 509–518.

Stuart R B (1967) Behavioural control of overeating. Behaviour Research and Therapy 5: 357–365.

Stunkard A J (1985) Behavioural management of obesity. Medical Journal of Australia 142 suppl: S13–S20.

Stunkard A J, Brownell K D (1980) Work-site treatment for obesity. American Journal of Psychiatry 137: 252–253.

Stunkard A J, Craighead L W, O'Brien R (1980) The treatment of obesity: a controlled trial of behaviour therapy, pharmacotherapy and their combination. Lancet i: 1045–1047.

Stunkard A J, Sorensen T I A, Hanis C, Teasdale T W, Chakraborty R, Schull W J, Schulsinger F (1986a). An adoption study of human obesity. New England Journal of Medicine 314: 193–198

Stunkard A J, Stinnett J L, Smoller J W (1986b) Psychological and social aspects of surgical treatment of obesity. American Journal of Psychiatry 143: 417–429.

Sveger T (1978) Does overnutrition or obesity during the first year affect weight at age four? Acta Paediatrica Scandinavica 67: 465–468.

Tanner J M (1965) Radiographic studies of body composition in children and adults. In: Brozek J, ed. Human Body Composition. Oxford, Pergamon Press, 211–236.

Tappy L, Buckert A, Griessen M, Golay A, Jequier E, Felber J (1986) Effect of trestatin, a new inhibitor of pancreatic alpha-amylase, on starch metabolism in man. International Journal of Obesity 10: 185–192.

Tewksbury D A, Lohrenz F N (1970) Circadian rhythm of urinary aminoacid excretion in fed and fasted states. Metabolism 19: 363–371.

Thomas P H, Hofmann A F (1973) A simple calculation of the lithogenic index of bile: expressing biliary lipid composition on rectangular coordinates. Gastroenterology 65: 698–700.

Thompson J K, Jarvie G J, Lahey B B, Cureton K J (1982) Exercise and obesity: etiology, physiology and intervention. Psychological Bulletin 91: 55–79.

Tokunaga K, Matsuzawa Y, Ishakawa K, Tarui S (1983) A novel technique for the determination of body fat by computed tomography. International Journal of Obesity 7: 437–445.

Trovati M, Carta Q, Cavalot F, Vitali S, Banaudi C, Lucchina P G, Fiocchi F, Emanualli G, Lenti G (1984) Influence of physical training on blood glucose control, glucose tolerance, insulin secretion, and insulin action in non-insulin-dependent diabetic patients. Diabetes Care 7: 416–420.

Tschegg E, Sigmund A, Veitl V, Schmid P, Irsigler K (1979) An isothermic, gradient-free, whole-body calorimeter for long-term investigations of energy balance in man. Metabolism 28: 764–770.

Turner W T, Cohn S (1975) Total body potassium and 24 h creatinine excretion in healthy males. Clinical Pharmacology and Therapeutics 18: 405–412.

Udall J N, Garrison G G, Vaucher Y, Walson P D, Morrow G (1978) Interaction of maternal and neonatal obesity. Pediatrics 62: 17–21.

Vague J (1953) La differenciation sexuelle humaine: ses incidences en pathologie. Paris, Masson, 386pp

Van Gaal L F, Snyders D, De Leeuw I H, Bekaert J L (1985) Anthropometric and calorimetric evidence for the protein sparing effects of a new protein supplemented low calorie preparation. American Journal of Clinical Nutrition 41: 540–544.

Van Graan C H, Wyndham C H (1964) Body surface area in human beings. Nature (Lond.) 204:998.

Van Itallie T B, Yang M-U (1984) Cardiac dysfunction in obese dieters: a potentially lethal complication of rapid, massive weight loss. American Journal of Clinical Nutrition 39: 695–702.

Van Sonsbeek J L A (1985) The Dutch by height and weight, differences in height and under- and overweight in adults. Maandbericht Gezondheidsstatist 6: 5–18.

van Staveren W A, de Boer J O, Burema J (1985) Validity and reproducibility of a dietary history method estimating the usual food intake during one month. American Journal of Clinical Nutrition 42: 554–559.

van Stratum P, Lussenburg R N, van Wezel L A, Vergroesen A J, Cremer D (1978) The effect of dietary carbohydrate: fat ration on energy intake by adult women. American Journal of Clinical Nutrition 31: 206–212.

Velasquez M T, Hoffmann R G (1985) Overweight and obesity in hypertension. Quarterly Journal of Medicine 54: 205–212.

Viste A, Bjornestad E, Opheim P, Skarstein A, Thunold J, Hartveit F, Eide G E, Eide T J, Soreide O. (1986) Risk of carcinoma following gastric operations for benign disease: an historical cohort study of 3470 patients. Lancet ii: 502–505.

Waaler H Th (1984) Height, weight and mortality: the Norwegian experience. Acta Medica Scandinavica Supplement 679, 56pp

Wadden T A, Stunkard A J (1985) Social and psychological consequences of obesity. Annals of Internal Medicine 103: 1062–1067.

Wadden T A, Stunkard A J (1986) Controlled trial of a very low calorie diet, behavior therapy, and their combination in the treatment of obesity. Journal of Consulting and Clinical Psychology 54: 482–488.

Wadden T A, Stunkard A J, Brownell K D (1983) Very-low-calorie diets: their efficacy, safety and future. Annals of Internal Medicine 99: 675–684.

Wadden T A, Stunkard A J, Brownell K D, Day S C (1985) Comparison of two very-low-calorie diets: protein-sparing-modified fast versus protein-formula-liquid diet. American Journal of Clinical Nutrition 41: 533–539.

Wadden T A, Stunkard A J, Brownell K D, Van Itallie T B (1984) The Cambridge Diet. Journal of the American Medical Association 252: 897–898.

Warnes C A, Roberts W C (1984) The heart in massive (more than 300 pounds or 136 kilograms) obesity: analysis of 12 patients studied at necropsy American Journal of Cardiology 54: 1087–1091.

Warwick P M, Garrow J S (1981) The effect of addition of exercise to a regimen of dietary restriction on weight loss, nitrogen balance, resting metabolic rate and spontaneous physical activity in three obese women in a metabolic ward. International Journal of Obesity 5: 25–32.

Warwick P M, Toft R, Garrow J S (1978) Individual variation in energy expenditure. International Journal of Obesity 2:396.

Waterston J A, Gilligan B S (1986) Wernicke's encephalopathy after prolonged fasting. Medical Journal of Australia 145: 154–155.

Webb P, Annis J F (1983) Adaptation to overeating in lean and overweight women. Human Nutrition: Clinical Nutrition 37C: 117–131.

Webb P, Annis J F, Troutman S J (1972) Human calorimetry with a water-cooled garment. Journal of Applied Physiology 32: 412–418.

Webster J D, Garrow J S (1985) Creatinine excretion over 24 hours as a measure of body composition or of completeness of urine collection. Human Nutrition: Clinical Nutrition 39C: 101–106.

Webster J D, Hesp R, Garrow J S (1984) The composition of excess weight in obese women estimated by body density, total body water and total body potassium. Human Nutrition: Clinical Nutrition 38C: 299–306.

Webster J D, Welsh G, Pacy P J, Garrow J S (1986) Description of a human direct calorimeter, with a note on the energy cost of clerical work. British Journal of Nutrition 55: 1–6.

Wechsler J G, Wenzel H, Swobodnik W, Ditschuneit H (1984) Nitrogen balance studies during modified fasting. Postgraduate Medical Journal 60: Suppl 3, 66–73.

Weinsier R L, Norris D J, Birch R, Bernstein R S, Wang J, Yang M-U, Pierson R N, Van Itallie T B (1985) The relative contribution of body fat and fat pattern to blood pressure level. Hypertension 7: 578–585.

Weir JB deV (1949) New methods for calculating metabolic rate with special reference to protein metabolism. Journal of Physiology (Lond) 109: 1–9.

Weissman C, Damask M C, Askanazi J, Rosenbaum S H, Kinney J M (1985) Evaluation of a non-invasive method for the measurement of metabolic rate in humans. Clinical Science 69: 135–141.

Weits T, van der Beek E J, Wedel M (1986) Comparison of ultrasound and skinfold caliper measurements of subcutaneous fat tissue. International Journal of Obesity 10: 161–168.

Welle S L, Campbell R G (1983) Normal thermic effect of glucose in obese women. American Journal of Clinical Nutrition 37: 87–92

Welle S L, Campbell R G (1986) Decrease in resting metabolic rate during rapid weight loss is reversed by low dose thyroid hormone treatment. Metabolism 35: 289–291.

Werner I, Hambraeus L, Thoren L (1985) Relationship between weight reduction and state of malabsorption after jejuno-ileal bypass for excessive obesity. Human Nutrition: Applied Nutrition 39A: 95–100.

Westerterp K R, Schoffelen P F M, Saris W H M, ten Hoor F (1985) Measurement of energy expenditure using doubly labelled water, a validation study. In: van Es A J H, ed. Human energy metabolism: physical activity and energy expenditure measurements in epidemiological research based on direct and indirect calorimetry. EUR-NUT Report No 5, Wageningen, Netherlands, 129–131.

Whitelaw A G L (1976) Influence of maternal obesity on subcutaneous fat in the newborn. British Medical Journal i: 985–986.

Whiting M J, Hall J C, Iannos J, Roberts H G, Watts J McK (1984) The cholesterol saturation of bile and its reduction by chendeoxycholic acid in massively obese patients. International Journal of Obesity 8: 681–688.

Widdowson E M (1936) A study of English diets by theindividual method. Part I. Men. Journal of Hygiene (London) 36: 269–292.

Widdowson E M, Dickerson J W T (1960) The effect of growth and function on the chemical composition of soft tissues. Biochemical Journal 77: 30–43.

Widdowson E M, McCance R A, Spray C M (1951) The chemical composition of the human body. Clinical Science 10: 113–125.

Wilson J H P, Lamberts S W J (1979) Nitrogen balance in obese patients receiving a very low calorie liquid formula diet. American Journal of Clinical Nutrition 32: 1612–1616.

Womersley J, Durnin J V G A (1977) A comparison of the skinfold method with extent of 'overweight' and various weight-height relationships in the assessment of obesity. British Journal of Nutrition 38: 271–284.

Woo R, Garrow J S, Pi-Sunyer F X (1982a) Effect of exercise on spontaneous calorie intake in obesity. American Journal of Clinical Nutrition 36: 470–477.

Woo R, Garrow J S, Pi-Sunyer F X (1982b) Voluntary food intake during prolonged exercise in obese women. American Journal of Clinical Nutrition 36: 478–484.

Woo R, O'Connell M, Horton E S, Danforth E Jr (1985) Changes in resting metabolism with increased intake and exercise. American Journal of Clinical Nutrition 41:859.

Woo R, Pi-Sunyer F X (1985) Effect of increased physical activity on voluntary intake in lean women. Metabolism 34: 836–841.

World Health Organisation European Collaborative Group (1986) European collaborative trial of multifactorial prevention of coronary heart disease: final report on the 6-year results. Lancet i: 869–871.

Worsley A, Coonan W, Leitch D, Crawford D (1984) Slim and obese children's perceptions of physical activities. International Journal of Obesity 8: 201–212.

Wursch P, Del Vedova S, Koellreutter B (1986) Cell structure and starch nature as key determinants of the digestion rate of starch in legume. American Journal of Clinical Nutrition 43: 25–29.

Wyndham C H, Williams C G, Loots S H (1968) Reactions to cold, Journal of Applied Physiology 24: 282–287.

Wyrwicka W (1976) The problem of motivation in feeding behaviour. In: Novin D, Wyrwicka W, Bray G A, eds. Hunger: Basic Mechanisms and Clinical Implications. New York, Raven Press, 203–213.

Yang M U, Van Itallie T B (1984) Variability in body protein loss during protracted severe caloric restriction: role of triiodothyronine and other possible determinants. American Journal of Clinical Nutrition 40: 611–622.

Yudkin J (1958) This Slimming Business. London, MacGibbon & Kee, 191pp

Yudkin J (1974) The low-carbohydrate diet. In: Burland W L, Samuel P D, Yudkin J, eds. Obesity. Edinburgh, Churchill Livingstone, 271–280.

Zack F M, Harlan W R, Leaverton P E, Cornoni-Huntley J (1979) A longitudinal study of body fatness in childhood and adolescence. Journal of Pediatrics 95: 126–130.

Zed C, James W P T (1986a) Dietary thermogenesis in obesity: fat feeding at different energy intakes. International Journal of Obesity 10: 391–406.

Zed C, James W P T (1986b) Dietary thermogenesis in obesity: response to carbohydrate and protein meals: the effect of beta-adrenergic blockade and semistarvation. International Journal of Obesity 10: 391–406.

Zuntz N (1897) Ueber den Stoffverbrauch des Hundes bei Muskelarbeit. Pfluger Archiv fur Physiologie 68: 191–211.

Author Index

Subject Index

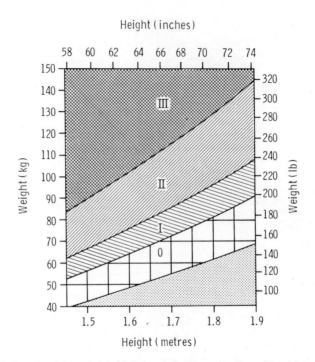

Fig. 1.1 Relation of weight to height defining desirable range (0), and grades I, II and III obesity, marked by boundaries W/H^2 = 25–29.9, 30–40, and over 40 respectively